Development of Oral Cancer

Ala-Eddin Al Moustafa
Editor

Development of Oral Cancer

Risk Factors and Prevention Strategies

Springer

Editor
Ala-Eddin Al Moustafa
Department of Basic Medical Science
Qatar University/College of Medicine
Doha
Qatar

ISBN 978-3-319-48053-4 ISBN 978-3-319-48054-1 (eBook)
DOI 10.1007/978-3-319-48054-1

Library of Congress Control Number: 2017945404

Printed on acid-free paper

This Springer imprint is published by Springer Nature
The registered company is Springer International Publishing AG
The registered company address is: Gewerbestrasse 11, 6330 Cham, Switzerland

Preface

Oral cancer is one of the most common noncommunicable diseases worldwide with an estimated 300,000 new cases and 145,000 deaths in 2012. Oral cancers occur in increased frequency especially in developing countries compared to developed ones. The etiology of human oral cancer varies, but a wide range of risk factors can be determined such as gene mutations, environmental conditions, and lifestyle including tobacco use and excessive alcohol consumption, in addition to physical inactivity. Based on the importance of this topic for human life especially in developing countries, I feel it is my duty to present this book which addresses different aspects of oral cancer as a preventive step toward the alleviation of the malignancy. Thus, I am thankful to all the authors who have joined me in this project and enriched the subject with their valuable contributions. The findings of these chapters are very interesting and contribute to our understanding of the complexity of human oral carcinogenesis and its predominant risk factors, in addition to outlining important prevention strategies to fight this disease.

This book comprises 12 chapters which cover the most important topics related to human oral cancer. The first chapter aims to provide a synopsis of the epidemiology of oral cancer globally and to highlight the main characteristics of this disease, which was elegantly described by Dr. Kujan. The second chapter was written by Drs. Al-Dewik and Qoronfleh in which the authors review the most common molecular genetic alterations at the genomic, epigenetic, and transcriptomic levels. They outline changes in tumor suppressor genes, oncogenes, genomic instability, mitochondrial DNA mutations, noncoding RNAs, and loss of heterozygosity in human oral cancer. Chapter 3 describes the causes and diagnosis of oral cancer and its treatment by designing novel drugs for human cancers in general and oral cancer in particular; this chapter was tackled by Dr. Khan. Chapter 4 discusses one of the most important risk factors for human oral cancer which is smoking wherein Drs. Abro and Pervez review the role of different types of tobacco use in human oral cancer. Chapter 5 reviews another major risk factor of human oral cancer which is alcohol intake; in this chapter Dr. Kujan and his colleagues discuss stylishly the role of alcohol-containing mouthwashes and its contribution to the increased risk of oral cancer development. In Chap. 6 the authors describe the presence and role of high-risk human papillomaviruses and Epstein-Barr virus in human oral cancer; more significantly, Dr. Al Moustafa and his colleagues discuss the cooperation outcome of these viruses in human oral carcinogenesis. In Chap. 7, Dr. Jaloudi and his colleagues review the role of bacterial and fungal infection in the global incidence of human oral cancers. In Chap. 8, Drs. Pervez and Abro review the role of chewing habits in human oral carcinogenesis. Chapter 9 describes the outcome of qat chewing and mate consumption in human oral diseases including cancer; this chapter was written by Kassab and Dr. Al Moustafa. Chapter 10 elucidates the concept behind photodynamic diagnosis/therapy along with their elements and cell death mechanisms; additionally, it provides a glimpse at the status of this technique from a clinical point of view; this work is presented by Dr. Abdel Gaber. Chapter 11 was prepared by Drs. Bawadi and Faris, and it outlines the important role of nutrition in human oral carcinogenesis; in addition, this chapter discusses the power of nutrition as a possible oral cancer prevention tool. Finally, Dr. Malki and his colleagues focus on prevention strategies in Chap. 12; they elaborate and expand on common risk factors and how to decrease chances of developing oral cancer.

We believe that the chapters presented in this volume provide a global overview of different approaches in understanding risk factors and prevention strategies of human oral cancer. They are intended to update scientists in the field about novel developments and provide a knowledge base for medical students, clinicians, and researchers contemplating to engage in this area of scientific research. Nevertheless, it should be noted that this book is not an exhaustive repertoire of all known human oral cancer risks. Rather, we admittedly made subjective choices to illustrate the diversity of these factors and their instrumental role in human oral cancer.

Doha, Qatar Ala-Eddin Al Moustafa

Contents

Human Oral Cancer (Epidemiology and Characteristic)

1

Omar Kujan

1.1 Introduction

Oral cancer is a major health burden particularly in the developing world where most of the cases are diagnosed [1]. More than 300,000 new patients are estimated to be diagnosed with oral and oropharyngeal cancer in 2012, and 50% of these cases will die annually [2]. The WHO International Statistical Classification of Diseases (ICD-10) defined oral and oropharyngeal cancer as the malignancy emerging from the anatomic sites that correspond to the rubrics C00–C10 of the ICD-10 [3]. Specifically, the involved oral anatomic subsites include the lips, buccal mucosa, alveolar ridge and gingiva, retromolar trigone, anterior two-thirds of the tongue (anterior to the circumvallate papillae), floor of the mouth and hard palate. The oropharynx (middle part of the pharynx) consists of the soft palate, base (or posterior one-third) of the tongue, palatine tonsils, palatoglossal folds, valleculae and posterior pharyngeal wall. Traditionally oral cancer was sometimes used to designate head and neck cancer that genuinely covers wider anatomical region with more heterogeneous nature. Though, for the purpose of this chapter, lip/mouth and oropharyngeal cancers have been combined and termed as oral and oropharyngeal cancer (OPC). Also, the cases originated from either nasopharynx or other pharynxes were excluded to distinguish it from the head and neck cancer. Squamous cell carcinoma is the most common type of malignancy that is diagnosed in the oral and oropharyngeal region with more than 95% [4].

The data presented in this chapter are mainly derived from GLOBOCAN database which is a project governed by the International Agency for Research on Cancer

O. Kujan
School of Dentistry/Oral Health Centre of Western Australia, The University of Western Australia, 17 Monash Avenue, Nedlands, WA 6009, Australia

Faculty of Dentistry, Hama University, Hama, Syrian Arab Republic
e-mail: omar.kujan@uwa.edu.au

A.-E. Al Moustafa (ed.), *Development of Oral Cancer*,
DOI 10.1007/978-3-319-48054-1_1

(IARC) to provide contemporary estimates of the incidence of mortality and prevalence from major types of cancer, at national level, for 184 countries of the world [5].

An international variation in the OPC prevalence rates exists and that corresponds to significant heterogeneity in trends by subsite, country and sex [6]. For example, oral and oropharyngeal cancer is ranked the 11th most common prevalent cancer among the top 20 malignancy in the body for both genders, all ages [7]. Whereas, the head and neck cancer is ranked the seventh most common type of malignancy with over 600,000 new cases diagnosed per annum [8]. Interestingly, oral cancer is the third most common type of cancer in India, where it is, in fact, ranked the most common type of cancer among male Indian [9]. Moreover, two-thirds of the diagnosed oral cancer cases are reported globally in low-to-middle-income countries literally the Southeast region of Asia [7]. This increasing incidence is mainly due to the social habit of chewing areca nut/betel quid in addition to the traditional major risk factors of tobacco and alcohol consumptions and, increasingly, infection with high-risk types of human papillomavirus (HPV) [4].

This chapter aimed to provide a synopsis of the epidemiology of oral cancer globally and to highlight the major characteristics.

1.2 Oral Cancer Epidemiology

1.2.1 Incidence and Mortality

According to the most recent GLOBOCAN estimates, worldwide in 2012, there were approximately 300,373 new cases of lip/oral cavity cancer (age-standardized rate [age standardized to the world population] or ASR [W], 4.0 per 100,000). The estimated age-standardized incidence, prevalence and mortality rates of oral cancer also vary among countries in different regions (Figs. 1.1–1.3) [5].

Notably, the highest estimated ASR (W) of oral and oropharyngeal cancer is found in the World Health Organization (WHO) Southeast Asian region (6.4 per 100,000), followed by the WHO European region (4.6 per 100,000), the WHO Eastern Mediterranean region (4.6 per 100,000), the WHO Americas region (4.1 per 100,000), the WHO African region (2.7 per 100,000) and the WHO Western Pacific region (2.0 per 100,000). Worldwide mortality estimates for 2012 include an ASR (W) of 2.7 per 100,000 for oral and oropharyngeal cancer [5]. Surprisingly, the highest ever incidence of OPC is found in Melanesia (ASR (W) 22.9 per 100,000 in men and 16.0 per 100,000 in women) [5].

Figure 1.4 shows the ASR rates of incidence and 5-year prevalence of OPC estimated in 2012 of the highest 20 countries over the world where India is the highest.

In the United States, based on the database of the Surveillance, Epidemiology, and End Results (SEER), it is estimated that more than 30,000 new cases of oral cancer are to be diagnosed in the United States in 2016, with 6500 deaths attributable to the disease sharing a 3.4% of the whole cancer burden [10]. In other words, the ASR incidence of OPC is 15.6 per 100,000 for male and 6.1 per 100,000 for female [10, 11] Tables 1.1 and 1.2.

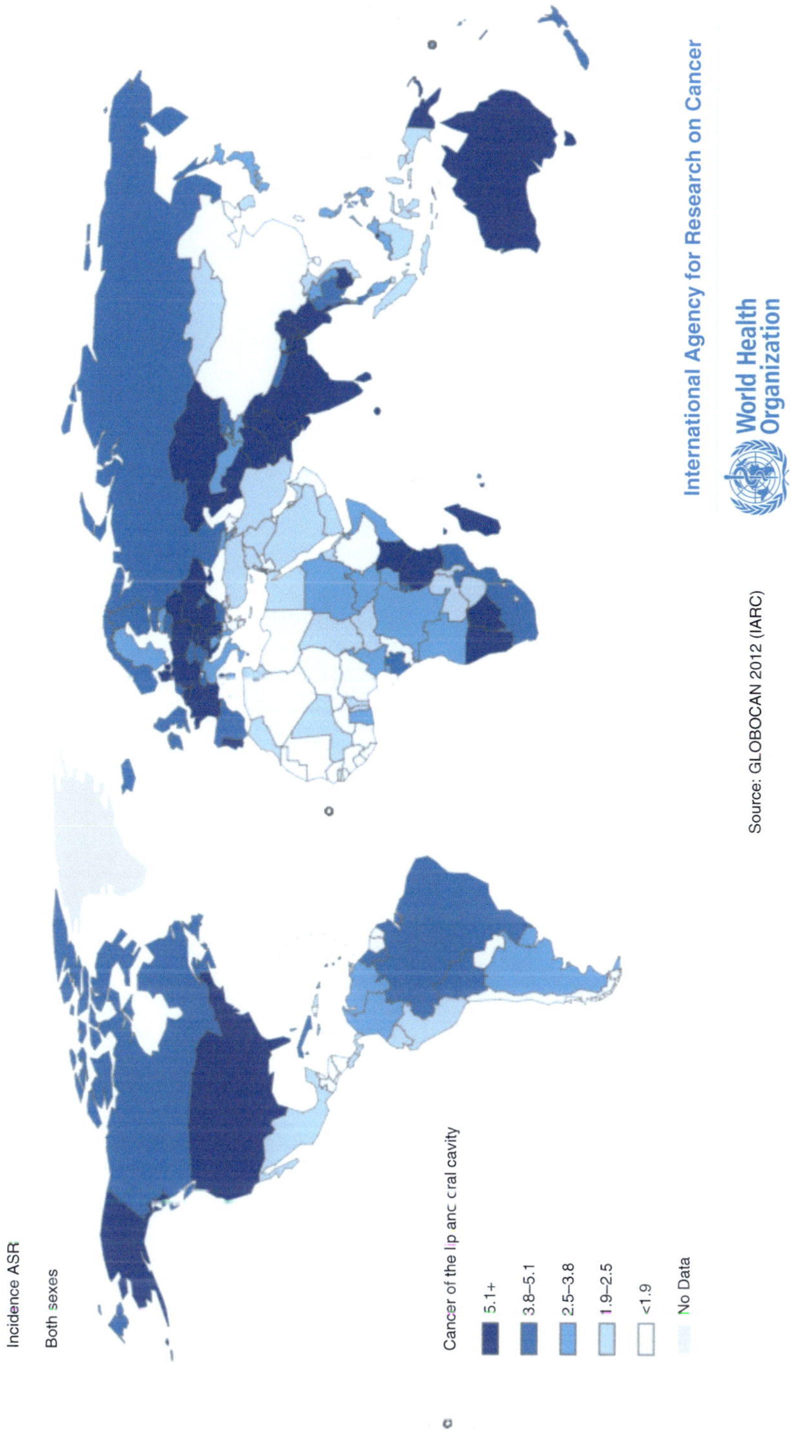

Fig. 1.1 Global map of age-standardized incidence rates of oral cancer in both sexes and all ages, data derived from GLOBOCAN 2012

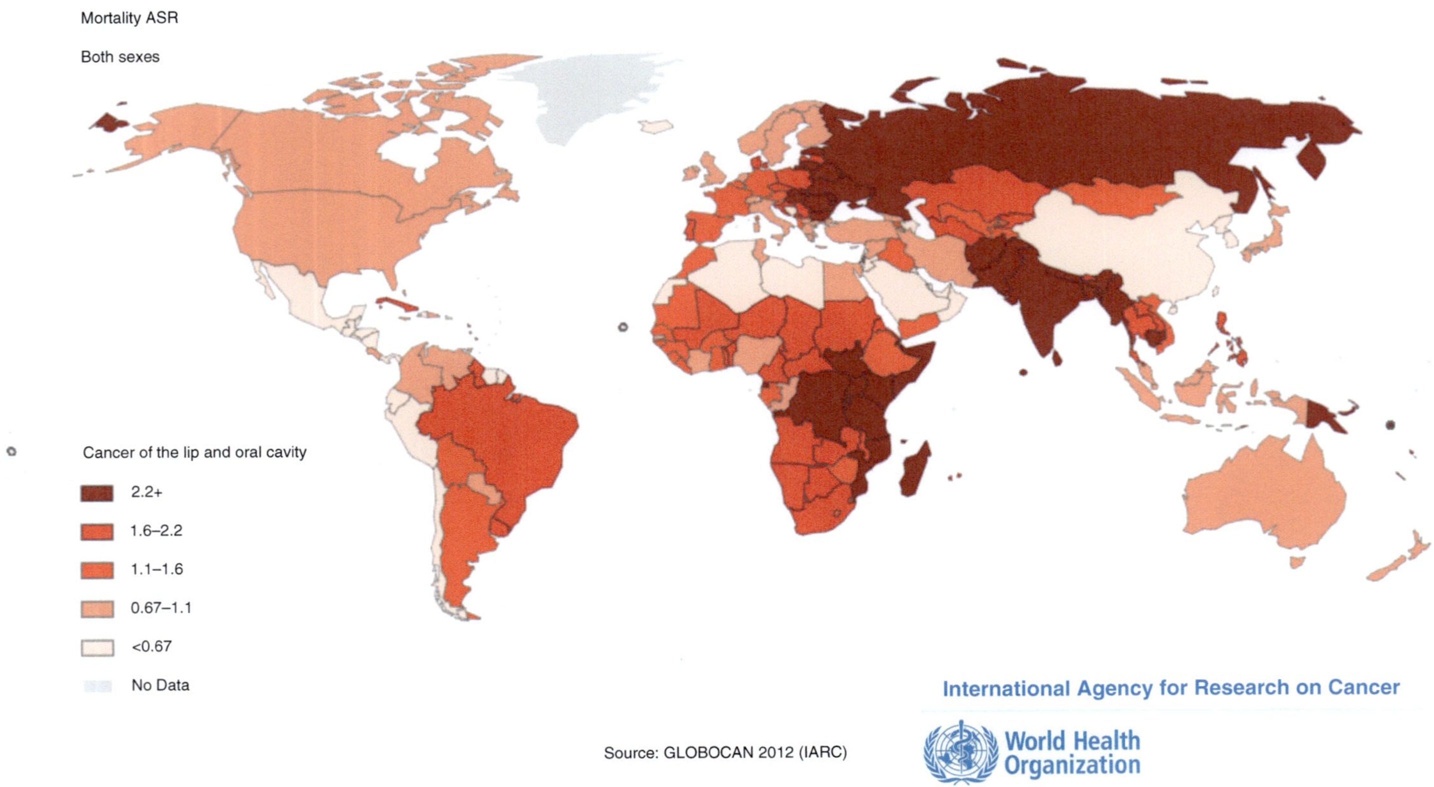

Fig. 1.2 Global map of age-standardized mortality rates of oral cancer in both sexes and all ages, data derived from GLOBOCAN 2012

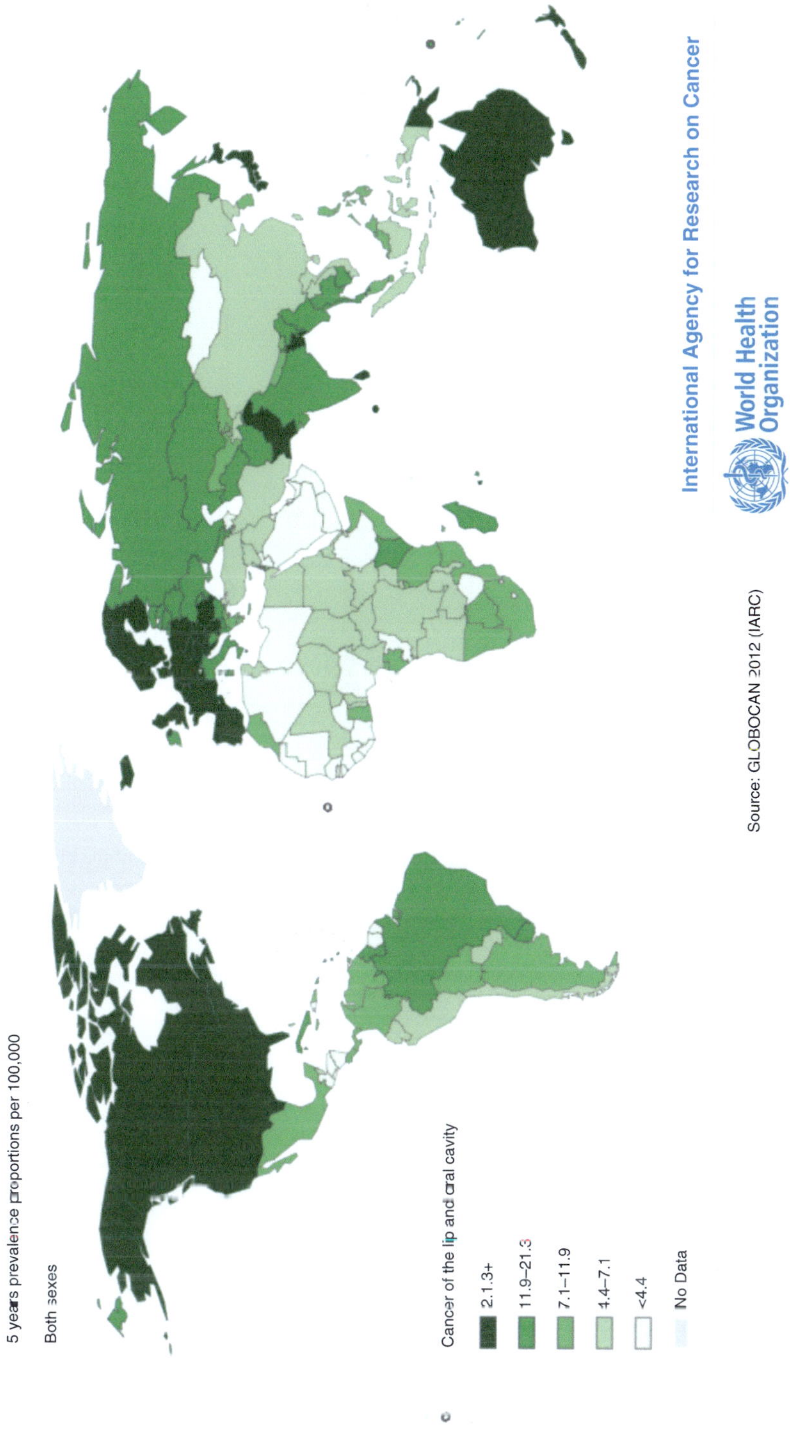

Fig. 1.3 Global map of age-standardized prevalence rates of oral cancer in both sexes and all ages, data derived from GLOBOCAN 2012

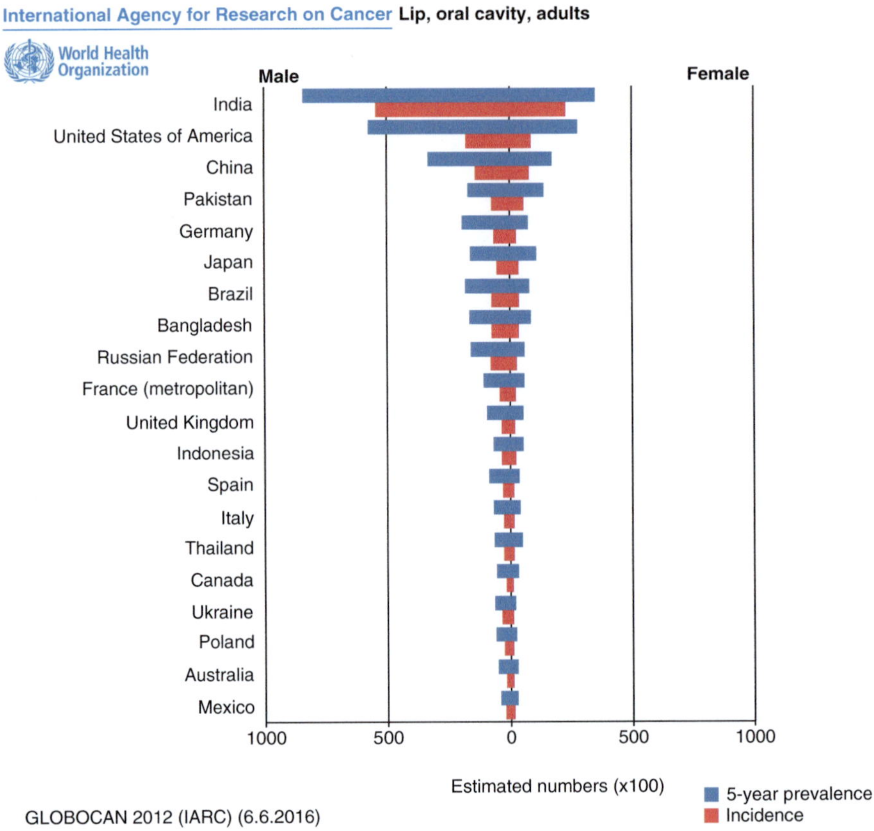

Fig. 1.4 The incidence and mortality of head and neck cancer estimated in 2012 of the highest 20 countries over the world

Table 1.1 Estimated incidence of lip, oral cavity and oropharyngeal cancer worldwide (all ages, both sexes), data derived from GLOBOCAN 2012

Population	Numbers	Crude rate	ASR (W)[a]	Cumulative risk
World	300,373	4.3	4.0	0.45
More developed regions	100,823	8.1	4.7	0.54
Less developed regions	199,550	3.4	3.7	0.42
Very high human development	92,338	8.0	4.8	0.54
High human development	45,734	4.4	3.8	0.45
Medium human development	121,240	3.4	3.3	0.38
Low human development	40,954	3.1	5.2	0.59
WHO African region (AFRO)	13,484	1.5	2.7	0.30
WHO Americas region (PAHO)	49,200	5.2	4.1	0.48

Table 1.1 (continued)

Population	Numbers	Crude rate	ASR (W)[a]	Cumulative risk
WHO East Mediterranean region (EMRO)	20,681	3.3	4.6	0.52
WHO European region (EURO)	65,933	7.3	4.6	0.53
WHO Southeast Asian region (SEARO)	103,464	5.6	6.4	0.73
WHO Western Pacific region (WPRO)	47,524	2.6	2.0	0.22
Middle East and Northern Africa (MENA)	7855	1.8	2.2	0.25

[a]ASR (W): Age-standardized rate to the world population

Table 1.2 Estimated mortality of lip, oral cavity and oropharyngeal cancer worldwide (all ages, both sexes), data derived from GLOBOCAN 2012

Population	Numbers	Crude rate	ASR (W)[a]	Cumulative risk
World	145,353	2.1	1.9	0.22
More developed regions	33,313	2.7	1.4	0.16
Less developed regions	112,040	1.9	2.1	0.24
Very high human development	26,970	2.3	1.2	0.14
High human development	19,615	1.9	1.6	0.19
Medium human development	73,503	2.1	2.0	0.23
Low human development	25,238	1.9	3.3	0.39
WHO African region (AFRO)	8530	1.0	1.8	0.20
WHO Americas region (PAHO)	12,803	1.3	1.0	0.12
WHO East Mediterranean region (EMRO)	10,997	1.8	2.5	0.30
WHO European region (EURO)	25,202	2.8	1.7	0.19
WHO Southeast Asian region (SEARO)	65,734	3.5	4.1	0.48
WHO Western Pacific region (WPRO)	22,068	1.2	0.9	0.09
IARC membership (24 countries)	81,929	3.1	2.6	0.29
Middle East and Northern Africa (MENA)	3154	0.7	0.9	0.10

[a]ASR (W): Age-standardized rate to the world population

In just India, over 100,000 cases of oral cancer are diagnosed annually, and the numbers are on the increase [5, 12, 13], while France has the highest incidence rate of oropharyngeal cancer [1].

1.2.2 Age and Gender

Oral and oropharyngeal cancers are considered to be the disease of elderly, while most of the cases of oral cancer occur between 50 and 75 years of age [4]. Table 1.3 shows the estimated ASR incidence of oral cancer in age grouping compared to all

Table 1.3 Estimated ASR incidence of oral cancer in age grouping compared to all cancers excluding non-melanoma skin cancer, data derived from Globocan 2012 for all sexes

Cancer	Total	0–14	15–39	40–44	45–49	50–54	55–59	60–64	65–69	70–74	75+	ASR (W)
All cancers excl. non-melanoma skin cancer	14,067,894	8.8	37.5	138.8	220.9	338.2	489.1	683.9	895.8	1114.4	1544.0	182.0
Lip, oral cavity	300,373	0.1	0.9	3.7	6.1	9.5	12.7	15.7	18.3	20.3	23.4	4.0

Table 1.4 Projected incidence for lip/oral cavity cancer (2012–2035)

Year	Estimated number of new cancers (all ages)	Male	Female	Both sexes
2012		198,975	101,398	300,373
	Ages <65	128,866	56,401	185,267
	Ages > = 65	70,109	44,997	115,106
2035		327,537	167,360	494,897
	Ages <65	181,507	77,866	259,373
	Ages > = 65	146,030	89,494	235,524
	Demographic change	128,562	65,962	194,524
	Ages <65	52,641	21,465	74,106
	Ages > = 65	75,921	44,497	120,418

Data derived from GLOBOCAN 2012

cancers excluding non-melanoma skin cancer. The mean age at presentation of this cancer is in the fifth and early sixth decades in Asian populations, compared to the seventh and eighth decades in North American populations [14, 15]. More recent, younger patients at the age of diagnosis were more reported [16]. For example, a study in Asia found that about 17% of the younger patients are below 40 years of age or at least in the fourth decade of their life [12] Table 1.4.

In a pooled analysis of case-control studies by the International Head and Neck Cancer Epidemiology Consortium, adults aged 45 years and younger exhibited a higher proportion of oral tongue cancers compared with adults older than 45 years (16% in women/11% in men versus 10.3% in women/5.9% in men, respectively). Also in that study, the associations of smoking and drinking with oral cavity cancer were weaker in young adults compared with older adults (ever-smokers/odds ratio [OR], 1.91 for young adults versus 2.18 for older adults; ever-drinkers/OR, 1.24 for young adults versus 1.61 for older adults) [16].

Considering all the age groups, men are more affected than women with a male to female (m/f) ratio ranging from 1.45 to 10.5 depending on the geography [12, 17–23]. For example, in Japan, the m/f ratio of OPC is 1.45 [17], 1.5 in Pakistan [18], 1.9 in Iran [24], 2.2–2.4 in the United States [25] and the highest of 10.5 in Taiwan [20]. However, a reverse gender ratio was reported in Thailand and India (Bangalore) where male to female ratio is 1:1.56 and 1:2.0, respectively [26, 27].

1.2.3 Site

It is well accepted that risk factors in a particular geographical region predominately define the site of occurrence. The tongue is the most common site for intraoral cancer among European, North American and Asian countries, amounting to 40–50% of oral cancers [4, 8, 28]. The next most common site is buccal mucosa where it is predominant among Asian populations due to areca nut/tobacco chewing habits in addition to gingiva [4, 8, 12]. Other sites include the lip, floor of the mouth and hard and soft palate and tonsils [4, 8]. In Australia, lip cancer was found to be the leading anatomical site in both sexes amounting to 36% of all OPC cases, of which 90% were diagnosed at the lower lip [29].

Remarkably, several studies have highlighted the tongue as the predominant site of oral cancer among young patients of 45 years or below [30–33].

1.2.4 Trends and Variations

Clearly, the changes in the use of the primary risk factors for oral cancer have over time and across countries influenced the trends in incidence and mortality rates [8, 14]. The decrease in smoking prevalence since the 1970s has been mirrored by a decline in the number of newly diagnosed tobacco-associated cancers [34]. Studies have shown that rates of oral cavity cancer increased among both men and women in some European countries but were stable or decreased in some of Asian countries and rates decreased for men and women in Canada and the United States. Rates of oropharyngeal cancer also increased among both men and women in a number of European nations and the United States [6, 8, 35–38].

Geography played an important role in the changing the face of the oral cancer statistics. Notably, varied trends in incidence rates of OPC across countries regarding subsite and sex were reported and more likely are due to the geographic differences in the prevalence of known OPC risk factors, such as tobacco and alcohol consumption and high-risk HPV infection [6, 8, 35–39]. Clearly, the increased rates of oropharyngeal cancers have strongly linked to the role of HPV infection that has risen in many economically developed countries where tobacco use has declined [4, 6, 35, 40–44]. Furthermore, a population-based SEER study found that the lifetime risk of second primary cancer in the head and neck in patients with cervical cancer was higher than in the general population, with a standardized incidence ratio (SIR) of 1.7, suggesting a significant role of HPV [45]. Likewise, the Swedish Family Cancer Database followed 135,386 women from 1958 to 1996 who were initially diagnosed with cervical carcinoma, for the occurrence of second primary cancers in the upper aerodigestive tract, as well as first primary cancers among their husbands [46]. This study revealed that female patients with cervical cancer had elevated risks for second cancers in the upper aerodigestive tract; for patients with in situ disease, the overall SIR was 1.68 (1.10–2.43), compared with females with invasive cervical cancer, who had an overall SIR of 2.45 (1.05–4.98). Husbands of cervical cancer patients also had elevated SIRs of cancers of the upper aerodigestive tract, suggesting a strong link to HPV [46].

Intriguingly, Chaturvedi et al. [35]. examined the trends in incidence rates of oral and oropharyngeal cancer using population-based registry data assembled by the Cancer Incidence in Five Continents (CI5) data system between 1983 and 2002 [35]. In men, substantial increases in OPC were observed among younger birth cohorts in most countries with significantly increasing overall incidence, resulting in the increasing incidence being statistically significantly stronger at ages younger than 60 years. More interestingly, among women, incidence significantly increased during the same period from 1983 to 2002 in Europe (Denmark, Estonia, France, the Netherlands, Slovakia, the United Kingdom, Italy and Spain) [35].

Another study by Simard et al. [6] assessed the trends in the rates of head and neck cancer incidence from 1983–1987 to 1998–2002. Their results similarly demonstrated increased rates of oral cancer among men and women in some European and Asian countries (Czech Republic, Slovak Republic, Denmark, Estonia, Finland, the United Kingdom and Japan). The largest increases were among men in Finland (RR = 1.61, 95% CI, 1.39–1.86) and women in Spain (RR = 2.23, 95% CI, 1.73–2.88). In France and Italy, rates declined among men but increased among women. Oral cavity incidence rates declined among men and women in many Asian countries as well as in Canada and the United States. Oropharyngeal cancer rates increased among both men and women in a number of European countries (Belarus, Czech Republic, Denmark, Finland, Iceland, Latvia, Norway and the United Kingdom), whereas they declined in some Asian countries. The largest increase in oropharyngeal rates was among Brazilian men [6].

In the United States, over the last three decades, a decline shaft in the incidence and mortality of oral cancer was reported. This observation was found irrespective of gender or ethnic background, but disparities remain where African-American males continue to have a higher incidence of oropharyngeal carcinomas compared to white patients [11, 47]. In Japan during the period between the years 1965 and 1999, fourfolds of increased incidence of OPC were observed in all sexes [14].

In Australia during the period from 1982 to 2008, an increased annual rate of 3.2% of the base of tongue cancers was observed [29].

The dramatic change in oropharyngeal cancer was the observation of an increased incidence in adults younger than 45 years of age, particularly base of the tongue and tonsil [48].

1.2.5 2035 Projection

A projected analysis of the proposed incidence and mortality burden of oral and oropharyngeal cancer was attempted using the GLOBOCAN, 2012. It shows that the OPC cases will have at least 40% increase in both incidence and mortality for both sexes, all ages (Figs. 1.5a and 1.6a). Remarkably, these increases will be demarcated in patients with an age of fewer than 65 years old (Tables 1.5 and 1.6). At the same time, it seems male will be more affected than female (Figs. 1.5b and 1.6b).

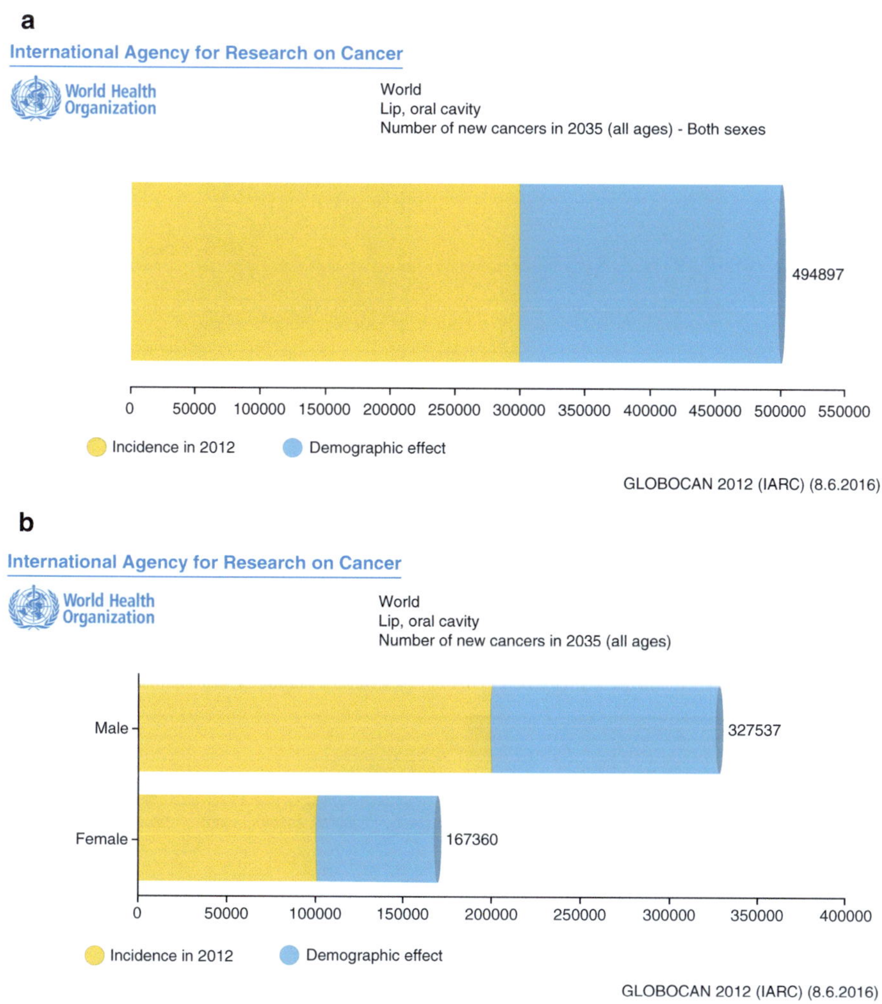

Fig. 1.5 (**a**) Crude incidence projections for lip/oral cavity cancer in all ages and both sexes (2012–2035). Data extracted from GLOBOCAN 2012. (**b**) Crude incidence projections for lip/oral cavity cancer in all ages (2012–2035). Data extracted from GLOBOCAN 2012

1.2.6 Survival

Several factors contribute to the overall survival rate of particular cancer. However, lymph node involvement, tumour size and socioeconomic status are the main prognostic factors [7, 8]. In the case of oral and oropharyngeal cancer, the overall 5-year survival rate has remained unchanged during the last 40 years with less than 50%. The best outcome is observed in lip carcinoma with an overall survival of over 90%. Overall, the prognosis is severely influenced by regional lymph node involvement. For early, localized stage I cancer, the 5-year survival exceeds 80% and falls to less than 15% in advanced disease stage IV [8].

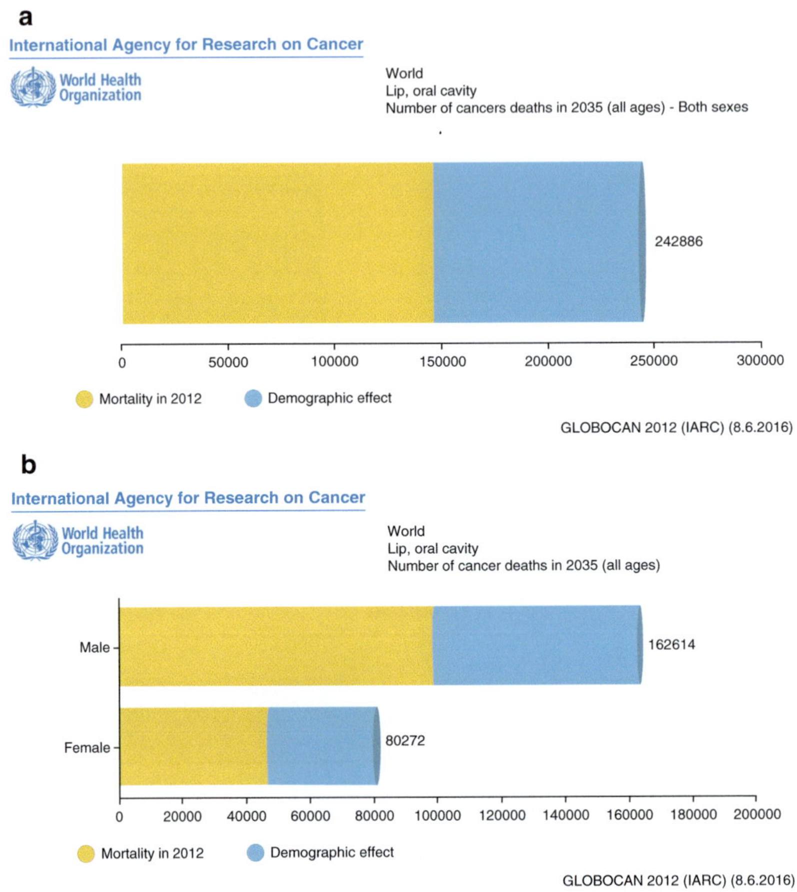

Fig. 1.6 (**a**) Crude mortality projections for lip/oral cavity cancer in all ages and both sexes (2012–2035). Data extracted from GLOBOCAN 2012. (**b**) Crude mortality projections for lip/oral cavity cancer, all ages (2012–2035). Data extracted from GLOBOCAN 2012

Table 1.5 Projected deaths for lip/oral cavity cancer (2012–2035)

Year	Estimated number of cancer deaths (all ages)	Male	Female	Both sexes
2012		97,940	47,413	145,353
	Ages <65	61,407	24,064	85,471
	Ages > = 65	36,533	23,349	59,882
2035		162,614	80,272	242,886
	Ages <65	86,436	33,838	120,274
	Ages > = 65	76,178	46,434	122,612
	Demographic change	64,674	32,859	97,533
	Ages <65	25,029	9774	34,803
	Ages > = 65	39,645	23,085	62,730

Data derived from GLOBOCAN 2012

Table 1.6 Urgent referral guidelines for head and neck cancer

Clinical signs and symptoms
• Hoarseness persisting for more than 6 weeks
• Ulceration of oral mucosa persisting for more than 3 weeks
• Oral swellings persisting for more than 3 weeks
• All red or red and white patches of the oral mucosa
• Dysphagia persisting for more than 3 weeks
• Unilateral nasal obstruction, particularly when associated with purulent discharge
• Unexplained tooth mobility not associated with periodontal disease
• Unresolving neck masses for more than 3 weeks
• Cranial neuropathies
• Orbital masses

(Adopted from Head and Neck Cancer: Multidisciplinary Management Guidelines) [90]

In the United States, a substantial improvement in the overall 5-year survival rate of OPC cases between 1973 and 2006 was reported in all age groups except for patients aged ≥75 years for tonsillar carcinoma, carcinoma of the tongue and carcinoma of the oral cavity [25]. The current overall 5-year survival rate in the United States is nearly 65% [25, 49], whereas around 50% in Europe [50]. However, a wider range between 32 and 54% is reported in low-to-middle-income countries (India, China, Republic of Korea, Pakistan, Singapore and Thailand [7, 51].

1.3 Clinical Characteristics

Oral cavity cancers are mostly preceded by a group of lesions which are termed "potentially oral malignant disorders" that are mainly white and red lesions on clinical presentation. Oral leukoplakia traditionally has been defined as "a white patch or plaque that cannot be characterized clinically or pathologically as any other disease (i.e. excluding pseudomembranous candidiasis, lichen planus, tobacco pouch keratosis, nicotine stomatitis, oral hairy leukoplakia, etc.)" [52, 53]. Histopathologically, leukoplakias exhibit squamous epithelium with hyperkeratosis and/or acanthosis and with or without dysplasia. Interestingly, epithelial dysplasia in leukoplakic lesions ranges from 16 to 39% [54]. Furthermore, a particular type of progressive multifocal leukoplakia exists and is called proliferative verrucous leukoplakia (PVL). It is usually associated with high rate of malignant transformation to either squamous cell cancer or verrucous carcinoma [55]. Erythroplakia is defined as "a velvety red patch that cannot be characterized clinically or pathologically as any other definable disease" [52–54, 56, 57]. Contrary to leukoplakia, almost all true erythroplakias will show evidence of high-grade dysplasia, carcinoma in situ or invasive carcinoma [57]. Most importantly, the risk of dysplasia or carcinoma is higher for leukoplakias at the lateral borders of the tongue and floor of the mouth compared to those in other oral sites [54, 56]. A list of the clinical signs and symptoms that warrant urgent referrals for suspicion of malignancy is presented in Table 1.6.

Carcinoma of the lip is the most common type of tumour in head and neck region, and it accounts nearly 25–30% of oral cavity cancer [58–60]. Generally, white men, 50–80 years of age, are mostly affected. The lower lip is the favourite site with 85–95% of all lip cancers. The upper lip and the commissures are lesser primary sites affected with an overall range of 2–7% and 1–4%, respectively [60]. It seems that the areas with high solar radiation and UV exposure associated with tobacco use have a higher incidence of lip cancer. For example, lip cancer is the most common type of head and neck cancer in Australia [29]. High incidence was also reported in the South American countries particularly the tropical regions where the sun exposure is too high in addition to areas in Canada, Spain and Eastern Europe [60]. In a high proportion of lip cancer cases, it was preceded by actinic cheilitis. Clinically, most of the cancer cases presented as a non-healing ulcer or rapidly growing exophytic mass [58]. Lip cancer is characterized by the best 5-year survival rate of oral cancer which is 85–90% with minimal lymphatic cervical metastasis with less 4% [4, 58, 59].

Cancer of the tongue accounts to 40–50 of all oral cancer cases in the Western world where the lateral surfaces and base of the tongue are mostly affected [4, 8, 61]. Tobacco and alcohol consumptions are primary risk factors for tongue carcinomas; however, HPV is the major risk factor for base of tongue tumours [62, 63]. The malignant cases of the anterior two-thirds of the tongue are detected earlier than those in the third posterior part [61]. The typical presentation of anterior two-thirds of tongue cancer is painless indurated ulcer on the lateral borders, though base of tongue cancers is more sort of ulcerative-infiltrative type. Most of the cases developed silently to be sizable when first diagnosed. Tongue carcinomas tend to send metastases to the cervical lymph nodes where prognosis is relatively poor [61].

Carcinomas of the buccal mucosa are mostly located in the posterior and widely seen in patients who chew areca nut/tobacco [64, 65]. It is the commonest type of oral cancer among Asian populations [8]. Buccal mucosa cancer is characterized by high recurrence and poor prognosis [65, 66]. Nair et al. [64] compared between two large cohorts of tongue and buccal mucosa squamous cell carcinomas using several clinical and histopathological parameters in one hospital in India. Tongue cancer was more prevalent in younger patients compared to buccal mucosa cancer where the mean age for tongue and buccal mucosa cancers was 48 and 51, respectively. The male to female ratio was found in buccal mucosa (3.26:1) higher than that of tongue cancers (2.51:1). 60% of tongue cases were diagnosed at an early stage (T1 + T2), while 18% of buccal mucosa cancers were diagnosed at this similar stage. Tongue carcinomas have shown more cases with poor differentiation and perineural invasion compared to those of the buccal mucosa [64].

Interestingly, cancer of the floor of the mouth is more often seen in men than women marking a ration 2.6:1 with age around 60 years. There is a predilection for incidence at anterolateral regions and tendance to send metastases via the lymphatic drainage to cervical lymph nodes correlating with poor prognosis. Nearly 25–30% of the T1–T2 floor of mouth carcinomas are diagnosed with occult lymph nodal involvement. Shafer and Waldron [67] firstly provided evidence that floor of mouth white and red lesions manifest either severe dysplasia, carcinoma in situ or invasive carcinoma 21 and 95%, respectively.

Carcinomas of the hard palate and gingiva are relatively rare and less seen than the other intraoral sites like the tongue or buccal mucosa, accounting 10% of all intraoral cancers [68–71]. Hard palate cancer is mostly seen in patients with reverse smoking habits [70]. Interestingly, gingival carcinomas are more often seen in the mandible than the maxilla [72]. Both hard palate and gingiva cancers share similar clinical and pathological characteristics. Both tumours show male predominance with a mean age of 64 [68, 69]. Yang et al. [68] showed that the incidence of occult node was 32.1% for the maxillary gingiva and 21.7% for the hard palate.

Soft palate and tonsil are the most common sites of oropharyngeal cancers [4, 17]. Both are linked to HPV infection predominantly type 16 that is attributed to the recent increase in the burden of oropharyngeal squamous cell carcinomas [6, 35, 73]. Most of tonsillar carcinoma patients are diagnosed at advanced stage [74]. In a long-term follow-up during the period 1970–1990 of a large cohort of 640 patients, with tonsillar carcinomas treated with radical radiotherapy, high mortality rate with recurrent disease was observed [75]. Notably, they reported a 5-year cause-specific survival of 40% for the whole cohort. In other words, the probability of death due to disease was much higher than the probability of death due to other causes [75].

Depending on the tumour location and size, like other oropharyngeal cancers, the symptoms of soft palate carcinomas are dictated. However, pain in the ear, trismus, bleeding from the mouth and feeling a lump in the throat are suggestive for soft palate cancers [76].

More interestingly, Ang et al. [77] provided strong evidence that HPV tumour status is an independent prognostic factor for overall survival and progression-free survival among patients with oropharyngeal squamous cell carcinomas. They found that patients with HPV-positive cancer had better overall survival and progression-free survival than patients with HPV-negative cancer.

1.4 Early Detection and Prevention of Oral Cancer

Early detection of the preliminary process of carcinogenesis enables conservative therapeutic approaches to a brief recovery and a more favourable prognosis. Prevention is better than cure. Oral cancer is a preventable disease.

1.4.1 Primary Prevention

Cancer prevention aims to reduce the likelihood of cancer occurrence by avoiding the cancer risk factors. Cancer of the lip and oral cavity has multiplicative effects of risk factors: tobacco product consumption either smoking or chewing/smokeless forms, areca nut/betel quid, alcohol beverages drinking or HPV infections [7]. Population-based preventive campaigns with the aim of reducing or eliminating tobacco, alcohol or areca nut/betel quid use should be encouraged and implemented

[7]. These measures have a great potential in diminishing the burden of oral cancer particularly in the low economic regions where most oral cancer cases are diagnosed. HPV vaccination has shown promising results in decreasing its prevalence. Additionally, changing lifestyle or eating habits by having regular physical exercises and a healthy diet may help to reduce the risks for developing OPC. It is evident that the incidence of lip cancers may be reduced by applying measure for sun exposure protection [8].

Cessation of tobacco smoking has decreased the risk of OPC development by one-half (50%) within 5 years [78]. Furthermore, a person requires 20 years of cigarette quitting arriving at the same level as for a person who never smoked [78, 79]. Likewise, 5 years of drinking cessation was associated with a reduction of around 15% in the alcohol-related elevated risk of OPC [80].

1.4.2 Secondary Prevention (Screening)

There is substantial scope for prevention and early detection of cancer through screening. It is remarkably important to distinguish screening from case finding. Screening is defined as "a public health service in which members of a defined population, who do not necessarily perceive they are at risk of, or are already affected by a disease or its complications, are asked a question or offered a test, to identify those individuals who are more likely to be helped than harmed by further tests or treatment to reduce the risk of a disease or its complications" [81]. The main objective of screening tests is to identify early disease or risk factors for disease to a great number of apparently healthy individuals [82]. The aim of a diagnostic test is to establish the presence (or absence) of disease as a basis for treatment decisions in symptomatic or screen-positive individuals (confirmatory test) [82]. Screening programmes for cervical cancer have resulted in a reduction of morbidity and mortality of invasive cervical lesions [83], and breast cancer screening has also resulted in reduced mortality [84]. Moreover, screening studies have provided useful information regarding the natural history of the screened cancer [85]. However, screening for oral cancer and precancer is more controversial. The challenge with oral cancer screening is the lack of a reliable evidence to support implementing population-based screening programmes [86]. Heavy users of tobacco and alcohol, elderly men with poor diet and low socioeconomic status, are defined as a high-risk population for developing OPC [47]. Opportunistic screening for high-risk groups, by offering a screening test when a patient attends a clinic for some other, unrelated reason, for example, patients attending general dental or medical offices, is advocated [87–89].

Conclusions

Malignant tumours that originate from the oral and oropharyngeal region are predominantly squamous cell carcinomas where age-standardized rates of incidence and mortality are higher in the developing world than the developed. They share common risk factors of tobacco and alcohol consumptions, areca nut chewing, the role of high-risk human papillomavirus and poor diet. The lip, lateral surfaces of the tongue and floor of mouth are most affected. Varied trends in the epidemiology of oral and oropharyngeal cancer were observed in the last three decades where it has declined in some areas and increased in others. Human papillomavirus has been attributed to the recently increased trend of oropharyngeal cancer cases over the world. Poor cancer registries in the developing countries shadow the real lifetime global epidemiological picture of oral and oropharyngeal cancer that is potentially worse than it is now due to unfortunately underreporting issues. Efforts are needed to improve the cancer registries on national population levels to improve the understanding of the statistics and associated disparities of oral and oropharyngeal cancer and hopefully to better control this fatal disease. Primary and secondary preventions are still considered the most efficient modes for combating the increasing burden of oral cancer worldwide. Conventional oral examination along with the patient's history risk stratification associated with an objective histopathological evaluation of a biopsy taken from a suspicious lesion is still the gold standard for the early detection of oral cancer. The nature of dental practice provides greater patient access to oral care providers compared with physicians. Periodic recall visits are an opportunity to establish an oral cancer surveillance programme in clinical practice.

Conflict of Interest No potential conflict of interest is declared.

References

1. Forman D, Bray F, Brewster DH, Gombe Mbalawa C, Kohler B, Piñeros M, et al., editors. Cancer incidence in five continents, vol. X. Lyon: International Agency for Research on Cancer; 2014.
2. Ferlay J, Soerjomataram I, Dikshit R, Eser S, Mathers C, Rebelo M, et al. Cancer incidence and mortality worldwide: sources, methods and major patterns in GLOBOCAN 2012. Int J Cancer. 2015;136(5):E359–86.
3. Organisation WH. International statistical classification of diseases and related health problems- 10th revision: 2016: WHO Publications; 2011. Available from: http://www.who.int/classifications/icd/en/.
4. Chi AC, Day TA, Neville BW. Oral cavity and oropharyngeal squamous cell carcinoma--an update. CA Cancer J Clin. 2015;65(5):401–21.
5. GLOBOCAN 2012 v1.0, Cancer Incidence and Mortality Worldwide: IARC CancerBase No. 11 [Internet]. Lyon, France: International Agency for Research on Cancer; 2013. Available from: http://globocan.iarc.fr, accessed on 05/05/2016. [Internet]. 2013.
6. Simard EP, Torre LA, Jemal A. International trends in head and neck cancer incidence rates: differences by country, sex and anatomic site. Oral Oncol. 2014;50(5):387–403.
7. Sankaranarayanan R, Ramadas K, Amarasinghe H, Subramanian S, Johnson N. Oral cancer: prevention, early detection, and treatment. In: Gelband H, Jha P, Sankaranarayanan R, Horton S, editors. Cancer: disease control priorities, vol. 3. 3rd ed. Washington DC: The International Bank for Reconstruction and Development/The World Bank; 2015.
8. Warnakulasuriya S. Global epidemiology of oral and oropharyngeal cancer. Oral Oncol. 2009;45(4–5):309–16.

9. Coelho KR. Challenges of the oral cancer burden in India. J Cancer Epidemiol. 2012;2012:701932.
10. Siegel RL, Miller KD, Jemal A. Cancer statistics, 2016. CA Cancer J Clin. 2016;66(1):7–30.
11. Torre LA, Sauer AM, Chen MS Jr, Kagawa-Singer M, Jemal A, Siegel RL. Cancer statistics for Asian Americans, Native Hawaiians, and Pacific Islanders, 2016: converging incidence in males and females. CA Cancer J Clin. 2016;66(3):182–202.
12. Krishna Rao SV, Mejia G, Roberts-Thomson K, Logan R. Epidemiology of oral cancer in Asia in the past decade--an update (2000–2012). Asian Pac J Cancer Prev. 2013;14(10):5567–77.
13. Gupta B, Ariyawardana A, Johnson NW. Oral cancer in India continues in epidemic proportions: evidence base and policy initiatives. Int Dent J. 2013;63(1):12–25.
14. Gupta B, Johnson NW, Kumar N. Global epidemiology of head and neck cancers: a continuing challenge. Oncology. 2016;91(1):13–23.
15. Rettig EM, D'Souza G. Epidemiology of head and neck cancer. Surg Oncol Clin N Am. 2015;24(3):379–96.
16. Toporcov TN, Znaor A, Zhang ZF, Yu GP, Winn DM, Wei Q, et al. Risk factors for head and neck cancer in young adults: a pooled analysis in the INHANCE consortium. Int J Epidemiol. 2015;44(1):169–85.
17. Ariyoshi Y, Shimahara M, Omura K, Yamamoto E, Mizuki H, Chiba H, et al. Epidemiological study of malignant tumors in the oral and maxillofacial region: survey of member institutions of the Japanese Society of Oral and Maxillofacial Surgeons, 2002. Int J Clin Oncol. 2008;13(3):220–8.
18. Bhurgri Y. Cancer of the oral cavity – trends in Karachi South (1995–2002). Asian Pac J Cancer Prev. 2005;6(1):22–6.
19. Halboub ES, Al-Anazi YM, Al-Mohaya MA. Characterization of Yemeni patients treated for oral and pharyngeal cancers in Saudi Arabia. Saudi Med J. 2011;32(11):1177–82.
20. Chiang CT, Hwang YH, Su CC, Tsai KY, Lian Ie B, Yuan TH, et al. Elucidating the underlying causes of oral cancer through spatial clustering in high-risk areas of Taiwan with a distinct gender ratio of incidence. Geospat Health. 2010;4(2):230–42.
21. Guneri P, Cankaya H, Yavuzer A, Guneri EA, Erisen L, Ozkul D, et al. Primary oral cancer in a Turkish population sample: association with sociodemographic features, smoking, alcohol, diet and dentition. Oral Oncol. 2005;41(10):1005–12.
22. Sherin N, Simi T, Shameena P, Sudha S. Changing trends in oral cancer. Indian J Cancer. 2008;45(3):93–6.
23. Rajkumar T, Sridhar H, Balaram P, Vaccarella S, Gajalakshmi V, Nandakumar A, et al. Oral cancer in Southern India: the influence of body size, diet, infections and sexual practices. Eur J Cancer Prev. 2003;12(2):135–43.
24. Mirzaei M, Hosseini SA, Ghoncheh M, Soheilipour F, Soltani S, Soheilipour F, et al. Epidemiology and trend of head and neck cancers in Iran. Glob J Health Sci. 2016;8(1):189–93.
25. Pulte D, Brenner H. Changes in survival in head and neck cancers in the late 20th and early 21st century: a period analysis. Oncologist. 2010;15(9):994–1001.
26. Franceschi S, Bidoli E, Herrero R, Munoz N. Comparison of cancers of the oral cavity and pharynx worldwide: etiological clues. Oral Oncol. 2000;36(1):106–15.
27. Kruaysawat W, Aekplakorn W, Chapman RS. Survival time and prognostic factors of oral cancer in Ubon Ratchathani Cancer Center. J Med Assoc Thail. 2010;93(3):278–84.
28. Khalili J. Oral cancer: risk factors, prevention and diagnostic. Exp Oncol. 2008;30(4):259–64.
29. Ariyawardana A, Johnson NW. Trends of lip, oral cavity and oropharyngeal cancers in Australia 1982–2008: overall good news but with rising rates in the oropharynx. BMC Cancer. 2013;13:333.
30. Manuel S, Raghavan SK, Pandey M, Sebastian P. Survival in patients under 45 years with squamous cell carcinoma of the oral tongue. Int J Oral Maxillofac Surg. 2003;32(2):167–73.
31. Komolmalai N, Chuachamsai S, Tantiwipawin S, Dejsuvan S, Buhngamongkol P, Wongvised C, et al. Ten-year analysis of oral cancer focusing on young people in northern Thailand. J Oral Sci. 2015;57(4):327–34.
32. Llewellyn CD, Linklater K, Bell J, Johnson NW, Warnakulasuriya S. An analysis of risk factors for oral cancer in young people: a case-control study. Oral Oncol. 2004;40(3):304–13.

33. Mallet Y, Avalos N, Le Ridant AM, Gangloff P, Moriniere S, Rame JP, et al. Head and neck cancer in young people: a series of 52 SCCs of the oral tongue in patients aged 35 years or less. Acta Otolaryngol. 2009;129(12):1503–8.
34. Petersen PE. Oral cancer prevention and control--the approach of the World Health Organization. Oral Oncol. 2009;45(4–5):454–60.
35. Chaturvedi AK, Anderson WF, Lortet-Tieulent J, Curado MP, Ferlay J, Franceschi S, et al. Worldwide trends in incidence rates for oral cavity and oropharyngeal cancers. J Clin Oncol. 2013;31(36):4550–9.
36. Boyle P, Ferlay J. Cancer incidence and mortality in Europe, 2004. Ann Oncol. 2005;16(3):481–8.
37. Garavello W, Bertuccio P, Levi F, Lucchini F, Bosetti C, Malvezzi M, et al. The oral cancer epidemic in central and eastern Europe. Int J Cancer. 2010;127(1):160–71.
38. Sturgis EM, Cinciripini PM. Trends in head and neck cancer incidence in relation to smoking prevalence: an emerging epidemic of human papillomavirus-associated cancers? Cancer. 2007;110(7):1429–35.
39. Anantharaman D, Muller DC, Lagiou P, Ahrens W, Holcatova I, Merletti F, et al. Combined effects of smoking and HPV16 in oropharyngeal cancer. Int J Epidemiol. 2016;45(3): 752–61.
40. Herrero R, Castellsague X, Pawlita M, Lissowska J, Kee F, Balaram P, et al. Human papillomavirus and oral cancer: the International Agency for Research on Cancer multicenter study. J Natl Cancer Inst. 2003;95(23):1772–83.
41. Gillison ML, Chaturvedi AK, Anderson WF, Fakhry C. Epidemiology of human papillomavirus-positive head and neck squamous cell carcinoma. J Clin Oncol. 2015;33(29):3235–42.
42. Gooi Z, Chan JY, Fakhry C. The epidemiology of the human papillomavirus related to oropharyngeal head and neck cancer. Laryngoscope. 2016;126(4):894–900.
43. Maxwell JH, Grandis JR, Ferris RL. HPV-associated head and neck cancer: unique features of epidemiology and clinical management. Annu Rev Med. 2016;67:91–101.
44. Anantharaman D, Gheit T, Waterboer T, Abedi-Ardekani B, Carreira C, McKay-Chopin S, et al. Human papillomavirus infections and upper aero-digestive tract cancers: the ARCAGE study. J Natl Cancer Inst. 2013;105(8):536–45.
45. Rose Ragin CC, Taioli E. Second primary head and neck tumor risk in patients with cervical cancer--SEER data analysis. Head Neck. 2008;30(1):58–66.
46. Hemminki K, Dong C, Frisch M. Tonsillar and other upper aerodigestive tract cancers among cervical cancer patients and their husbands. Eur J Cancer Prev. 2000;9(6):433–7.
47. Conway DI, Petticrew M, Marlborough H, Berthiller J, Hashibe M, Macpherson LM. Socioeconomic inequalities and oral cancer risk: a systematic review and meta-analysis of case-control studies. Int J Cancer. 2008;122(12):2811–9.
48. Saman DM. A review of the epidemiology of oral and pharyngeal carcinoma: update. Head Neck Oncol. 2012;4:1.
49. Ringash J. Survivorship and quality of life in head and neck cancer. J Clin Oncol. 2015; 33(29):3322–7.
50. Sant M, Allemani C, Santaquilani M, Knijn A, Marchesi F, Capocaccia R, et al. EUROCARE-4. Survival of cancer patients diagnosed in 1995-1999. Results and commentary. Eur J Cancer. 2009;45(6):931–91.
51. Sankaranarayanan R, Swaminathan R, Brenner H, Chen K, Chia KS, Chen JG, et al. Cancer survival in Africa, Asia, and Central America: a population-based study. Lancet Oncol. 2010;11(2):165–73.
52. Warnakulasuriya S, Johnson NW, van der Waal I. Nomenclature and classification of potentially malignant disorders of the oral mucosa. J Oral Pathol Med. 2007;36(10):575–80.
53. Bouquot JE. Oral leukoplakia and erythroplakia: a review and update. Pract Periodontics Aesthet Dent. 1994;6(6):9–17. quiz 9
54. Napier SS, Speight PM. Natural history of potentially malignant oral lesions and conditions: an overview of the literature. J Oral Pathol Med. 2008;37(1):1–10.
55. Cabay RJ, Morton TH Jr, Epstein JB. Proliferative verrucous leukoplakia and its progression to oral carcinoma: a review of the literature. J Oral Pathol Med. 2007;36(5):255–61.

56. Neville BW, Day TA. Oral cancer and precancerous lesions. CA Cancer J Clin. 2002; 52(4):195–215.
57. Reichart PA, Philipsen HP. Oral erythroplakia--a review. Oral Oncol. 2005;41(6):551–61.
58. Biasoli ER, Valente VB, Mantovan B, Collado FU, Neto SC, Sundefeld ML, et al. Lip cancer: a clinicopathological study and treatment outcomes in a 25-year experience. J Oral Maxillofac Surg. 2016;74(7):1360–7.
59. Dominguez-Gordillo A, Esparza-Gomez G, Garcia-Jimenez B, Cerero-Lapiedra R, Casado-Gomez I, Romero-Lastra P, et al. The pattern of lip cancer occurrence over the 1990–2011 period in public hospitals in Madrid, Spain. J Oral Pathol Med. 2016;45(3):202–10.
60. Moore S, Johnson N, Pierce A, Wilson D. The epidemiology of lip cancer: a review of global incidence and aetiology. Oral Dis. 1999;5(3):185–95.
61. Moore SR, Johnson NW, Pierce AM, Wilson DF. The epidemiology of tongue cancer: a review of global incidence. Oral Dis. 2000;6(2):75–84.
62. Pezzuto F, Buonaguro L, Caponigro F, Ionna F, Starita N, Annunziata C, et al. Update on head and neck cancer: current knowledge on epidemiology, risk factors, molecular features and novel therapies. Oncology. 2015;89(3):125–36.
63. Dok R, Nuyts S. HPV positive head and neck cancers: molecular pathogenesis and evolving treatment strategies. Cancer. 2016;8(4):41.
64. Nair S, Singh B, Pawar PV, Datta S, Nair D, Kane S, et al. Squamous cell carcinoma of tongue and buccal mucosa: clinico-pathologically different entities. Eur Arch Otorhinolaryngol. 2016;273(11):3921–8.
65. Fang QG, Shi S, Li ZN, Zhang X, Liua FY, Xu ZF, et al. Squamous cell carcinoma of the buccal mucosa: analysis of clinical presentation, outcome and prognostic factors. Mol Clin Oncol. 2013;1(3):531–4.
66. DeConde A, Miller ME, Palla B, Lai C, Elashoff D, Chhetri D, et al. Squamous cell carcinoma of buccal mucosa: a 40-year review. Am J Otolaryngol. 2012;33(6):673–7.
67. Shafer WG, Waldron CA. Erythroplakia of the oral cavity. Cancer. 1975;36(3):1021–8.
68. Yang X, Song X, Chu W, Li L, Ma L, Wu Y. Clinicopathological characteristics and outcome predictors in squamous cell carcinoma of the maxillary gingiva and hard palate. J Oral Maxillofac Surg. 2015;73(7):1429–36.
69. Mourouzis C, Pratt C, Brennan PA. Squamous cell carcinoma of the maxillary gingiva, alveolus, and hard palate: is there a need for elective neck dissection? Br J Oral Maxillofac Surg. 2010;48(5):345–8.
70. Chung CK, Rahman SM, Lim ML, Constable WC. Squamous cell carcinoma of the hard palate. Int J Radiat Oncol Biol Phys. 1979;5(2):191–6.
71. Rautava J, Luukkaa M, Heikinheimo K, Alin J, Grenman R, Happonen R-P. Squamous cell carcinomas arising from different types of oral epithelia differ in their tumor and patient characteristics and survival. Oral Oncol. 2007;43(9):911–9.
72. Fitzpatrick SG, Neuman AN, Cohen DM, Bhattacharyya I. The clinical and histologic presentation of gingival squamous cell carcinoma: a study of 519 cases. Oral Surg Oral Med Oral Pathol Oral Radiol. 2012;114(4):509–15.
73. Shiboski CH, Schmidt BL, Jordan RC. Tongue and tonsil carcinoma: increasing trends in the U.S. population ages 20–44 years. Cancer. 2005;103(9):1843–9.
74. Frisch M, Hjalgrim H, Jaeger AB, Biggar RJ. Changing patterns of tonsillar squamous cell carcinoma in the United States. Cancer Causes Control. 2000;11(6):489–95.
75. Bachar GY, Goh C, Goldstein DP, O'Sullivan B, Irish JC. Long-term outcome analysis after surgical salvage for recurrent tonsil carcinoma following radical radiotherapy. Eur Arch Otorhinolaryngol. 2010;267(2):295–301.
76. Leemans CR, Engelbrecht WJ, Tiwari R, Deville WL, Karim AB, van der Waal I, et al. Carcinoma of the soft palate and anterior tonsillar pillar. Laryngoscope. 1994;104(12):1477–81.
77. Ang KK, Harris J, Wheeler R, Weber R, Rosenthal DI, Nguyen-Tan PF, et al. Human papillomavirus and survival of patients with oropharyngeal cancer. N Engl J Med. 2010; 363(1):24–35.
78. Samet JM. The health benefits of smoking cessation. Med Clin North Am. 1992;76(2):399–414.

79. Cully M. Public health: the benefits and challenges of smoking cessation. Nat Rev Cardiol. 2013;10(3):117.
80. Franceschi S, Levi F, Dal Maso L, Talamini R, Conti E, Negri E, et al. Cessation of alcohol drinking and risk of cancer of the oral cavity and pharynx. Int J Cancer. 2000;85(6):787–90.
81. Department of Health UK. Second Report of the UK National Screening Committee. London: 2000.
82. Lewis G, Sheringham J, Bernal JL, Crayford T. Mastering public health: a postgraduate guide to examinations and revalidation. 2nd ed. Boca Raton: CRC Press; 2014.
83. Gramer DW. The role of cervical cytology in the declining morbidity and mortality of cervical cancer. Cancer. 1974;34:2018–27.
84. Fletcher SW, Black W, Harris R, Rimer BK, Shapiro S. Report of the international workshop on screening for breast cancer. J Natl Cancer Inst. 1993;85(20):1644–56.
85. Jatoi I. Breast cancer screening. New York: Chapman & Hall; 1997.
86. Kujan O, Glenny AM, Duxbury J, Thakker N, Sloan P. Evaluation of screening strategies for improving oral cancer mortality: a Cochrane systematic review. J Dent Educ. 2005;69(2):255–65.
87. Iyer S, Thankappan K, Balasubramanian D. Early detection of oral cancers: current status and future prospects. Curr Opin Otolaryngol Head Neck Surg. 2016;24(2):110–4.
88. Sankaranarayanan R, Ramadas K, Thara S, Muwonge R, Thomas G, Anju G, et al. Long term effect of visual screening on oral cancer incidence and mortality in a randomized trial in Kerala, India. Oral Oncol. 2013;49(4):314–21.
89. Brocklehurst P, Kujan O, O'Malley LA, Ogden G, Shepherd S, Glenny AM. Screening programmes for the early detection and prevention of oral cancer. Cochrane Database Syst Rev. 2013;11:CD004150.
90. Roland N, Paleri V, editors. Head and neck cancer: multidisciplinary management guidelines. 4th ed. London: ENT UK; 2011.

Novel Developments in the Molecular Genetic Basis of Oral Squamous Cell Carcinoma (OSCC)

2

Nader I Al-Dewik and M. Walid Qoronfleh

2.1 Introduction

Consumption of tobacco, alcohol, and other carcinogenic products makes oral cancer the most prevalent malignancy. More than 95% of the carcinomas of the oral cavity represent squamous cell type. Oral carcinogenesis is a highly complex, multistep process. In the last two decades, our understanding and knowledge of the underlying molecular genetic anomalies of oral squamous cell carcinoma (OSCC) has been unprecedentedly expanded due to the novel discoveries as the result of the breakthroughs in genomics technology.

In this chapter, we will focus on the most important and common molecular genetic alterations at the genomic, epigenetic, and transcriptomic levels and study changes in tumor suppressor genes (TSGs), oncogenes, gene expression, cell surface receptors, epigenetic and chromosomal instability and copy number variation (genomic instability), mitochondrial DNA (mtDNA) mutations, telomeres and telomerase, microsatellite instability and alteration and noncoding RNA, and loss of heterozygosity (LOH) in OSCC.

OSCC genetic changes are divided into two groups: (1) dominant inheritance changes most often arising in proto-oncogenes, in particular, TSGs, resulting in

N.I. Al-Dewik (✉)
Qatar Medical Genetics Center (QMGC), Interim Translational Research Institute (iTRI), HMC, P.O. Box 3050, Doha, Qatar

Faculty of Health and Social Care Sciences, Kingston University, St George's University of London, London, UK
e-mail: NALDEWIK@hamad.qa

M.W. Qoronfleh
Biotechnology Development Department, Qatar Biomedical Research Institute (QBRI), Hamad bin Khalifa University (HBKU), P.O. Box 34110, Doha, Qatar
e-mail: wqoronfleh@qf.org.qa

A.-E. Al Moustafa (ed.), *Development of Oral Cancer*,
DOI 10.1007/978-3-319-48054-1_2

gain of function, and (2) recessive inheritance changes, mutations most commonly observed in the growth-inhibitory signaling pathway genes or generally in TSGs, causing the loss of function.

2.2 Transcriptional Factors

The cell division gene types responsible for cancer are proto-oncogenes and tumor suppressor genes. In human cancer, transcription factors (TFs) are usually deregulated in the cells. Therefore, they represent an attractive target for therapy. TFs participate in the regulation of some 19-signal pathways that are highly conserved and are thought to be involved in cancer [1].

2.3 Tumor Suppressor Genes or Anti-oncogenes

Tumor suppressor genes (TSGs) (loss of function) slow the growth of cells, i.e., inhibit cell proliferation. Thus, the TSGs function to protect a normal cell transformation into malignant cell. TSGs include caretaker genes (cell cycle genes, DNA repair genes, p53 gene), gatekeeper genes (apoptosis genes, APC gene, RB gene), and landscaper genes (extracellular matrix proteins, adhesion molecules, growth factors) [2, 3].

Inactivation or loss of function of the TSGs has been very well documented in oral cancer. Several studies showed that mutations are more frequent in tumor suppressor genes rather than oncogenes in oral cancer. So far, several TSGs, namely, (1) p53; (2) FAT; (3) cyclin-dependent kinase inhibitor 2A (CDKN2A) p16, p21, and p27 and retinoblastoma RB1; (4) deleted in oral cancer-1 (DOC-1); (5) MTNR1A; (6) thrombospondin 1 (TSP-1); (7) PTEN; and (8) Bcl-2 and caspase-3, have showed tumor suppressor activity in malignant oral keratinocytes [4, 5].

In TP53, the majority of mutations are missense which occurs in the DNA-binding domain (DBD) cluster from exons 5–8; several hotspot regions in the DBD contain approximately 63% changes resulting in avoiding binding to DNA, while frameshift and nonsense mutations are distributed similarly throughout the gene. LOH in the exon 4 of the p53 gene at chromosome 17 (17p) has been also associated with oral cancer. In addition, the most predominant mutations in the FAT1 (4q35) are homozygous deletion which is found in 80% (hotspot regions in exons 1 and 4) of primary oral cancers; nonsense and frameshift mutations and mutated FAT1 promote tumor cell growth via sustained β-catenin shuttle to the nucleus [6–11].

On the other hand, in the cell cycle genes such as CDKN2A and RB1, the pattern of mutations that inactivate cell cycle inhibitors is significantly different; deletion, frameshifts, nonsense mutations, and splice site changes along with epigenetic changes (hypermethylation) were all reported in CDKN2A and mutations and deletion in RB1 [5, 8].

Deleted in oral cancer-1 (DOC-1) has been discovered in animal model of oral cancer and proposed as novel TSG in the development of oral cancer. Two genetic changes such as LOH and mutations lead to a reduction of its expression and protein production. Interestingly, in oral cancer cell lines, homozygous deletion of melatonin receptor 1 A (MTNR1A) and slicing of its expression were also noted implying that MTNR1A is disabled in OSCC potentially contributing to oral carcinogenesis [5, 12].

Several reports showed that thrombospondin 1 (TSP-1) possesses tumor suppressor function, and reducing the expression of TSP-1 is associated with loss of control of angiogenesis processes in malignant keratinocytes in oral cancer [5].

PTEN is a member of phosphatase which acts via dephosphorylating PI3K signaling. Study of 133 OSCC cases concluded that PTEN protein expression downregulation may play a role in tumorigenesis of OSCC [13].

Recent evidence suggests a role for apoptotic oncoproteins such as Bcl-2 and caspase-3 in OSCCS. Overexpression of these proteins seems to correlate with promoting the progression of oral cancer [14].

2.4 Proto-oncogenes and Oncogenes

Numerous oncogenes have been found to be implicated in oral carcinogenesis. For instance, Ras is one of the most frequently activated oncogene in OSCC. When Ras is activated, it switches on other proteins that ultimately trigger genes involved in cell growth, differentiation, and survival. Mutated Ras gene was also found to produce permanently activated Ras protein. Other proteins such as the transcription factor Myc that participates in cell cycle progression, cell growth and differentiation, apoptosis, cell metabolism, and adhesion are found to be mutated and activated in oral cancer [15–17].

POK erythroid myeloid ontogenic (Pokemon) factor, which is known to be upregulated in several cancers, and its oncogenic activity were elucidated when overexpressed in cooperation with other oncogenes. However, Sartini et al. showed that Pokemon factor was found to be downregulated in OSCC when compared to normal tissue suggesting that it could play an oncosuppressive activity in the early phase of tumor growth [18, 19].

Recently, in two published articles by Liu Peiqi et al. and Shuaimei Xu, the authors established a relationship between the overexpression of RSF3S and DJ-1 and OSCC carcinogenesis and progression. They also showed that inhibition of RSF3S expression caused Snail and N-cadherin suppression in cell culture and reduced DJ-1 expression. This correlated with decreased proliferation and invasion capability of cancer cells. Therefore, SRSF3 and DJ-1 may be utilized either as a biomarker or a therapeutic target of OSCC [20, 21].

Kozaki and his colleagues showed that phosphatidylinositol 3-kinase (PI3K) mutations and amplification are found in 10–20% OSCC patients. Mutations seem to be frequent in advanced stages, while the frequency of amplification is similar among all other stages [22]. Another study from Malaysia confirmed the above findings and stated that oncogenic mutations are less frequent/rare in OSCC when compared to other common tumors. The mutations in this cohort of patients were documented on *PIK3CA* and *HRAS* 1 corroborating other reports [23].

2.5 Gene Expression

Several studies showed differential gene expression in oral carcinogenesis, for example, Sumino et al. identified 15 candidate genes using large-scale gene expression profiling (microarray—Human V4.0 OpArrays) that were constantly upregulated or downregulated at the expression level during oral carcinogenesis. Ten genes have been identified to be significantly overexpressed (ACTG2, APOC1, FCGR3A, ISG15, NRIP2, PZP, RAPGEF6, SLC29A3, STMN3, and SYT10), and five genes were significantly downexpressed (FMO1, NUCB2, OMA1, TMPRSS1B, and FAM149A). Some of these genes can be also utilized as prognostic markers for oral cancer [24]. Another older study by Chakraborty et al. that utilized differential display RT-PCR has identified a separate set of eight genes that are significantly overexpressed and downexpressed in OSCC: five genes, GLTP, PCNA, RBM28, C17orf75, and DIAPH1, and three genes, TNKS2, PAM, and TUBB2C, respectively [25]. Both research groups obtained clinical samples from oral cancer patients from Japan and China, respectively. A larger microarray study (Affymetrix GeneChip® Human Genome U133 Plus 2.0 Array) from the USA including 167 primary tumors showed that 71 genes were significantly and consistently up- or downregulated. Out of these 71 genes, 20 genes were associated with progression-free survival [26].

Oliveira-Costa et al., on the other hand, identified four unique sets of genes expressed among OSCC stages (utilizing Agilent two-color microarray-based gene expression), which include 58 differentially expressed genes; RUNX family genes and zinc finger proteins were found to be overexpressed and downexpressed, respectively, that for the first were implicated in oral carcinogenesis and could potentially be novel targets in OSCC. An updated article by the same group revealed a correlation between PD-L1 and tumor size and lymph node metastasis, HOXB9 and tumor size, BLNK and perineural invasion, and ZNF813 and perineural invasion in circulating tumor cells (CTCs) [27].

A group from Fred Hutchinson Cancer Research Center, USA, using Affymetrix GeneChip® Human Genome U133 Plus 2.0 Array was able to identify potentially early-detection biomarkers for the invasive OSCC; 131 differentially expressed genes were identified (119 OSCC for patients and 35 for controls). Four genes—laminin-gamma2 chain (LAMC2), collagen type IV alpha1 chain (COL4A1), collagen type I alpha1 chain (COL1A1), and peptidylarginine deiminase (type 1 chain PADI1)—were found to distinguish OSCC from controls [28].

Obviously, performing experiments with different technologies and methodologies yields variable results. It seems that a diverse set of genes are being identified with minimal overlap. The discrepancies might be attributed to geographic distribution, genetic background of patients, or etiological factors involved in oral carcinogenesis.

A meta-analysis of Gene Expression Omnibus database was conducted by Thanaphum Osathanon and documented upregulation of genes in Notch signaling pathway, namely, *JAG1*, *JAG2*, *ADAM17*, *NCSTN*, *PSEN1*, *NCOR2*, *NUMB*, *DVL3*,

HDAC1, and HDAC2, and these genes were successfully downregulated by Notch signaling inhibitors in vitro. Yet, these Notch genes were not identified in the previous studies [29].

2.6 Cell Surface Receptors

Several surface receptors have been found to be dysregulated in OSCC. For instance, reduced TGF-beta cell surface receptors correlated with disease progression [30], while expression of Toll-like receptors (TLRs) reduced the antitumor response, such as suppressive cytokines and suppressive regulatory T cells (Tregs) [31].

The expression of several matrix metalloproteinases (MMPs) was also found to be upregulated in OSCCs. However, its exact mechanism in OSCC carcinogenesis is still elusive. One possible mechanism based on observations in OSCC cell lines is that high MMP concentrations reduce natural killer (NK) cell-mediated cytotoxicity [32].

Silva et al. established a relationship between ErbB2, fatty acid synthase (FAS), and Ki-67 with the pathological features of tongue squamous cell carcinoma (TSCC) and showed that localization of ErbB2 at the cell surface of malignant oral keratinocytes is related to FAS expression, while its intracytoplasmic localization is associated with TSCC [33].

Mahendra et al. found that the level of expression of epidermal growth factor receptor (EGFR) in the premalignant lesion is an indicator predicting the neoplastic potential of dysplastic tissues further suggesting that EGFR may serve as a biological marker to identify high-risk subgroups and guide prophylactic therapy [34].

2.7 Epigenetic Changes

Epigenetic changes such as DNA methylation and histone modification are heritable modification in gene activity without any change in the DNA sequence. Accumulating evidence suggests that DNA methylation, histone modifications, and altered expression of miRNAs induce OSCC tumorigenesis.

The major epigenetic modification of tumors is methylation (genome-wide hypomethylation and promoter hypermethylation); even histone modifications are tightly associated with DNA methylation. Thus, malignant transformation is due to DNA-repairing gene inactivation.

Hypermethylated genes in OSCC cover broad cellular processes comprising cell cycle control (p16, p15), DNA repair (MGMT and hMLH1), apoptosis (p14, DAPK, p73, and RASSF1A), Wnt signaling (APC, WIF1, RUNX3), and cell-cell adhesion (E-cadherin). Typically, genes that are hypermethylated and silenced in cancer cells reside in chromosome regions commonly showing loss of heterozygosity. This event may provide a selective growth advantage to OSCC cells leading to tumor neo-angiogenesis and enhanced metastatic ability. Furthermore, promoter methylation is a form of silencing of tumor suppressor genes in OSCC, and this phenomenon is well documented [35]. It appears that methylation is an early event in oral carcinogenesis. Ha and Califano epigenetic work identified four important genes: CDKN2A, CDH1, MGMT, and DAPK1 [36]. Moreover, DNA methylation comparison of healthy oral mucosa and OSCC discovered that the 5hmC was lost in OSCC [37]. A separate study found that FHL1 downregulation in OSCC was induced by DNA methylation in the promoter region rather than histone deacetylation or DNA mutation [38, 39].

2.8 Chromosomal Instability and Copy Number Variation

Several copy number variations (CNVs) have been identified in oral cancer. CNAs can be divided into two categories: (1) amplification (the most frequently amplified CNAs were located on chromosome regions: 8p11.23–p11.22 (80%), 7q34 (52 and 72%), 20p13 (61%), 6p21.32 (59%), 14q31.3–q32.33 (57%), 11q23.3–q25 (57%), 20p13–p12.3 (54%), 14q21.3–q31.1 (54%), 9q13–q34.3 (54%), 1q21.3–q22 (54%), 8q11.1–q24.4 (54%), 11q11 (52%), 2p22.3 (52%), and 20q11.21–q13.33 (52%)) and (2) deletion (the most frequently deleted chromosome region was located on 3q26.1 (54%)) (Fig. 2.1). The same results were also confirmed from cell lines of oral cancer [40, 41].

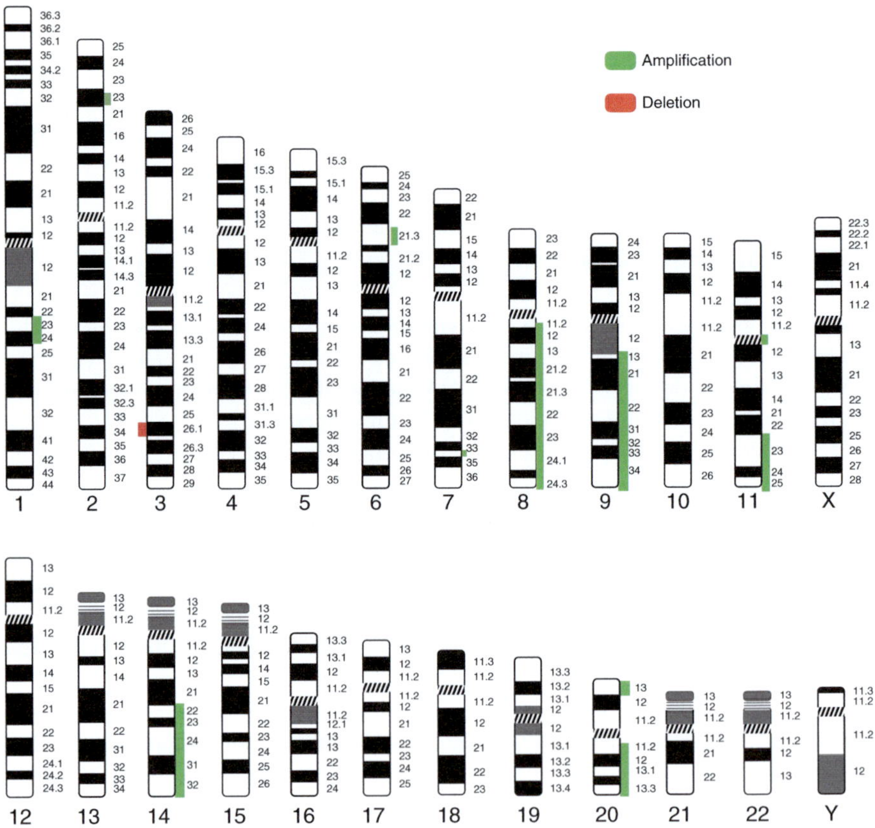

Fig. 2.1 The most common CNVs in OSCC

2.9 mtDNA Mutation

The machinery repair mechanisms of damage in mtDNA are less vigorous than DNA in nuclear compartments due to the high susceptibility of mtDNA to oxidative stress/damage resulting from its respiratory chain when compared to the nuclear genome.

Alteration of mtDNA may lead to a mutant protein resulting in transformation of normal cells to cancer. These mtDNA changes have been documented in OSCC; however, the exact molecular mechanisms in which mtDNA changes contribute to oral carcinogenesis remain unclear.

Yuan et al. identified several changes that ranged from point mutations and deletions to insertion mutations in the D-loop region of mtDNA in a quarter of 30 OSCC cases showing diverse clinical presentations such as tongue, soft palate, floor of the mouth, oropharyngeal, and lip cancer [42, 43]. Mondal et al. identified several D-loop hotspot mutations in Indian OSCC patients via whole mitochondrial sequencing [44].

Kloss-Brandstatter found that there are shared mtDNA mutations/variants between benign and cancerous tissue as well as between primary tumor and metastatic lymph node with higher-frequency mutations in cancerous cells. The percentage of mutation heteroplasmy is higher in lymph node metastases from the primary tumor [45]. Uzawa et al. were able to identify that those OSCC patients with high mtDNA mutations in both serum and tissue samples have higher recurrence rates and worse prognosis [46].

2.10 Telomeres and Telomerase

Telomeres are TTAGGG hexanucleotides located at the ends of human chromosomes. Biologically, they act to protect the chromosome ends from deterioration or from fusion with the adjacent chromosomes. In normal cells, telomere length is shortened in each cell division leading to cell death after certain cell division cycles. However, abnormal cells get immortalized due to increased activities of protein called telomerase which maintain the telomere length.

In oral cancer, it is well documented that the telomerase activities are increased and are associated with dysplasia severity. Two studies showed that the length of telomeres and telomerase activation and overexpression are associated with poor prognosis from clinical point of view and disease recurrence with poor survival rate [47, 48].

2.11 Microsatellite Instability and Alteration

Genetic hypermutability resulting from damaged DNA mismatch repair is termed microsatellite instability (MI). These indels of base pair changes that occur in specific microsatellite regions are significant features of OSCC. Ashazila et al. showed that MI status is associated significantly with tumor stage and differentiation in 50

OSCCs [49]. Lin et al. documented that MI and microsatellite alteration (MA) occur in 95% and 35% of OSCC, respectively [50].

Mahale and Saranath, on the other hand, showed that MI and MA are also associated with betel-induced OSCC among Indian subcontinent patients [51]. Furthermore, Shin et al., [52] suggested that MI plays an important role also in the oral cancer pathogenesis in Koreans.

2.12 Noncoding RNA

The lack of understanding of carcinogenesis could be attributed to the fact that the majority of cancer genomic studies have focused mainly on genomic alterations in the minute portion 2% of the human genome encoding protein overlooking studying the large portion of the genome, i.e., the 70% of the genome that is transcribed into the noncoding RNA (ncRNA). Nonetheless, several studies nowadays have started to focus on and study comprehensively ncRNA via extensively profiling these ncRNAs at different cellular stages such as transcription, genomic, and epigenetic levels to provide novel insight into ncRNAs in cancers. As it turns out, some ncRNAs practically incorporate into several important cell proliferation pathways, and aberrant ncRNA expression may have some role in sustaining self-proliferative signaling in cancer cells, and their contribution to cancer initiation and progression has been recently more appreciated.

2.13 MicroRNA (miRNA)

miRNAs are short, single-stranded (SS) RNA moieties about 20–22 nucleotides in length regulating gene expression via 3′ end binding of the untranslated region (3-UTR) of the complementary mRNA sequence causing gene silencing and protein suppression. Substantial evidence suggests that abnormal expression of miRNAs leads to carcinogenesis development, including OSCC [18, 19]. Experiments implicated a small number of impaired miRNAs as being either oncogenes or tumor suppressors affecting the disease initiation, progression, and metastasization [53–56]. Analysis of two studies (one was carried out in primary cell line and the other used human tissue for the most part) revealed no miRNAs in common. This could be attributed either to the sample source or to the choice of the molecular method (Table 2.1).

In animal models, OSCC of Syrian hamsters was treated with 5% 7,12-dimethylbenz[a]anthracene (DMBA) in acetone (immunosuppressor). Five microRNAs (has-miR-21, -200b, -221, -338, and mmu-miR-762) were significantly upregulated, and 12 microRNAs (hsa-miR-16, -26a, -29a, -124a, -125b, -143, -145, -148b, -155, -199a, -203, and mmu-miR-126-5p) were downregulated in cancer tissues [59]. These miRNAs bear no resemblance to findings in human cell lines or tissue from patients.

Table 2.1 Comparison of miRNA expression in cell lines and human tissue samples

miRNA expression	Sample source	Technology	References
Upregulated hsa-miRNA-572, -214, -563, -637, -628, -191, -210, -498, -373, -98, -148b, -15a, -148-a, -200a, -30b, -429, -7, hsa-let-7e, -7i, and -7g Downregulated hsa-miRNA-122a, -565, -195, -30e–5p, -374, -19a, -101, -424, -29b, -186, -141, -320, -422b, -22, -331 and -197	OSCC cell line cultured under hypoxia condition	Microarray	[57]
Upregulated miR-184, -34c, -137, -372, -124a, -21, -124b, -31, -128a, -34b, -154, -197, -132, -147, -325, -181c, -198, -155, -30a–3p, -338, -17-5p, -104, -134, and -213 Downregulated miR-133a, -99a, -194, -133b, -219, -100, -125b, -26b, -138, -149, -195, -107 and -139	Tongue squamous cell carcinoma	RT-PCR	[58]

Other studies stressing miRNAs' clinical utility are presented in Table 2.2. While these biomarker candidates have not been validated, they offer the prospect to employ in oral cancer detection, risk assessment, and monitoring.

2.14 Long Noncoding RNAs (lncRNAs)

Long noncoding RNAs (lncRNAs) are a novel class of noncoding RNAs characteristically more than 200 nucleotides in size. Nowadays, lncRNAs have wide-ranging biological functions from cell signaling to serving as molecular decoys and to guiding ribonucleoprotein complexes into specific chromatin sites or participating as scaffolds in the formation of complexes. So far, several lncRNAs have been linked to OSCC pathogenesis [79, 80]. A study by Gibb et al. profiled the expression of more than 300 lncRNAs in OSCC and has found that more than half of the lncRNAs are aberrantly expressed suggesting that lncRNAs play an important role in disease initiation and progression [81].

Recently, Yang et al. showed that lncRNA urothelial carcinoma-associated 1 (UCA1) is dysregulated in OSCC and the UCA1 expression levels were found to be clearly overexpressed in tongue squamous cell carcinoma tissues and are associated with lymph node metastasis and TNM stage. Knocking down UCA1 not only inhibited OSCC proliferation and metastasis but also induced apoptosis in vitro and in vivo, which could be attributed to the regulatory role of lncRNA UCA1 in Wnt/β--catenin signaling [82]. In 2014, Fang et al. reported that metastasis-associated lung adenocarcinoma transcript 1 (MALAT-1) is upregulated, while MEG3 is reduced in TSCCs. Meanwhile, UCA1 expression increased in TSCCs and correlated with

Table 2.2 Biomarker candidates in OSCC from tissue, cell lines, and blood plasma

miRNA	Targets	Significance in OSCC	References
OSCC tissues			
et-7g	MYC	Associated with hypoxia, local control, neck control, distant metastases, disease-specific survival	[57, 60]
miRNA-218	SP1	A predictor for disease-free survival and disease-specific survival	[60]
miRNA-363	PDPN	Stimulates tumor invasion and lymph node metastasis	[61]
OSCC tissue, cell lines			
miRNA-9	CXCR4	Reduces cell proliferation and invasion Controls cell cycle	[62]
miRNA-21	TPM1, PTEN, RECK	Facilitates anchorage-independent growth Enhances cell proliferation Enhances chemosensitivity/chemoresistance Overexpression associated with reduced survival and disease progression	[58, 59, 63–67]
miRNA-125b	ICAM2, TP53	Decreases cell proliferation, the prediction marker of neck control	[58–60, 63–65, 68]
miRNA-126	VEGFA	Decreases migration and invasion, regulates VEGFA expression	[69]
miRNA-194	AGK, cyclin D1, p21	Decreases cell proliferation, controls cell cycle	[58, 63, 64, 70, 71]
miRNA-203	Yes-1	Elevated the nuclear condensation and apoptosis	[59, 71, 72]
miRNA-491-5p	GIT1	Reduces migration/invasion, metastasis, and focal adhesions	[73]
miRNA-506	GATA6	Reduces proliferation, migration, and invasion	[72]
OSCC cell lines			
miRNA-17	ITGb8	Reduces migration and invasion, the prediction marker of survival	[74]
miRNA-101	EZH2	Downregulation associated with hypoxia Inhibits EMT, migration, and invasion	[57, 75]
miRNA-134	WWOX	Enhances the proliferation and migration Enhances invasion and anchorage-independent growth Enhances xenographic tumorigenesis	[76]
miRNA-137	CDK6, E2F6	Reduces the proliferation	[71]
miRNA-153	SNAI1, ZEB2	Reduces epithelial-mesenchymal transition and tumor metastasis	[77]
OSCC tissues and blood plasma			
miRNA-181	p27 and bcl-2	Stimulates lymph node metastasis and vascular invasion	[78]

tumor lymph node metastasis. High expression level of UCA1 may serve as a prognostic indicator in lymph node metastasis in TSCC. [83].

In 2015, Wu et al. documented that HOTAIR was expressed in OSCC tumor compared with normal tissues, and the expression was greater in lymph node metastasis compared to non-lymph node metastasis revealing that the expression is greatly correlated with the clinical stage, lymph node metastasis, and histological differentiation in OSCC. Furthermore, the survival study revealed that OSCC patients with high HOTAIR expression level had significantly reduced disease-free survival and overall survival rates. Functional studies of HOTAIR on OSCC cell lines indicated that silencing of HOTAIR significantly reduced cell proliferation and colony formation, increased cell invasion and migration, and induced apoptosis [84]. Additionally, an inverse correlation was found between HOTAIR and E-cadherin levels in OSCC tissues and cell lines. This confirms HOTAIR direct contribution to E-cadherin regulation via binding to EZH2 and H3K27me3 where the complex binds E-cadherin promoter [84].

Gao group, on the other hand, was able to document eight differentially expressed lncRNAs. Six lncRNAs—lnc-PPP2R4-5, lnc-SPRR2D-1, lnc-MAN1A2-1, lnc-FAM46A-1, lnc-MBL2-4:1, and lnc-MBL2-4:3—were overexpressed, and two lncRNAs, namely, lnc-AL355149.1 1 and lnc-STXBP5-1, were downregulated. Interestingly, the extensive downregulation of lnc-AL355149.1-1 is associated with disease progression, and the expression could be reversed after treatment with 5-fluorouracil and paclitaxel [85].

Conclusion and Perspective

Oral squamous cell carcinoma (OSCC) global frequency and mortality are on the rise. Due to late diagnosis of oral cancer, prognosis is discouraging. The poor prognosis of OSCC has intensified the field's research efforts in prevention and early detection of this disease. Early-stage detection not only improves prognosis but also increases the survival rate and enhances patient life quality. Advances in the understanding of the molecular basis of oral cancer should help in the identification of new biomarkers and open new horizons for therapy. Studying the carcinogenic process of the oral cancer would allow the identification of new diagnostic and/or prognostic markers, thus providing a promising basis for the application of more rational, targeted, and efficient therapies. Different treatment modalities are being used to address OSCC such as surgery, radiotherapy, and chemotherapy. Novel chemotherapy compounds have taken on a vital role to battle oral cancer. Agents from the antimetabolite or platinum classes are regarded as the foundation for chemotherapy. Combination therapy and synergy treatment with chemotherapy and radiotherapy is one of the mainly accepted methods for oral cancer treatment. More recently, the monoclonal antibody cetuximab is being explored as an agent to treat OSCC. The drug target is EGFR; such targeted therapeutic approach is more likely to be successful in the long run. lncRNAs arrest gene expression and disease progression, thus making them a new class of targets for drug discovery though not without novel challenges. As of June 2016, there are few miRNAs in clinical development; however, to the authors' knowledge, none are in oral cancer. Future developments in the realms of nanotechnology may also contribute to oral cancer treatment.

The use of appropriate in vitro and in vivo experimental models is critical to advancing our understanding of disease progression and therapeutic response. While in vitro models are highly valuable, in vivo models are more pertinent and effective in dissecting malignancy development.

Another way to combat oral cancer is education. Global studies have shown that the sense of awareness regarding oral cancer and its signs and symptoms among the general population is deficient. Public awareness programs are necessary tools to fight oral cancer at all levels in terms of diagnosis, risk management, and treatment monitoring.

References

1. Nebert DW. Transcription factors and cancer: an overview. Toxicology. 2002;181–182:131–41.
2. Kinzler KW, Vogelstein B. Cancer-susceptibility genes. Gatekeepers and caretakers. Nature. 1997;386(6627):761–3.
3. Michor F, Iwasa Y, Nowak MA. Dynamics of cancer progression. Nat Rev Cancer. 2004;4(3):197–205.
4. Ram H, et al. Oral cancer: risk factors and molecular pathogenesis. J Maxillofac Oral Surg. 2011;10(2):132–7.
5. Jurel SK, et al. Genes and oral cancer. Indian J Hum Genet. 2014;20(1):4–9.
6. Nakaya K, et al. Identification of homozygous deletions of tumor suppressor gene FAT in oral cancer using CGH-array. Oncogene. 2007;26(36):5300–8.
7. Morris LG, et al. Recurrent somatic mutation of FAT1 in multiple human cancers leads to aberrant Wnt activation. Nat Genet. 2013;45(3):253–61.
8. Riaz N, et al. Unraveling the molecular genetics of head and neck cancer through genome-wide approaches. Genes Dis. 2014;1(1):75–86.
9. Kim KT, Kim BS, Kim JH. Association between FAT1 mutation and overall survival in patients with human papillomavirus-negative head and neck squamous cell carcinoma. Head Neck. 2016;38(Suppl 1):E2021–9.
10. Glazer CA, et al. Applying the molecular biology and epigenetics of head and neck cancer in everyday clinical practice. Oral Oncol. 2009;45(4–5):440–6.
11. Sakai E, et al. The p53 tumor-suppressor gene and ras oncogene mutations in oral squamous-cell carcinoma. Int J Cancer. 1992;52(6):867–72.
12. Nakamura E, et al. Frequent silencing of a putative tumor suppressor gene melatonin receptor 1 a (MTNR1A) in oral squamous-cell carcinoma. Cancer Sci. 2008;99(7):1390–400.
13. Kurasawa Y, et al. PTEN expression and methylation status in oral squamous cell carcinoma. Oncol Rep. 2008;19(6):1429–34.
14. Arya V, Singh S, Daniel MJ. Clinicopathological correlation of bcl-2 oncoprotein expression in oral precancer and cancer. J Oral Biol Craniofac Res. 2016;6(1):18–23.
15. Murugan AK, Munirajan AK, Tsuchida N. Ras oncogenes in oral cancer: the past 20 years. Oral Oncol. 2012;48(5):383–92.
16. Shah NG, et al. Prognostic significance of molecular markers in oral squamous cell carcinoma: a multivariate analysis. Head Neck. 2009;31(12):1544–56.
17. Pérez-Sayáns M, et al. What real influence does the proto-oncogene c-myc have in OSCC behavior? Oral Oncol. 2011;47(8):688–92.

18. Sartini D, et al. Pokemon proto-oncogene in oral cancer: potential role in the early phase of tumorigenesis. Oral Dis. 2015;21(4):462–9.
19. Maeda T, et al. Role of the proto-oncogene Pokemon in cellular transformation and ARF repression. Nature. 2005;433(7023):278–85.
20. Peiqi L, et al. Expression of SRSF3 is correlated with carcinogenesis and progression of oral squamous cell carcinoma. Int J Med Sci. 2016;13(7):533–9.
21. Xu S, et al. DJ-1 is upregulated in oral squamous cell carcinoma and promotes oral cancer cell proliferation and invasion. J Cancer. 2016;7(8):1020–8.
22. Kozaki K-I, et al. PIK3CA mutation is an oncogenic aberration at advanced stages of oral squamous cell carcinoma. Cancer Sci. 2006;97(12):1351–8.
23. Zanaruddin SN, et al. Common oncogenic mutations are infrequent in oral squamous cell carcinoma of Asian origin. PLoS One. 2013;8(11):e80229.
24. Sumino J, et al. Gene expression changes in initiation and progression of oral squamous cell carcinomas revealed by laser microdissection and oligonucleotide microarray analysis. Int J Cancer. 2013;132(3):540–8.
25. Chakraborty S, et al. Gene expression profiling of oral squamous cell carcinoma by differential display rt-PCR and identification of tumor biomarkers. Indian J Surg Oncol. 2010;1(4): 284–93.
26. Lohavanichbutr P, et al. Gene expression in uninvolved oral mucosa of OSCC patients facilitates identification of markers predictive of OSCC outcomes. PLoS One. 2012;7(9):e46575.
27. Oliveira-Costa JP, et al. Gene expression patterns through oral squamous cell carcinoma development. FASEB J. 2013;27(Suppl 1):lb473.
28. Chen C, et al. Gene expression profiling identifies genes predictive of oral squamous cell carcinoma. Cancer Epidemiol Biomark Prev. 2008;17(8):2152–62.
29. Osathanon T, Nowwarote N, Pavasant P. Expression and influence of Notch signaling in oral squamous cell carcinoma. J Oral Sci. 2016;58(2):283–94
30. Paterson IC, et al. Decreased expression of TGF-beta cell surface receptors during progression of human oral squamous cell carcinoma. J Pathol. 2001;193(4):458–67.
31. Rich AM, et al. Toll-like receptors and cancer, particularly oral squamous cell carcinoma. Front Immunol. 2014;5:464.
32. Lee BK, et al. A high concentration of MMP-2/gelatinase a and MMP-9/gelatinase B reduce NK cell-mediated cytotoxicity against an oral squamous cell carcinoma cell line. In Vivo. 2008;22(5):593–7.
33. Silva SD, et al. ErbB2 and fatty acid synthase (FAS) expression in 102 squamous cell carcinomas of the tongue: correlation with clinical outcomes. Oral Oncol. 2008;44(5):484–90.
34. Mahendra A, et al. Epidermal growth factor receptor protein: a biological marker for oral precancer and cancer. J Dent Surg. 2014;2014:7.
35. Gasche JA, Goel A. Epigenetic mechanisms in oral carcinogenesis. Future Oncol. 2012;8(11):1407–25.
36. Ha PK, Califano JA. Promoter methylation and inactivation of tumour-suppressor genes in oral squamous-cell carcinoma. Lancet Oncol. 2006;7(1):77–82.
37. Jawert F, et al. Loss of 5-hydroxymethylcytosine and TET2 in oral squamous cell carcinoma. Anticancer Res. 2013;33(10):4325–8.
38. Koike K, et al. High prevalence of epigenetic inactivation of the human four and a half LIM domains 1 gene in human oral cancer. Int J Oncol. 2013;42(1):141–50.
39. Mascolo M, et al. Epigenetic dysregulation in oral cancer. Int J Mol Sci. 2012;13(2): 2331–53.
40. Vincent-Chong VK, et al. Genome wide analysis of chromosomal alterations in oral squamous cell carcinomas revealed over expression of MGAM and ADAM9. PLoS One. 2013;8(2):e54705.
41. Castagnola P, et al. Genomic DNA copy number aberrations, histological diagnosis, oral subsite and aneuploidy in OPMDs/OSCCs. PLoS One. 2015;10(11):e0142294.
42. Sun Y, et al. Screening of the gene mutation in D-loop region of mitochondrial DNA in oral squamous cell carcinoma. Zhonghua Kou Qiang Yi Xue Za Zhi. 2013;48(5):285–7.
43. Yuan RT, et al. Gene mutations in the D loop region of mitochondrial DNA in oral squamous cell carcinoma. Mol Med Rep. 2015;11(6):4496–500.

44. Mondal R, Ghosh SK. Accumulation of mutations over the complete mitochondrial genome in tobacco-related oral cancer from northeast India. Mitochondrial DNA. 2013;24(4):432–9.
45. Kloss-Brandstatter A, et al. Validation of next-generation sequencing of entire mitochondrial genomes and the diversity of mitochondrial DNA mutations in oral squamous cell carcinoma. PLoS One. 2015;10(8):e0135643.
46. Uzawa K, et al. Circulating tumor-derived mutant mitochondrial DNA: a predictive biomarker of clinical prognosis in human squamous cell carcinoma. Oncotarget. 2012;3(7):670–7.
47. Sainger RN, et al. Clinical significance of telomere length and associated proteins in oral cancer. Biomark Insights. 2007;2:9–19.
48. Chen HH, et al. Expression of human telomerase reverse transcriptase (hTERT) protein is significantly associated with the progression, recurrence and prognosis of oral squamous cell carcinoma in Taiwan. Oral Oncol. 2007;43(2):122–9.
49. Ashazila MJ, et al. Microsatellite instability and loss of heterozygosity in oral squamous cell carcinoma in Malaysian population. Oral Oncol. 2011;47(5):358–64.
50. Lin SC, et al. Frequent microsatellite alterations of chromosome locus 4q13.1 in oral squamous cell carcinomas. J Oral Pathol Med. 2005;34(4):209–13.
51. Mahale A, Saranath D. Microsatellite alterations on chromosome 9 in chewing tobacco-induced oral squamous cell carcinomas from India. Oral Oncol. 2000;36(2):199–206.
52. Shin K.-H, et al. Prevalence of microsatellite instability, inactivation of mismatch repair genes, p53 mutation, and human papillomavirus infection in Korean oral cancer patients. Int J Oncol. 2002;21(2):297–302(6).
53. Sun K, Lai EC. Adult-specific functions of animal microRNAs. Nat Rev Genet. 2013;14(8):535–48.
54. Tang G, et al. Construction of short tandem target mimic (STTM) to block the functions of plant and animal microRNAs. Methods. 2012;58(2):118–25.
55. Kloosterman WP, Plasterk RH. The diverse functions of microRNAs in animal development and disease. Dev Cell. 2006;11(4):441–50.
56. Ambros V. The functions of animal microRNAs. Nature. 2004;431(7006):350–5.
57. Hebert C, et al. High mobility group A2 is a target for miRNA-98 in head and neck squamous cell carcinoma. Mol Cancer. 2007;6:5.
58. Wong TS, et al. Identification of pyruvate kinase type M2 as potential oncoprotein in squamous cell carcinoma of tongue through microRNA profiling. Int J Cancer. 2008;123(2):251–7.
59. Yu T, et al. The expression profile of microRNAs in a model of 7,12-dimethyl-benz[a]anthracene-induced oral carcinogenesis in Syrian hamster. J Exp Clin Cancer Res. 2009;28:64.
60. Peng SC, et al. MicroRNAs MiR-218, MiR-125b, and let-7g predict prognosis in patients with oral cavity squamous cell carcinoma. PLoS One. 2014;9(7):e102403.
61. Sun Q, et al. Dysregulated miR-363 affects head and neck cancer invasion and metastasis by targeting podoplanin. Int J Biochem Cell Biol. 2013;45(3):513–20.
62. Yu T, et al. MicroRNA-9 inhibits the proliferation of oral squamous cell carcinoma cells by suppressing expression of CXCR4 via the wnt/beta-catenin signaling pathway. Oncogene. 2014;33(42):5017–27.
63. Wong TS, et al. Mature miR-184 and squamous cell carcinoma of the tongue. ScientificWorldJournal. 2009;9:130–2.
64. Wong TS, et al. Mature miR-184 as potential oncogenic microRNA of squamous cell carcinoma of tongue. Clin Cancer Res. 2008;14(9):2588–92.
65. Ramdas L, et al. miRNA expression profiles in head and neck squamous cell carcinoma and adjacent normal tissue. Head Neck. 2009;31(5):642–54.
66. Jung HM, et al. Keratinization-associated miR-7 and miR-21 regulate tumor suppressor reversion-inducing cysteine-rich protein with kazal motifs (RECK) in oral cancer. J Biol Chem. 2012;287(35):29261–72.
67. Gee HE, et al. Hsa-mir-210 is a marker of tumor hypoxia and a prognostic factor in head and neck cancer. Cancer. 2010;116(9):2148–58.

68. Shiiba M, et al. MicroRNA-125b regulates proliferation and radioresistance of oral squamous cell carcinoma. Br J Cancer. 2013;108(9):1817–21.
69. Sasahira T, et al. Downregulation of miR-126 induces angiogenesis and lymphangiogenesis by activation of VEGF-A in oral cancer. Br J Cancer. 2012;107(4):700–6.
70. Chi H. miR-194 regulated AGK and inhibited cell proliferation of oral squamous cell carcinoma by reducing PI3K-akt-FoxO3a signaling. Biomed Pharmacother. 2015;71:53–7.
71. Kozaki K, et al. Exploration of tumor-suppressive microRNAs silenced by DNA hypermethylation in oral cancer. Cancer Res. 2008;68(7):2094–105.
72. Deng L, Liu H. MicroRNA-506 suppresses growth and metastasis of oral squamous cell carcinoma via targeting GATA6. Int J Clin Exp Med. 2015;8(2):1862–70.
73. Huang WC, et al. miRNA-491-5p and GIT1 serve as modulators and biomarkers for oral squamous cell carcinoma invasion and metastasis. Cancer Res. 2014;74(3):751–64.
74. Chang CC, et al. MicroRNA-17/20a functions to inhibit cell migration and can be used a prognostic marker in oral squamous cell carcinoma. Oral Oncol. 2013;49(9):923–31.
75. Zheng M, et al. Snail and slug collaborate on EMT and tumor metastasis through miR-101-mediated EZH2 axis in oral tongue squamous cell carcinoma. Oncotarget. 2015;6(9): 6797–810.
76. Liu CJ, et al. miR-134 induces oncogenicity and metastasis in head and neck carcinoma through targeting WWOX gene. Int J Cancer. 2014;134(4):811–21.
77. Xu Q, et al. Downregulation of miR-153 contributes to epithelial-mesenchymal transition and tumor metastasis in human epithelial cancer. Carcinogenesis. 2013;34(3):539–49.
78. Yang CC, et al. miR-181 as a putative biomarker for lymph-node metastasis of oral squamous cell carcinoma. J Oral Pathol Med. 2011;40(5):397–404.
79. Pan YF, et al. Role of long non-coding RNAs in gene regulation and oncogenesis. Chin Med J. 2011;124(15):2378–83.
80. Denaro N, et al. Non coding RNAs in head and neck squamous cell carcinoma (HNSCC): a clinical perspective. Anticancer Res. 2014;34(12):6887–96.
81. Gibb EA, et al. Long non-coding RNAs are expressed in oral mucosa and altered in oral premalignant lesions. Oral Oncol. 2011;47(11):1055–61.
82. Yang YT, et al. Long non-coding RNA UCA1 contributes to the progression of oral squamous cell carcinoma by regulating the WNT/beta-catenin signaling pathway. Cancer Sci. 2016;107(11):1581–9.
83. Fang Z, et al. Increased expression of the long non-coding RNA UCA1 in tongue squamous cell carcinomas: a possible correlation with cancer metastasis. Oral Surg Oral Med Oral Pathol Oral Radiol. 2014;117(1):89–95.
84. Wu Y, et al. Long non-coding RNA HOTAIR promotes tumor cell invasion and metastasis by recruiting EZH2 and repressing E-cadherin in oral squamous cell carcinoma. Int J Oncol. 2015;46(6):2586–94.
85. Gao W, Chan JY, Wong TS. Long non-coding RNA deregulation in tongue squamous cell carcinoma. Biomed Res Int. 2014;2014:405860.

Oral Cancer: After the Completion of the Human Genome Project

3

A. Hameed Khan

3.1 Gene Profiling: (A Personal Journey)

This chapter describes the rationale for gene profiling leading to gene expression leading to diagnosis (identification of mutated genes) and to treatment (development of novel drugs to shut off mutated genes). Gene expression profiling measures the amount of mRNA which is produced by normal as well as abnormal or cancer cells. The amount of mRNA measures the progress of a disease. Several hundred genes are expressed simultaneously. We have expression of good as well as bad gene profiles. Gene profiling identifies which gene is functioning normally to produce healthy cells. For developing treatment or cure, we are also interested in identifying mutated genes whose expression produces bad proteins causing abnormal growth resulting in cancers.

Oral and lung cancers are usually caused by chewing and smoking tobacco products. (See my lectures on **Smoking and Cancer**—https://www.facebook.com/hameed.khan.7773/notes). Tobacco contains dozens of carcinogenic chemicals, and the major culprit is nicotine which is considered as one of the most addictive chemicals. Some studies showed that it is more addictive than many known narcotics such as marijuana, opiates, and heroin. Oral cancer (OC) is caused by chemicals released by chewing tobacco. Most football players chew tobacco. Smoking burns tobacco generating more aromatic amines which are known carcinogens. Nitrosamines bind to DNA-producing mutations. Mutated DNAs code for wrong amino acids which cause abnormal growth. In addition to chemicals from tobacco products, mutations are also caused by radiations, chemical pollutions (heavy metal particles), genetic inheritance, or viral infections. As mutation begins in a single biological molecule,

A. Hameed Khan, Ph.D.
NCMRR (National Center for Medical Rehabilitation Research), National Institutes of Health (NIH), Bethesda, MD, USA
e-mail: Hameedkhan111@Comcast.net

A.-E. Al Moustafa (ed.), *Development of Oral Cancer*,
DOI 10.1007/978-3-319-48054-1_3

it is called a point mutation. To study changes in genetic profile of a single cell, we examine the entire genome of a single cell. As cells grow rapidly, mistakes in DNA replications are most likely to occur such as deletion, insertion, or inversion of nucleotide sequence. Such mutations are responsible for major diseases. Mutations in the oral cavity are responsible for causing oral cancer. More than 90% of cancers of the oral cavity and oropharynx are squamous cell carcinomas, and verrucous carcinoma is a type of squamous cell carcinoma that makes up to less than 5% of all oral cancers. In addition, there are several types of salivary gland cancers including adenoid cystic carcinoma, mucoepidermoid carcinoma, and polymorphous low-grade adenocarcinoma. Tonsils and base of the tongue tissues also develop lymphomas.

Sequencing the genomes of these cancers and comparing their genomes with the normal cell genomes (by GWAS or genome-wide association studies) will identify the responsible mutations with great accuracy and precision. Once the mutation sites on a specific chromosome are identified, the next logical step is to develop treatment by designing drugs to shut off those genes. In addition, our oral cavity is home to hundreds of known microbial life forms. Almost 400 microorganisms have been identified in our mouth so far [1], and only few are responsible for causing infections. Infectious microflora of the oral cavity could be treated with either antibiotics or vaccines.

To understand the basis of all diseases, we must read and understand our genome as our normal book of life, the total genetic information that makes up our personal genome, and the changes that make it abnormal which are responsible for causing diseases including cancers especially OC. Our genome carries the total genetic information that makes us. That is how the story of our book of life begins: as we all know, we are the product of the loving union of our parents. Our mother's egg receives our father's sperm, and we are conceived. The fertilized egg carries complete information to make us. More than 70 years ago, the Nobel Laureate, Erwin Schrödinger, examined, for comparison, the fertilized egg of a human, mouse, and monkey under a microscope. He observed that all fertilized eggs look exactly the same, and yet the first fertilized egg carries the instructions to make a man, the second carries the information to make a mouse, and the third carries the information to make a monkey. He postulated that there exists a secret code within those fertilized eggs; he called that secret code as the script code (now known as Genetic Code). He stated that if we break the genetic code, we would be able to unlock the secret of life. If we unlock the secret of life, we would be able to create new life forms carrying instructions to create new food, new fuel, and new medicine to treat every disease known to mankind.

DNA is a storehouse of information and is made of the four nucleotide bases, and they are adenine (A), thymine (T), guanine (G), and cytosine (C). According to Crick's central dogma, the information flows from the DNA which is transcribed into RNA which is translated in ribosome into proteins. RNA is converted into an active form and is transcribed into RNA (or messenger RNA) by converting thymine to active form uracil (U) and from a double-stranded DNA to a single-stranded RNA and where the sugar deoxyribose is replaced by sugar ribose. The RNA is translated by ribosome into proteins.

Gene expression begins in ribosome when a four-letter genetic text is converted to a three-letter codon. By comparing gene profiles of normal genes with mutated genes, one can identify with precision and accuracy the exact location of a mutated nucleotide responsible for causing the disease. Comparing gene profiles is an excellent diagnostic method which helps us design drugs to specifically shut off the mutated genes.

Seventy years ago in the above experiment, Schrödinger was using such a poor-resolution microscope that we don't even use in our high school today. Instead, we have electron microscope today. We can magnify the same fertilized egg to a million times of its original size, almost the size of a house. What we observe inside the fertilized egg is very analogous to the house. The house has a kitchen; the cell has a nucleus. Suppose your kitchen has a shelf which contains 46 volumes of cookbooks which contain 24,000 recipes which carry instructions to cook food for your breakfast, lunch, and dinner. The nucleus in the fertilized egg contains 46 chromosomes (23 from our mother and 23 from our father), which carry 24,000 chapters called genes. Genes are units of inheritance which code for all 20 amino acids. Hundreds of amino acids join together to form a protein, and thousands of proteins interact to make a cell. Millions of cells interact to make an organ, and several organs interact to make a man or a mouse or a monkey.

If the cookbooks in your kitchen is written in the English language, it uses 26 letters, but the book of life of all living creatures is written in 4 letters, and they are A, T, G, and C. These are the initials of four chemicals called nucleotides (adenine, thymine, guanine, and cytosine) which are found in the nucleus of all living cells. Nucleotides are made of sugar ribose (deoxyribose in DNA and ribose in RNA), a phosphate group and one of the four nitrogen bases, two purines, and two pyrimidines, and the thymine is converted to uracil in RNA. These molecules are found in the nucleus of all living cells from a tiny blade of grass to a mighty elephant including man, mouse, and monkey. The total genetic information to make any living creature is based on the above four-letter text and, out of these four letters, only a three-letter codon which carries the genetic code for an amino acid (such as GUU which is for amino acid valine, GCU which is for alanine, GAA which is for glutamine, etc.) which is the building block for all proteins. Sixty-four codons code for 20 amino acids, and codons for all 20 amino acids have been decoded. All living creatures use the same genetic code. A string of these nucleotides is called the DNA (deoxyribonucleic acid). Reading the number and the order of nucleotides is called genome sequencing.

In 1990, United States Congress authorized 3 billion dollars to NIH to decipher the entire human genome within 15 years that is the total genetic information that makes us human called the Human Genome Project. Thousands of scientists from 6 industrialized nations and 20 biomedical centers joined our effort, and within 13 years, the entire human genome was deciphered and published in the scientific journal *Nature* and linked to the website. If you have an access to a computer keyboard, then you have access to all that information.

We deciphered all 46 chromosomes. What surprise us most was that our genome contains six billion four hundred million nucleotide base pairs, and less than 2% of our genome contains genes which code for proteins. The other 98% of our genome contains switches, promoters, terminators, etc.

Before sequencing (determining the number and the order of the four nucleotide), it is essential to know how many genes are present in our genome. The Human Genome Project has identified the following genes on each chromosome. We found that the chromosome (1) is the largest chromosome carrying 263 million A, T, G, and C nucleotide bases and it has only 2610 genes. The chromosome (2) contains 255 million nucleotide bases and has only 1748 genes. The chromosome (3) contains 214 million nucleotide bases and carries 1381 genes. The chromosome (4) contains 203 million nucleotide bases and carries 1024 genes. The chromosome (5) contains 194 million nucleotide bases and carries 1190 genes. The chromosome (6) contains 183 million nucleotide bases and carries 1394 genes. The chromosome (7) contains 171 million nucleotide bases and carries 1378 genes. The chromosome (8) contains 155 million nucleotide bases and carries 927 genes. The chromosome (9) contains 145 million nucleotide bases and carries 1076 genes. The chromosome (10) contains 144 million nucleotide bases and carries 983 genes. The chromosome (11) contains 144 million nucleotide bases and carries 1692 genes. The chromosome (12) contains 143 million nucleotide bases and carries 1268 genes. The chromosome (13) contains 114 million nucleotide bases and carries 496 genes. The chromosome (14) contains 109 million nucleotide bases and carries 1173 genes. The chromosome (15) contains 106 million nucleotide bases and carries 906 genes. The chromosome (16) contains 98 million nucleotide bases and carries 1032 genes. The chromosome (17) contains 92 million nucleotide bases and carries 1394 genes. The chromosome (18) contains 85 million nucleotide bases and carries 400 genes. The chromosome (19) contains 67 million nucleotide bases and carries 1592 genes. The chromosome (20) contains 72 million nucleotide bases and carries 710 genes. The chromosome (21) contains 50 million nucleotide bases and carries 337 genes. Finally, the sex chromosome of all female called the (X) contains 164 million nucleotide bases and carries 1141 genes. The male sperm chromosome (Y) contains 59 million nucleotide bases and carries 255 genes.

If you add up all genes in the 23 chromosomes, they come up to 26,808 genes, and yet we keep on mentioning 24,000 genes. The remaining genes are called the pseudogenes. For example, millions of years ago, humans and dogs shared some of the same ancestral genes; we both carry the same olfactory genes. Since humans don't use these genes to smell for searching food, these genes are broken and lost their functions in humans, but we still carry them. We call them pseudogenes. Recently, some Japanese scientists have activated the pseudogenes; this work may create an ethical problem in the future as more and more pseudogenes are activated.

The above DNA nucleotide bases constitute the genetic map of the normal human being; what makes it abnormal and makes us sick are the mutations in the coding regions of the genome. As I said above, less than 2% of the genome codes for amino acids. Slightest damage to the coding regions of the four nucleotides A, T, G, and C either by radiations or chemical pollution or genetic inheritance or viral infection or by insertion, deletion, or inversion of the nucleotide bases code for wrong or abnormal amino acids results into diseases.

The basis of OC is that people who are chewing tobacco or inhaling burning tobacco by smoking (as in India) or chewing betel quid, betel nut, etc. (as in Taiwan) are causing major mutations in their genomes producing a host of chemicals which damage the normal function of the cells causing them to become abnormal or cancerous. To understand the molecular basis of cancers, we have to sequence the normal as well as cancer cell genomes for comparison.

The sequencing of the first human genome costs us about 3 billion dollars. The advent of third-generation sequencing machines has made sequence-based expression analysis increasingly popular. In addition, techniques of DNA microarray technology which measures the relative activity of previously identified target genes and sequence-based techniques, like serial analysis of gene expression, are also used for gene expression profiling and have lowered the cost of sequencing significantly. As third-generation sequencers are becoming available, it is expected that the sequencing of genomes will become cheaper and faster; the cost of sequencing will come down from 3 billion dollars to 1000 dollars per genome, and then it would be possible to sequence the genome of every man, woman, and child on Earth and place the data on a central data genome center for future use. Your personal genome can be placed on a microchip of the size of a penny which you could carry on person at all times. In case of medical emergency, the hospital emergency staff can help you instantly.

There are over 220 different types of tissues in our body. We will be able to sequence every tissue for the data center. From the central database, it would be possible to examine a single cell which is responsible for causing oral tumor (squamous cell) and sequence its genome. Using GWAS (genome-wide association studies), we align the sequence of the normal cell genome with the oral tumor cell genome. The computer will compare the two genomes letter by letter, word by word, sentence by sentence, gene by gene, and chromosome by chromosome. With great precision and accuracy, the computer will identify the exact location of the mutations.

In the future, we might be able to perform the gene therapy if the cancer is caused by a single mutation, removing the bad gene using the restriction enzymes (scissors to cut DNA) and replacing the bad gene with the good gene using the enzyme ligase. If the oral cancer is caused by multiple mutations, gene therapy will not work, but drug therapy will work. We design drugs to shut off genes responsible for oral cancer mutations.

After the completion of the Human Genome Project, the next logical step is determining the gene expression profile of the good as well as bad gene. Gene profiling identifies which gene is functioning normally to produce healthy cells. The next step is to separate the normal genes from the mutated genes. This step will identify the good genes which produce normal proteins that keep us healthy. The work of large-scale production of such proteins is best done by biotechnology firms. The next logical step is to isolate the good gene whose product protein could be used to treat diseases. One of the greatest intellectual achievements of the twenty-first century is the genetic engineering that is using biochemical scissors called restriction enzymes (more than 3000 restrictions enzymes have been discovered). In our chemical store at NIH, there are at least 300 restriction enzymes sitting on the shelves to be used for cutting out a single normal gene from the entire human genome, pasting (ligase) into a carrying vector (besides viruses, other vectors include plasmid, cosmid, phagemid, BAC or bacterial artificial chromosome, and YAC or yeast artificial chromosome to carry the largest gene called Duchamp muscular dystrophy which is 2.5 million base pairs long), and transferring into a replicating host (yeast or mammalian cells) cell to make billions of copies of the good proteins used to treat diseases. For example, genetic engineers cut, paste, and ligase a copy of a gene that codes for a specific protein. Scientists at Genentech, a biotechnology firm in California, were the first to produce insulin to treat over 300 million diabetics around the world. They are also producing clotting factor VIII to treat hemophilia.

The next step is to separate diseases caused by a single gene mutation versus multiple gene mutations such as cardiac diseases and cancers. Almost 3000 diseases are caused by a single mutated gene called the Mendelian diseases. The next logical step is to conduct the gene therapy that replaced the bad gene with the good gene. For example, W. French Anderson and Mike Blaese who are considered the fathers of gene therapy, while working at NIH, were responsible for using a virus as a vector (carrier) to replace the bad gene responsible for causing severe combined immunodeficiency (SCID) syndrome with the good gene and cure the SCID. Today, more than 5000 previously SCID children are free from the disease and living a normal life. At this time, dozens of clinical trials on gene therapy to treat various diseases are in progress.

While gene therapy is successful for Mendelian diseases to replace a single bad gene with the good gene, multiple genetically defective diseases such as cardiac diseases and cancers cannot be treated with gene therapy. The next step for multiple genetic defects is to develop drug therapy to treat such diseases. Two approaches were made: the first is to synthesize the analogs of metabolites of the four nucleotide bases to interfere with the normal function of the cancer cell to prevent its replication. The most successful example of using antimetabolite drugs to treat cancer is the synthesis of 5-fluorouracil and 6-mercaptopurine for treating childhood leukemia.

For shutting off multiple genetic defects, the most logical step is to shut off the gene replication by cross-linking both strands of DNA carrying multiple mutated genes. All living creatures are the product of the union of both parents. Each parent is donating one strand of DNA making double-stranded DNA in all living creatures except a few viruses which are single stranded.

3.2 Drug Design to Shut Off Bad Genes

Professor WCJ Ross, the director of the Chemistry Division of the Chester Beatty Cancer Research Institute of the Royal Cancer Hospital, a postgraduate medical center of the University of London, was the first person to develop a series of chemical compounds called nitrogen mustards, developed by Fritz Haber as chemical weapons used during WWI and WWII, to cross-link the double-stranded DNA to prevent its replication of multiple mutated genes along the double-stranded DNA. Ross made highly successful cross-linking drugs such as chlorambucil [2] (for treating chronic lymphocytic leukemia) and melphalan [3] (used for treating multiple myeloma and ovarian cancer). Although they are highly useful drugs, they are also highly toxic. Ross has done the pioneering work in developing a drug like melphalan to treat pharyngeal carcinoma.

Over decades, Ross made hundreds of derivatives of nitrogen mustard as cross-linking agents. All of his students were searching for dyes for all 220 tissues as coloring agents which could be used as carrier for nitrogen mustard to attack the tumor of that specific tissue. The rationale is that if a dye colors pharyngeal tissues, by attaching nitrogen mustard, we could attack the tumor of the pharynx. This rationale does work. Before the Human Genome Project, all drugs were developed by trial and error method. Finding a useful drug by trial and error is time-consuming and expensive. In rare cases, this approach turned out to be successful. We were developing derivatives of mustard to attack the tumors. A large number of nitrogen mustards were tested against a variety of investigational tumors in rats. One of the toughest tumors was the solid tumor called the Walker carcinoma 256 in rats. If a compound reduces the tumor growth of the Walker carcinoma 256, it is the most likely candidate to go for clinical trials.

While studying the mechanism of action of nitrogen mustard, Ross discovered that radio-labeled nitrogen mustard does not bind to both strands of DNA at the same time. First, one arm of nitrogen mustard binds to one strand of DNA and then followed by the second arm of the nitrogen mustard binds to the second strand of the DNA. He proposed that it goes through an intermediate mechanism. The two carbonium ions produced by nitrogen mustard are extremely reactive; while one attacks the N-7 nitrogen atom of guanine, the second arm attacks the nitrogen atom of the mustard itself forming a three-member aziridine ring which is opened by acid produced by tumor and attacks the second strand of the DNA cross-linking both strands. The intermediate aziridine was unstable in acidic biological fluid and could not be isolated.

You might wonder what have I accomplished and how my work is different from my colleagues. Under Professor Ross' supervision, I received my Ph.D. degree in organic chemistry from the University of London. I worked for almost 10 years in Ross' lab as a student and as a postdoctoral fellow and as his special assistant at the Chester Beatty Cancer Research Institute of the Royal Cancer Hospital, a post-graduate medical center of the University of London.

From Ross' study, I picked up the idea of binding to one strand of DNA by using the intermediate aziridine ring. Using dinitrophenyl as a dye which colors Walker carcinoma 256 solid tumor cells, I made over 100 aziridine analogs while working in the laboratory of Professor Ross for over a 10-year period. Aziridine derivatives are completely harmless to touch but highly toxic to animal tissues in acidic medium. As I said above, toxicity is measured as the ratio (chemotherapeutic index as C/I) of its effect on normal to abnormal cells. All cross-linking compounds have a therapeutic index C/I of 10 when tested against Walker carcinoma 256 in rats. All my dinitrophenyl aziridine compounds were tested against Walker carcinoma. One of my drugs, dinitrophenyl aziridine benzamide (CB 1954), showed the highest toxicity ever recorded to Walker carcinoma 256 cells. It has a C/I of 70, and it is 70 times more toxic to a cancer cell compared to a normal cell. Ross and I published a series of three classical papers describing the synthesis of over 100 dinitrophenyl aziridine compounds [4–6].

I translated the animal work to human when I moved from England to America when I was honored with a Fogarty International Fellowship Award to come to America to continue my work on aziridines at the National Cancer Institute (NCI) of the National Institutes of Health (NIH). NIH has been my home for over a quarter of a century. The mission of NIH is to conduct research, support research, and report research. Over the years, I participated in all its missions. At NCI, I worked in the Drug Development Branch where a major part of my work involved designing anticancer drugs.

We at NIH are working on the expression profiling of the bad genes or the mutated genes whose proteins are responsible for causing all 6000 diseases including cardiac disease and cancers. Our institute, NIH, is established to diagnose, prevent, and treat all diseases known to mankind. We are interested in developing drugs to treat cancers. Gene profiling of solid tumors is the most important. Designing drugs to stop the gene expression of solid tumors offers the greatest challenge.

Our group designed drugs which bind to DNA to shut off the gene expression of bad genes. By trial and error, we find a coloring dye which colors a specific tissue. Using these dyes as carriers, we attach DNA-binding aziridines, nitrogen mustards, or carbamates to attack the tumors of those tissues. These compounds have the ability to generate carbonium ions which preferentially attack the nucleotide guanine of the abnormal cell DNA shutting off the gene.

If a normal cell is attacked, we call the effect toxicity, but when the abnormal cells are attacked, a cure is observed. The ratio of toxicity to normal versus abnormal cell is measured as the chemotherapeutic or toxicity index or C/I. A higher C/I index means that the drug is more toxic to abnormal cells compared to normal cells. Most nitrogen mustards shut off genes by binding to both strands of DNA, and they are known as the cross-linking agents. They generally have a toxicity index (C/I) of 10.

At NCI, I abandoned the dinitrophenyl dye as a carrier for aziridine; instead I used quinone as a new carrier for aziridine moiety because quinone has the ability to cross the blood-brain barrier (BBB). I thought that if I could deliver the aziridine ring across the BBB, I should be able to attack brain tumor. I had already demonstrated that CB 1954 could inhibit the growth of solid tumor in rats. Using quinone as a carrier, I thought that I should be able to attack solid brain tumor like glioblastoma in humans. Over the years, I made 45 quinone aziridines for screening against CNS (central nervous system) tumors system [7–9]. All 45 aziridines are considered so valuable that they are patented by the US government. One of them [10] is AZQ (US Patent 4,146,622) which is undergoing extensive screening as CNS active drug for treating brain cancer for which I was honored with the "2004 NIH Scientific Achievement Award," one of America's highest awards in medicine.

Conclusion

Ethical Issues: Scientists in our group are working on different kinds of cancers. As I stated above, there are more than 220 different types of tissues, and they could all become cancerous. We are all working to cure those cancers. Unfortunately, there was no great enthusiasm for working on either OC or lung cancer. Such diseases are considered self-inflicting wounds. The users of tobacco products are addicted and frequently developed these types of cancers. Many scientists believe that all of us have free will. We have a right to live and we have a right to die. If you shoot in your foot, it will hurt you. Do we protect you from shooting yourselves? If you don't smoke or chew tobacco, you will not expose yourself to a host of carcinogens. Some of us believe that you are addicted to nicotine if we cure your OC and you still go back to chewing tobacco. How can we protect you from yourself? On the other hand, if you are one of those unfortunate persons who inherited a mutated gene or were exposed to radiations or heavy metal particles, you deserve all our help, and many of us have been designing drugs for treating oral and lung cancer for you.

Let me summarize what I have written so far. It is expected that the third-generation sequencing would bring the cost down to a $1000/genome. Sequencing of cancer genome is of utmost important because at lower cost, we can sequence the genomes of all OCs including oropharynx which are squamous cell carcinomas or verrucous carcinoma responsible for causing oral cavity cancer.

Sequencing could also include salivary gland cancers including adenoid cystic carcinoma, mucoepidermoid carcinoma, and polymorphous low-grade adenocarcinoma or lymphomas of the tonsils and base of the tongue tissues for GWAS comparison. We cannot only identify the chromosome number on which mutations are located but also the number of mutations responsible for causing cancer.

Once the mutation sites and chromosome number are identified, we can diagnose, prevent, and treat the OCs either by gene therapy if a single gene mutation is responsible for causing any of the above cancers or by drug therapy if multiple mutations are involved. As I stated above, W. French Anderson and his colleagues have successfully developed gene therapy for treating SCID (severe combined immunodeficiency syndrome), and we could use the same method to cut and paste and replace the bad gene with the good gene to treat those cancers. On the other hand, if cancer is caused by multiple mutations, we could use the method developed by Ross for cross-linking both strands of DNA. Using dyes specific to OC cells as carriers for nitrogen mustard, we could develop a new class of drugs which acts as cross-linking alkylating agents and which binds to both strands of DNA. On the other hand, you could also design drugs by using our method by attaching aziridines to oral cancer-specific dyes to shut off mutated genes by binding to a single strand of DNA. What would happen if we succeed, when next-generation sequencers that perform inexpensive and fast sequencing of genomes become available to researchers? On that moment, the dawn of a new day at long last will shine on all the members of medical staff for developing treatment for cancers.

References

1. The future of life by Edward O. Wilson, First Vintage Books Edition; 2003. p. 20.
2. Chlorambucil – CancerConnect News. CancerConnect News. Retrieved on 2015-12-21.
3. Melphalan Lancet. 370(9594):1209–18.
4. Cobb LM, Connors TA, Elson LA, Khan AH, Mitchley BCV, Ross WCJ, Whisson ME. 2,4-dinitro-5-ethyleneiminobenzamide (CB 1954): a potent and selective inhibitor of the growth of the Walker carcinoma 256. Biochem Pharmacol. 1969;18:1519–27.
5. Khan AH, Ross WCJ. Tumour-growth inhibitory nitrophenylaziridines and related compounds: structure-activity relationships. Part I. Chem Biol Interact. 1969/1970;1:27–47.
6. Khan AH, Ross WCJ. Tumour-growth inhibitory nitrophenylaziridines and related compounds: structure-activity relationships. Part II. Chem Biol Interact. 1971/1972;4:11–22.
7. Hameed Khan A, Driscoll JS. Active antitumor components in a decomposed amino sugar part 1, effect of sugar structure on activity. J Pharm Sci. 1975;64(2):295–9.
8. Hameed Khan A, Driscoll JS. Potential central nervous system antitumor agents: aziridinylbenzoquinones. Part I. J Med Chem. 1976;19(2):313–7.
9. Chou E, Hameed Khan A, Driscoll JS. Potential central nervous system antitumor agents: aziridinylbenzoquinones. Part II. J Med Chem. 1976;19:1302.
10. Driscoll JS, Hameed Khan A, Feng-e-Chou. Aziridinyl quinone: anti-transplanted tumor agents. Unites States Patent # 4,146,622, March 27, 1979.

Smoking and Oral Cancer

4

Brooj Abro and Shahid Pervez

4.1 Introduction

Tobacco smoking remains a major concern in public health and a widely known cause of many cancers and various other chronic conditions. It is by far the most important risk factor for developing cancer and causes even more deaths from other conditions, such as respiratory and vascular diseases [1]. About 6 million people die of tobacco smoke every year, which includes deaths due to direct tobacco use and exposure to secondhand smoke. Tobacco is used by more than a billion people worldwide, and about 80% are from middle- and low-income countries [2]. According to the World Health Organization's (WHO) report on mortality attributable to tobacco (2012), 12% of all deaths worldwide, of people aged 30 and above are due to tobacco. The association of tobacco smoke with oral cancer has been well established, and recently the precise genetic mutations caused by smoking leading to the development of cancer have also been delineated. Both forms of tobacco, smoked and smokeless, have been declared as carcinogenic to humans by the International Agency for Research on Cancer (IARC) [3].

4.2 History of Tobacco Usage

Since over a century, tobacco has emerged as an epidemic with its rapid spread and use among the world population [4]. It is believed that tobacco was used initially in tropical America as far back as 6000 BCE [5]. The tobacco plant belongs to the genus *Nicotiana*, and it can grow in a wide range of warm climates hence easy to

B. Abro (✉) • S. Pervez
Section of Histopathology, Department of Pathology & Laboratory Medicine, Aga Khan University Hospital, Karachi, Pakistan
e-mail: abro.brooj@gmail.com

A.-E. Al Moustafa (ed.), *Development of Oral Cancer*,
DOI 10.1007/978-3-319-48054-1_4

cultivate in most continents [5]. Tobacco gradually spread to other parts of the world, and was cultivated for its leaves to manufacture different products. The leaves were dried and processed to make cigarettes, cigars, and other forms that are chewable [6].

By the sixteenth and seventeenth century, tobacco had spread to parts of North America, Europe, Africa, and Asia [7]. Columbus's voyage has been noted by some sources to have led to the discovery of this plant and its introduction to European countries; however, some historians claim this isn't entirely true, and many Europeans didn't start using it until the late 1550s. Initially this plant was regarded as a herbal product and used as a medicine. In many European countries for over a period of 200 years, tobacco was known as a cure for all ailments, a panacea widely endorsed by physicians [7]. In 1560 Jean Nicot described some medical uses of tobacco, including cures for toothache, halitosis, cancer, etc. [8]. Tobacco started being produced commercially in North America in the 1600s, when farmers began cultivating it in Virginia and it became a major cash crop since then. By the 1800s it was being cultivated throughout the United States, Canada, India, China, and many other countries [7]. The nineteenth century is marked by developments that made the distribution of tobacco products easier, invention of the Bonsack machine in 1880 that made it possible to produce large amounts of cigarettes, spread of safety match that allowed the possibility of smoking tobacco anywhere, and the development of rail transportation making it easier to transport products to different places efficiently [9]. In the twentieth century, there was another major development that made tobacco smoking very easy. This was a new method of tobacco production by flue-curing that produced an inhalable smoke unlike the older version produced by air-curing that gave rise to smoke which was non-inhalable. This was one of the most important manufacturing strategies that made this product so popular and lead to increased incidence of lung cancer [10].

In the mid-twentieth century, the widespread use of tobacco became known as the tobacco epidemic [11]. Marketing and advertisement played a substantial role in promoting its use. The United States became one of the largest manufacturer and exporter of tobacco till the 1960s, after which the use declined due to growing evidence of the harmful effects of this product. On January 11, 1964, the first US Surgeon General's report was released by Luther L. Terry, M.D. This report highlighted the effects of smoking and concluded that it was related to the development of lung and laryngeal cancer and the most important cause of bronchitis [12]. This report was followed by initiation of advertising health warnings on tobacco products in the United States by 1967. This was a major event in history that led to widespread recognition of the health effects of tobacco and many quit tobacco smoking after that.

4.3 Cigarettes and Other Forms of Tobacco Preparations

Cigarettes are the most widely used tobacco products. They are manufactured from tobacco leaves shaped cylindrically and rolled in thin paper. One end is kept in the mouth, and the other end is used for burning, and the smoke produced is inhaled.

Cigarettes became more popular in the United States after the Civil War, and the mechanization during the nineteenth century helped promote the tobacco industry's growth and spread. After the US Surgeon General's report released in 1964, cigarette smoking gradually declined [13]. Among adult population in the United States during 1965, the prevalence was reported to be 42.4%, and in 2012 it fell to about 18% [14]. The use remained higher in men compared to women, and people living in poverty also had higher rates of smoking [13]. Even though cigarette use declined in the United States and Europe, the industry continued to have a good market in the developing countries, and it continues to be a profitable industry.

Other forms of smoked tobacco products include cigars, narghiles, and pipes. In smokeless forms, we have chewable tobacco (often combined with areca nut and used in betel quid in many Asian countries), snuff which is inhaled, and the newly developed products called e-cigarettes [15]. Pipe smoking is a very old form of smoking and more prevalent in Asia compared to Western countries. Cigars look a bit similar to cigarettes, are made of whole leaf tobacco, contain a larger concentration of tobacco than cigarettes, and are smoked without a filter [15]. Narghiles are a form of smoking thought to have originated in Central Asia. It consists of an apparatus that has a container for water and a chamber where tobacco is placed; a pipe is connected through a tube and placed in the mouth to smoke the tobacco. This form of smoking is also commonly called hookah and sheesha. It is very common in the Asian continent, in countries like India, Pakistan, Bangladesh, and also in the Arabian Peninsula. In these regions, it is readily available in restaurants and easily accessible to the younger population [15].

Smokeless tobacco is the oldest form of tobacco. It is used in betel quid preparations like "pan" (common use in Indian subcontinent) and another widespread product in Asia called "gutka." It is estimated that about 600 million people use this form of tobacco worldwide [15]. Snuff consists of powdered tobacco that is absorbed through the oral and nasal mucosa.

4.4 Composition and Carcinogenesis

As tobacco use spread among the world population and concerns about its health effects started to surface, many researchers went on to investigate the precise composition of tobacco, to figure out which chemicals were responsible for causing disease, especially cancer. Both forms of tobacco, smoked and smokeless, contain numerous chemicals that can play a significant role in the development or progression of cancers.

In cigarette smoking, the human cells are exposed to several thousand chemicals, 60 of which have been established as carcinogens [16]. The US Surgeon General's report in 2004 concluded that there is enough evidence to suggest that smoking has a causal relationship with the development of cancers in various organs including the oral cavity. The other organs stated in the report included lung, larynx, pharynx, esophagus, pancreas, bladder, kidney, cervix, stomach, and acute myeloid leukemia [17].

When a cigarette is smoked, two different compositions of smoke are released: at the mouth end and the burning side, the former known as mainstream smoke and the latter as sidestream smoke. In mainstream smoke about 4000 chemicals have been identified [18]. The IARC evaluated the carcinogens in mainstream smoke and identified about 11 compounds which were classified as IARC Group 1 human carcinogens. These included 2-naphthylamine, 4-aminobiphenyl, benzene, vinyl chloride, ethylene oxide, arsenic, beryllium, nickel compounds, chromium, cadmium, and polonium-210 [19–23].

Of the several compounds in tobacco smoke known to have carcinogenic properties, the potent carcinogenicity of PAHs (polycyclic aromatic hydrocarbons), i.e., benzo(a)pyrene and TSNAs (tobacco-specific nitrosamines), specifically 4-(methylnitrosamino)-l-(3-pyridyl)-l-butanone (NNK), has been researched in most detail [24]. A study published in 2013 investigated the effects of combusted vs noncombusted tobacco products on oral epithelial cells and concluded that the former has a much higher impact and results in more significant DNA damage [25].

The carcinogens in tobacco smoke cause damage to human cells through multiple mechanisms (Fig. 4.1). The various pathways influenced by harmful substances in tobacco ultimately lead to loss of mechanisms that control normal cell growth and division. This loss of normal cell growth can result from chemicals in tobacco binding to receptors leading to activation of protein kinase A and B, uptake by epithelial cells and hypermethylation at growth promoter sites which can cause inactivation of tumor suppressor genes, and direct damage to DNA by forming DNA adducts [16]. These changes in the cell can lead to precursor lesions, and constant exposure can result in subsequent development of cancer. There is enough evidence to support that the level of DNA adducts in tissues of smokers is significantly higher when compared to nonsmokers, indicating that this pathway is crucial in causing genetic damage and development of cancer in smokers. Chromosomal losses are also noted to be more common in cancers that occur in smokers when compared to nonsmokers [16]. A very recent study published in November 2016 investigated the precise genomic mutations in 17 different cancers linked to smoking. The researchers studied the differences in somatic mutations and DNA methylation in cancer tissues from smokers and nonsmokers. They observed a complex pattern of mutations such as base substitutions only present in cancers from smokers [26]. This study provided new insights into how smoking increases the risk of cancer in many organs by causing certain somatic mutations. One of the mutations discovered in this study leads to misreplication of damaged DNA, and many chemicals in tobacco cause DNA damage; hence, both these properties collaborate in creating a suitable environment of oncogenesis.

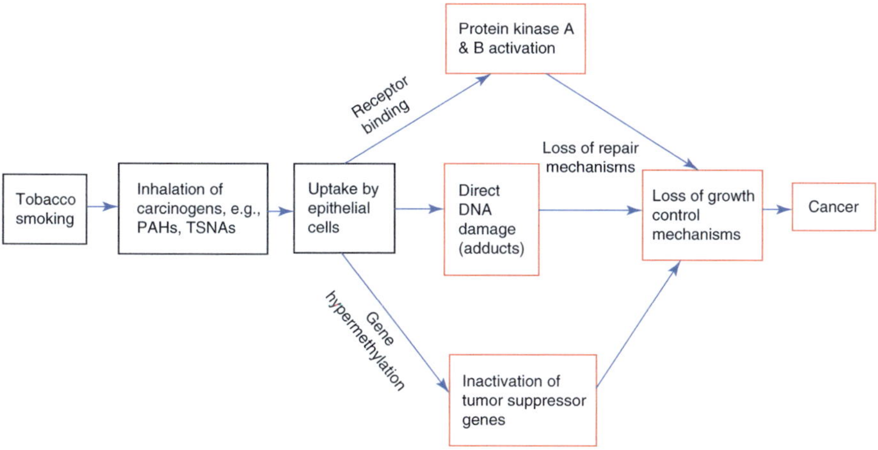

Fig. 4.1 Mechanisms of carcinogenesis by tobacco smoke. *PAHs* polycyclic aromatic hydrocarbons, *TSNAs* tobacco-specific nitrosamines

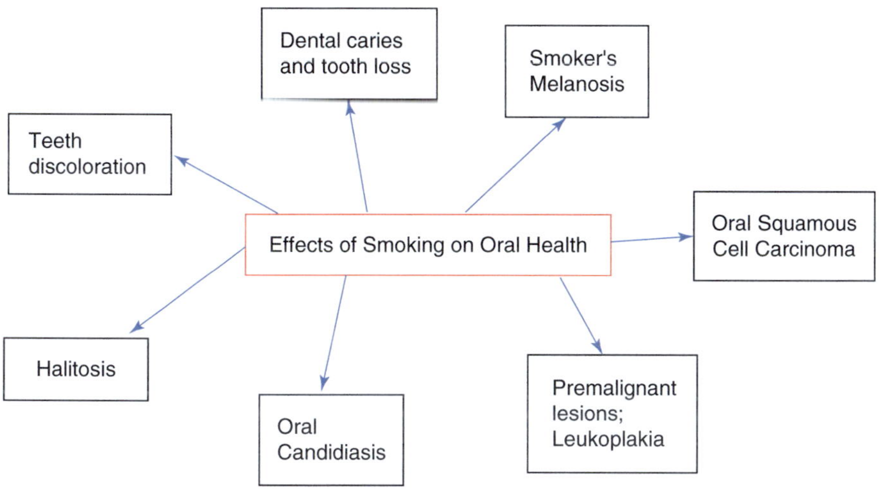

Fig. 4.2 Common oral conditions associated with smoking

4.5 Effects on Oral Health

There are well-established risks to oral health from smoking and chewing tobacco. It is a significant public health concern, and many individuals, especially in the developing world, are not aware of the implications of their smoking habits (Fig. 4.2).

4.5.1 Oral Hygiene and Aesthetics

Tobacco is known to cause staining of oral and lip mucosa, teeth, and dentures. Smokers tend to have a greater degree of teeth staining when compared to nonsmokers [27]. There is some evidence that the incidence of dental caries increases with use of tobacco products. A study identified tobacco smoking to significantly increase the risk of dental caries and tooth loss in elderly population [28]. Another study conducted in Sweden analyzed the risk of dental caries in teenagers and found to have increased prevalence among smokers although that does not necessarily apply a causal relationship [29]. Smoking also impacts smell and taste and is a common cause of halitosis [30].

4.5.2 Oral Mucosal Diseases: Nonmalignant

- **Nicotinic stomatitis**
- Frequent smoking can cause changes in the epithelium of the hard palate. The palate acquires a whitish color and can also have red dots scattered in the white background. This is not a premalignant condition and tends to resolve after smoking is discontinued [31]. A study in India found that it constitutes about 40% of all oral lesions in the elderly population [32].
- **Smoker's melanosis**
- Higher level of mucosal melanin pigmentation has been noted in heavy smokers [33]. This condition is also not a precursor of cancer and is reversible if the tobacco exposure is discontinued [34]. It does not require any treatment unless needed for aesthetic purposes [35].
- **Oral candidiasis**
- This is an infection of the oral cavity caused by a fungus, *Candida albicans*. Smoking along with other factors predisposes to this infection although the precise mechanism is not clearly known. Some older studies have reported that smoking increases the risk significantly [36, 37]. In HIV-positive individuals, smoking has been found to act as an independent risk factor for developing oral candidiasis [38].

4.5.3 Oral Premalignant Disorders

The effects on oral mucosa from tobacco smoking range from premalignant conditions to squamous cell carcinoma.

The most common premalignant condition is oral leukoplakia. It is defined as a whitish plaque on the oral mucosa that cannot be characterized by any other disease process [39]. Smoking increases the risk of leukoplakia by about six times [40]. Several studies have shown the propensity of leukoplakia to transform into dysplasia, and malignancy and the frequency of transformation range from about 15 to 30% [41–44]. Erythroplakia and submucosal fibrosis are other less common premalignant conditions; however, they are commonly associated with chewing smokeless tobacco over long periods of time [45, 46]. Out of all the premalignant conditions, progression to malignancy is highest in erythroplakia [47].

4.5.4 Oral Cancer

Out of the many cancers identified as a potential result of frequent smoking, oral cancer (OC) is a major one and is ranked as the 11th most common cancer worldwide [48]. It is most common in the Southeast Asia, overall ranking as the fifth common cancer in this region according to Globocan 2012. India, Pakistan, Bangladesh, and Sri Lanka are noted to have the highest incidence of OC. Squamous cell carcinoma (SCC) is the most common histological type, and the main etiologic factors identified for causing it are tobacco and alcohol [49, 50].

Tobacco has addictive and carcinogenic chemicals, the reason why it is consumed over prolonged periods of time increasing the likelihood of causing cancer. Nicotine is the primary chemical that causes addiction and thus making it difficult for smokers to quit. Nitrosamines, benzopyrenes, and aromatic amines promote cellular changes that are pro-carcinogenic [51].

When compared to nonsmokers, a smoker has three times higher risk of developing OC [52]. There is a dose-response relationship; the greater the number of years of tobacco exposure, the higher the risk of OC. The risk can be reduced with tobacco cessation and goes down by about 30% in the first 9 years post-cessation and about 50% in the years after that [53, 54]. Living in an environment with tobacco smoke has also shown to increase risk; there is an 87% higher risk in secondhand smokers to develop OC cancer when compared to people who have never been exposed to tobacco smoke [55]. Additionally, patients who have been treated for OC and continue to smoke have a six times higher risk of getting a second malignancy of the oropharynx [56, 57]. Individuals who smoke and consume alcohol have an even greater risk than the ones who consume either of these risk factors alone, because both these agents act synergistically to induce changes in favor of SCC [49, 58, 59].

OC develops over a course of many years, and many factors play a role at different stages of its progression. In many cases a premalignant lesion such as leukoplakia can be identified. If such premalignant lesions are identified, it should be used as an opportunity to warn and encourage the patient to quit smoking to reduce the potential of transformation to SCC. If a suspicious lesion in the oral cavity is identified that does not heal for a period of 3 weeks, a biopsy for pathological diagnosis should be done to rule out malignancy [60].

4.6 Prevention Strategies

Prevention can be achieved by two ways: creating awareness in the community to avoid and quit smoking and using screening methods in those who are at high risk to detect and treat the disease at an early stage.

Multiple steps have been taken by government and public health organizations to control the tobacco epidemic, which include adding health warnings to all tobacco products, using media to spread awareness on the harms of tobacco smoke, and banning its use in many public places. This has helped control smoking in developed countries; however, it is more difficult to implement these measures in the developing world, and smoking continues to be major health hazard. Continuous efforts from governments and public health policy makers are needed to control the widespread use of cigarettes. Since tobacco causes dependence and withdrawal effects on quitting, certain strategies are available to help smokers quit. At every clinical encounter, physicians should address the patient about harms of this habit and offer ways to help quit smoking. Counseling and behavior modification are a helpful initial step. Patients needing further support can also be offered pharmacotherapy for smoking cessation which includes nicotine replacement therapy: nicotine gum, nicotine inhaler, nicotine patch, and nicotine nasal spray [61]. For secondary prevention and identification of disease at an early stage, visual examination of the oral cavity has been approved as a useful screening method in high-risk individuals [62].

Conclusion

Tobacco is one of the world's leading causes of preventable death. Oral health is particularly affected by tobacco products, causing a wide range of problems such as halitosis, hyperpigmentation, increased susceptibility to infections, premalignant lesions, and oral squamous cell carcinoma. All these conditions can be easily prevented if tobacco is avoided. Physicians should encourage smoking cessation during clinic encounters, and visual screening should be used in high-risk individuals to assess for any suspicious and potentially malignant lesions.

References

1. Parkin DM, Bray F, Ferlay J, Pisani P. Estimating the world cancer burden: Globocan 2000. Int J Cancer. 2001;94(2):153–6.
2. WHO fact sheet, Tobacco, June 2016.
3. IARC Working Group on the Evaluation of Carcinogenic Risk to Humans. Tobacco Smoke and Involuntary Smoking. Lyon: International Agency for Research on Cancer; 2004. (IARC Monographs on the Evaluation of Carcinogenic Risks to Humans, No. 83.) Available from: https://www.ncbi.nlm.nih.gov/books/NBK316407/.
4. WHO: Tobacco. Geneva, World Health Organization, 2014.
5. Borio G. The Tobacco Timeline. http://archive.tobacco.org/History/Tobacco_History.html.
6. Haustein KO, Groneberg D. Tobacco or health? Physiological and social damages caused by tobacco smoking. 2nd ed. Berlin: Springer; 2010.
7. Loddenkemper R, Kreuter M. The tobacco epidemic, 2nd revised and extended edition. Progress in respiratory research, vol. 42. Basel: Karger; 2015. p. 1–18.
8. Mackenzie C. Sublime tobacco. London: Chatto & Windus; 1957.
9. Slade J. The tobacco epidemic: lessons from History. J Psychoactive Drugs. 1989;21(3):281–91.
10. Proctor R. Golden holocaust: origins of the cigarette catastrophe and the case for abolition. Oakland: University of California Press; 2012.

11. Brandt A. The cigarette century. The rise, fall, and deadly persistence of the product that defined America. New York: Basic Books; 2007.
12. History of the Surgeon General's Reports on Smoking and Health, compiled by the Office on Smoking and Health, National Center for Chronic Disease Prevention and Health Promotion, Centers for Disease Control and Prevention. Updated December 2006.
13. Mendez D, Warner KE, Courant PN. Has smoking cessation ceased? Expected trends in the prevalence of smoking in the United States. Am J Epidemiol. 1998;148(3):249–58.
14. Centers for Disease Control and Prevention: Cigarette Smoking in the United States. Atlanta, CDC, 2014. http://www.cdc.gov/tobacco/campaign/tips/resources/data/cigarette-smoking-in-united-states.html.
15. Viegas CA. Noncigarette forms of tobacco use. J Bras Pneumol. 2008;34:1069–73.
16. Centers for Disease Control and Prevention (US); National Center for Chronic Disease Prevention and Health Promotion (US); Office on Smoking and Health (US). Cancer. In: How tobacco smoke causes disease: the biology and behavioral basis for smoking-attributable disease: a report of the surgeon general. Atlanta: Centers for Disease Control and Prevention (US); 2010. Available from: https://www.ncbi.nlm.nih.gov/books/NBK53010/.
17. US Department of Health and Human Services. The health consequences of smoking: a report of the surgeon general. Atlanta: U.S. Department of Health and Human Services, Centers for Disease Control and Prevention, National Center for Chronic Disease Prevention and Health Promotion, Office on Smoking and Health; 2004.
18. Green CR, Rodgman A. The tobacco chemists' research conference; a half century of advances in analytical methodology of tobacco and its products. Recent Adv Tob Sci. 1996;22: 131–304.
19. IARC. IARC monographs on the evaluation of carcinogenic risks to humans, suppl. 7, overall evaluations of carcinogenicity: an updating of IARC monographs volumes 1 to 42. Lyon: IARC Press; 1987.
20. IARC. IARC monographs on the evaluation of carcinogenic risks to humans, vol. 49, chromium, nickel and welding. Lyon: IARC Press; 1990.
21. IARC. IARC monographs on the evaluation of carcinogenic risks to humans, vol. 58, beryllium, cadmium, mercury and exposures in the glass manufacturing industry. Lyon: IARC Press; 1993.
22. Hoffmann D, Hoffmann I. The changing cigarette: chemical studies and bioassays. In: Risks associated with smoking cigarettes with low machine-measured yields of tar and nicotine (Smoking and tobacco control monograph No. 13; NIH Publ. No. 02-5074). Bethesda: National Cancer Institute; 2001. p. 159–91.
23. IARC. IARC monographs on the evaluation of carcinogenic risks to humans, vol. 78, ionizing radiation. Part 2: Some internally deposited radionuclides. Lyon: IARC Press; 2001.
24. Engstrom PF, Clapper ML, Schnoll RA. Carcinogenic and genotoxic effects of tobacco constituents. In: Kufe DW, Pollock RE, Weichselbaum RR, et al., editors. Holland-Frei cancer medicine. 6th ed. Hamilton: BC Decker; 2003. Available from: https://www.ncbi.nlm.nih.gov/books/NBK12437/.
25. Gao H, Prasad GL, Zacharias W. Combusted but not smokeless tobacco products cause DNA damage in oral cavity cells. Environ Toxicol Pharmacol. 2014;37(3):1079–89. doi:10.1016/j.etap.2014.03.022.
26. Alexandrov LB, Ju YS, Haase K, Van Loo P, Martincorena I, Nik-Zainal S, Totoki Y, Fujimoto A, Nakagawa H, Shibata T, Campbell PJ, Vineis P, Phillips DH, Stratton MR. Mutational signatures associated with tobacco smoking in human cancer. Science. 2016;354(6312):618–22.
27. Asmussen E, Hansen EK. Surface discoloration of restorative resins in relation to surface softening and oral hygiene. Scand J Dent Res. 1986;94:174–7.
28. Jette AM, Feldman HA, Tennstedt SL. Tobacco use: a modifiable risk factor for dental disease in the elderly. Am J Public Health. 1993;83:1271–6.
29. Hirsch JM, Livian G, Edward S, et al. Tobacco habits among teenagers in the city of Göteborg, Sweden, and possible association with dental caries. Swed Dent J. 1991;15:117–23.
30. Fortier I, Ferraris J, Mergler D. Measurement precision of an olfactory perception threshold test for use in field studies. Am J Ind Med. 1991;20:495–504.

31. Agnihotri R, Gaur S. Implications of tobacco smoking on the oral health of older adults. Geriatr Gerontol Int. 2014;14(3):526–40.
32. Patil S, Doni B, Maheshwari S. Prevalence and distribution of oral mucosal lesions in a geriatric Indian population. Can Geriatr J. 2015;18(1):11–4.
33. Axeixt T, Hedin CA. Epidemiologic study of excessive oral melanin pigmentation with special reference to the influence of tobacco habits. Eur J Oral Sci. 1982;90(6):434–42.
34. Hedin C, Pindborg JJ, Axéll T. Disappearance of smoker's melanosis after reducing smoking. J Oral Pathol Med. 1993;22(5):228–30.
35. Monteiro LS, Costa JA, da Camara MI, et al. Aesthetic depigmentation of gingival smoker's melanosis using carbon dioxide lasers. Case Rep Dent. 2015;2015:510589.
36. Galai N, Park LP, Wesch J, et al. Effect of smoking on the clinical progression of HIV-1 infection. J Acquir Immune Defic Syndr Hum Retrovirol. 1997;14(5):451–8.
37. Abu-Elteen KH, Abu-Alteen RM. The prevalence of *Candida albicans* populations in the mouths of complete denture wearers. New Microbiol. 1998;21(1):41–8.
38. Shiboski CH, Shiboski SC. Smoking is an independent risk factor for the development of oral candidiasis (OC) in HIV-1 infected persons. J Evid Based Dent Pract. 2013;13(4):180–2.
39. Kramer IR, Lucas RB, Pindborg JJ, et al. WHO collaborating Centre for Oral Precancerous Lesions. Definition of leukoplakia and related lesions: an aid to studies on oral precancer. Oral Surg Oral Med Oral Pathol. 1978;46:518–39.
40. Van der Waal I. Potentially malignant disorders of the oral and oropharyngeal mucosa; terminology, classification and present concepts of management. Oral Oncol. 2009;45(4–5):317–23.
41. Shafer WB, Waldron CA. A clinical and histopathologic study of oral leukoplakia. Surg Gynecol Obstet. 1961;112:411–20.
42. Waldron CA, Shafer WG. Leukoplakia revisited: a clinicopathologic study of 3256 oral leukoplakias. Cancer. 1975;36:1386–92.
43. Pindborg JJ, Renstrup G, Poulsen HE, et al. Studies in oral leukoplakia. V. Clinical and histologic signs of malignancy. Acta Odont Scand. 1963;21:407–14.
44. Feller L, Altini M, Slabbert H. Pre-malignant lesions of the oral mucosa in a South African sample: a clinicopathologic study. J Dent Assoc S Afr. 1991;46:261–5.
45. Hashibe M, Mathew B, Kuruvilla B, Thomas G, Sankaranarayanan R, Parkin DM, Zhang ZF. Chewing tobacco, alcohol, and the risk of erythroplakia. Cancer Epidemiol Biomark Prev. 2000;9(7):639–45.
46. Arakeri G, Brennan PA. Oral submucous fibrosis: an overview of the aetiology, pathogenesis, classification, and principles of management. Br J Oral Maxillofac Surg. 2013;51(7):587–93.
47. Villa A, Villa C, Abati S. Oral cancer and oral erythroplakia: an update and implication for clinicians. Aust Dent J. 2011;56:253–6. doi:10.1111/j.1834-7819.2011.01337.x.
48. Bray F, Ren JS, Masuyer E, Ferlay J. Global estimates of cancer prevalence for 27 sites in the adult population in 2008. Int J Cancer. 2013;132(5):1133–45. doi:10.1002/ijc.27711.
49. Blot WJ, McLaughlin JK, Winn DM, Austin DF, Greenberg RS, Preston-Martin S, Bernstein L, Schoenberg JB, Stemhagen A, Fraumeni JF Jr. Smoking and drinking in relation to oral and pharyngeal cancer. Cancer Res. 1988;48(11):3282–7.
50. Blot WJ. Alcohol and cancer. Cancer Res. 1992;52(7 Suppl):2119s–23s.
51. Rivera C. Essentials of oral cancer. Int J Clin Exp Pathol. 2015;8(9):11884–94.
52. Gandini S, Botteri E, Iodice S, et al. Tobacco smoking and cancer: a meta-analysis (link is external). Int J Cancer. 2008;122(1):155–64.
53. Macfarlane GJ, Zheng T, Marshall JR, et al. Alcohol, tobacco, diet and the risk of oral cancer: a pooled analysis of three case-control studies. Eur J Cancer B Oral Oncol. 1995;31B(3):181–7.
54. Samet JM. The health benefits of smoking cessation. Med Clin North Am. 1992;76(2):399–414.
55. Lee YC, Marron M, Benhamou S, Bouchardy C, Ahrens W, Pohlabeln H, Lagiou P, Trichopoulos D, Agudo A, Castellsague X, Bencko V, Holcatova I, Kjaerheim K, Merletti F,

Richiardi L, Macfarlane GJ, Macfarlane TV, Talamini R, Barzan L, Canova C, Simonato L, Conway DI, McKinney PA, Lowry RJ, Sneddon L, Znaor A, Healy CM, McCartan BE, Brennan P, Hashibe M. Active and involuntary tobacco smoking and upper aerodigestive tract cancer risks in a multicenter case-control study. Cancer Epidemiol Biomark Prev. 2009;18(12):3353–61. doi:10.1158/1055-9965.EPI-09-0910.

56. Silverman S Jr, Shillitoe EF. Etiology and predisposing factors. In: Silverman Jr S, editor. Oral cancer. 4th ed. Hamilton: BC Decker Inc; 1998. p. 7–24.
57. Silverman S Jr, Griffith M. Smoking characteristics of patients with oral carcinoma and the risk for second oral primary carcinoma. J Am Dent Assoc. 1972;85:637–40.
58. McCoy GD, Wynder EL. Etiological and preventive implications in alcohol carcinogenesis. Cancer Res. 1979;39(7 Pt 2):2844–50.
59. Brugere J, Guenel P, Leclerc A, Rodriguez J. Differential effects of tobacco and alcohol in cancer of the larynx, pharynx, and mouth. Cancer. 1986;57(2):391–5.
60. Scully C, Bagan JV, Hopper C, Epstein JB. Oral cancer: current and future diagnostic techniques. Am J Dent. 2008;21(4):199–209.
61. Black JH 3rd. Evidence base and strategies for successful smoking cessation. J Vasc Surg. 2010;51(6):1529–37. doi:10.1016/j.jvs.2009.10.124.
62. Brocklehurst P, Kujan O, O'Malley LA, Ogden G, Shepherd S, Glenny AM. Screening programmes for the early detection and prevention of oral cancer. Cochrane Database Syst Rev. 2013;11:CD004150.

Alcohol and Oral Cancer

5

Omar Kujan, Abdulhameed Husain, and Camile S. Farah

5.1 Introduction

Alcohol consumption has long been recognised as one of the major risk factors for the development of oral cancer [1]. The establishment of the sole effect of alcohol on the oral mucosa and its link to the development of oral cancer have been considered a significant challenge, principally because alcohol consumption histories are difficult to verify, alter over time, both with respect to beverage type and quantity, and are frequently confounded by tobacco use [2]. This is further explained by the established joint effect of alcohol and tobacco in the development of head and neck cancers [2]. In addition, it can be difficult to obtain reliable information from patients about their alcohol intake where the data on alcohol ingestion is based on a highly subjective estimate provided by patients, and this can be due to the different drinking behaviours, e.g. some may 'binge' drink and others have a high daily intake. This chapter will discuss the epidemiological evidence for the role of alcohol in oral cancer, the topical and systemic effects of alcohol, alcohol-related oral carcinogenesis and the association between alcohol-containing mouthwashes and oral cancer risk. It will also outline the health benefits of alcohol moderation and cessation and its role in prevention of human oral cancer.

O. Kujan (✉) • A. Husain
School of Dentistry, University of Western Australia,
17 Monash Avenue, Nedlands, WA 6009, Australia
e-mail: omar.kujan@uwa.edu.au

C.S. Farah
School of Dentistry, University of Western Australia,
17 Monash Avenue, Nedlands, WA 6009, Australia

Australian Centre for Oral Oncology Research & Education, Nedlands, WA 6009, Australia

A.-E. Al Moustafa (ed.), *Development of Oral Cancer*,
DOI 10.1007/978-3-319-48054-1_5

5.2 Alcohol and Oral Cancer: Epidemiological Evidence

According to the global burden of disease project of the World Health Organisation (WHO) for the year 2000, 1.8 million deaths per year were attributed to alcohol consumption [3]. This accounts for approximately 3.2% of all deaths [3]. Alcohol consumption is believed to be increasing in regions of rapid economic growth. It is also claimed that alcohol consumption by women is rising [4]. Regular consumption of alcoholic beverages was estimated to be greater than 1.9 billion people worldwide in 2002, with an average daily consumption of 13 g of ethanol equivalent to one standard drink [4]. Given that a high number of these consumers are at high risk of alcohol abuse disorders, the International Agency for Research on Cancer (IARC) reviewed the available epidemiological evidence in 2007 [5]. They concluded that 'alcoholic beverages are carcinogenic to humans (Group 1)' and that 'the occurrence of malignant tumours of the oral cavity, pharynx, larynx, oesophagus, liver, colorectum, and female breast is causally related to alcohol consumption' [5, 6]. The agency has also classified that the ethanol contained within alcoholic beverages is 'carcinogenic to humans (Group 1)'. In light of these statements, chronic alcohol consumption can account for approximately 389,000 cases of cancer worldwide [5]. Alcohol consumption is a well-established risk factor for the development of oral squamous cell carcinoma (OSCC) [7]. Oral squamous cell carcinoma may present clinically in different forms (Fig. 5.1). The association between alcohol consumption and the development of OSCC was first explored in 1961, and, since then, epidemiologic studies and reviews have further investigated such an association [4, 8–26]. Several mechanisms have been suggested by which alcohol consumption results in an elevated risk of OSCC, and this will be discussed later in the chapter.

A meta-analysis of 42 case-control studies published by Tramacere in 2010 found the pooled relative risk for heavy drinking being 5.24 (95% CI, 4.36–6.30), compared to a relative risk for light drinking of 1.21 (95% CI, 1.10–1.33) [27].

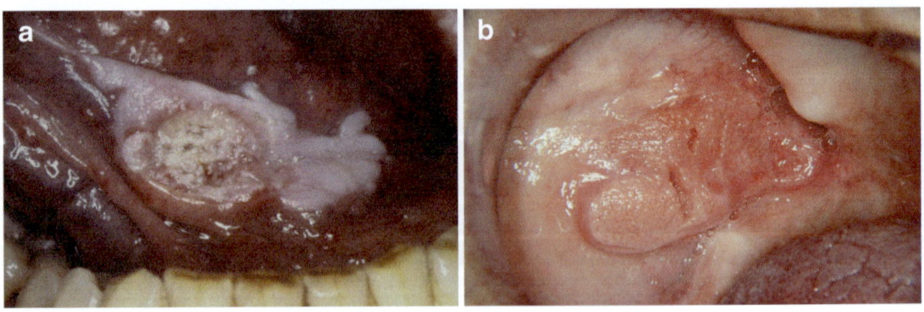

Fig. 5.1 Clinical presentation of oral squamous cell carcinoma. (**a**) Ulcerated white lesion on the ventral surface of the tongue in a heavy drinker and cigarette smoker 68-year-old female; biopsy proven moderately differentiated squamous cell carcinoma. (**b**) Ulcerated exophytic lesion with granular appearance on the right buccal mucosa in a heavy drinker and smoker 63-year-old male; biopsy proven moderately differentiated squamous cell carcinoma

Heavy drinking was defined as four or more drinks a day and light drinking was one drink or less a day. The findings have clearly demonstrated a dose-response relationship. In this context, the consumption of one drink a day was found to be significantly associated with an increased risk of oral cancer [11]. Similar results have been shown in a meta-analysis conducted by Bagnardi et al. in which one drink or less a day conferred a relative risk of 1.17 (95% CI, 1.06–1.29) [28]. Another large meta-analysis has concluded the same results with a relative risk of 1.26 (95% CI, 0.94–1.67) [29]. The cessation of alcohol consumption has been shown to reduce the risk of oral cancer development, and this has been evidenced in several studies [11, 13, 30]. Risk reduction following cessation would require more than 15 years to eliminate any elevated risk, and this would affirm the importance of long-term studies [31]. In addition, it has been noted that concentration of ethanol in alcoholic beverages acts as an independent risk factor for the development of OSCC. Studies have shown consistent findings in which an increase in the ethanol concentration accounts for an increased risk [11, 14, 26]. An example is a study investigating alcohol concentration and risk of oral cancer in Puerto Rico which found that strong spirits were associated with a 6.4 times increased risk compared to other alcoholic beverages [17]. Due to such findings, oral carcinogenesis can be better understood by investigating local effects of ethanol in the oral cavity.

When studying the epidemiology of alcohol and oral cancer, it is important to note that smoking acts as a strong cofactor. That said, studies have examined nonsmoking drinkers to establish alcohol use as an independent risk factor for OSCC [15, 32]. A meta-analysis conducted by Turati et al. found that the use of alcohol in nonsmokers conferred a relative risk of 1.32 (95% CI, 1.05–1.67) of developing OSCC and pharyngeal cancer [32]. Another finding was the increased risk in heavy drinkers.

Tobacco smoking is a well-established independent risk factor for the development of OSCC. When tobacco smoking is combined with alcohol consumption, synergistic effects produce a greater than multiplicative increase in the risk of developing OSCC compared to smoking or drinking independently [6, 9, 11, 13, 14, 19, 26, 33]. This was evidenced in the International Head and Neck Cancer Epidemiology Consortium (INHANCE) pooled analysis conducted by Hashibe et al. in 2009 where smoking and drinking together were associated with a greater than multiplicative increased risk of oral and pharyngeal cancer in 12,828 cases [16]. Local interactions between tobacco smoking and alcohol consumption account for the potentiation of carcinogens, and, consequently, the effects in the head and neck are observed.

5.3 Alcoholic Beverages and Weekly Consumption

In the context of the types of alcoholic beverages, controversy exists when reviewing their role in oral carcinogenesis. Several problems are encountered when looking at studies related to the type of beverage and OSCC risk due to the differences in terminology in alcohol measurements (standard drinks, units, gram ounces and whisky equivalents all features in the literature) in different studies in different countries around the world [2]. Another problem is that consumption by individuals is often not confined to one specific type of alcoholic beverage, and there can also be marked differences in alcohol content in different brands of the same alcoholic beverage group [25]. In addition, the type of alcoholic beverage has been regarded as significant, often with contrasting results. The main available beverage types include those that are home-made or locally produced in developing countries such as sorghum beer, palm wine or sugarcane spirits [34]. The IARC monograph focuses on beer, wine and spirits as the main beverage categories; however, a combination of two types must also be considered in the context of production methods and raw materials [35]. The Standard International Trade Classification (SITC) has four categories: wine from fresh grapes, cider and other fermented beverages, beer and distilled alcoholic beverages [35]. Regardless of the type of alcoholic beverage, each type was found to be associated with cancer risk; however, there was a strong association with drinking spirits [11]. This finding supplements results from a study mentioned earlier in which strong spirits were associated with a 6.4 times increased risk compared to other alcoholic beverages [17]. Further, the cancer risk was found to increase with increase in ethanol content of each beverage type [11]. It is important to note the amount of ethanol contained in a specific drink which can be measured by multiplying the amount of alcoholic beverage (200 mL wine) by the ethanol conversion factor. Although the latter measurement differs from country to country, the general figures for conversion factors for beer are 4–5, 12 vol% for wine and 40 vol% for distilled spirits. As an example the ethanol content in a 330 mL bottle of beer would be $330 \times 0.04 = 13.2$ mL ethanol. In light of this, the ethanol content in beer varies from 2.3% to more than 10 vol%. Wine accounts for a higher ethanol content, ranging from 8 to 15 vol%; however, light wines and non-alcoholic wines are available. Of the IARC categories, the highest ethanol content is contained in spirits which comprise up to 40 vol%; however, aperitifs contain around half that alcohol content [35]. Other types of alcoholic beverages have a significantly lower amount of ethanol content, and these could include alcopops, flavoured alcoholic beverages or ready-made beverages that contain 4–7 vol% [35].

Studies have shown that beer and wine have been implicated for a higher OSCC development risk over whisky, whilst beer and whisky have a higher relative risk of development of OSCC over wine, and the relative risk of whisky has been implicated over beer and wine [36–38]. The alcoholic strengths in many beverages differ from brand to brand, but most are in the range of 3–6%. In the USA, the average alcoholic strength of beers is 4.6 vol%, whereas, in the UK, the mean alcohol content of all beers is 4.1 vol% [39]. Specific alcoholic beverages have been shown to contain specific impurities or contaminants (such as *N*-nitrosodiethylamine) which can be carcinogenic and present in some beers and whisky and associated with an increased risk of OSCC [40]. In Brazil, the excess risks for oral cancer were evident with increased consumption of distilled sugarcane spirit [41]. Studies in Italy showed an excess risk for wine alone [42], or with other alcoholic beverages [43]. Multiple studies in Spain, Brazil and Puerto Rico have shown that alcohol concentration is a risk factor for oral cancer regardless of the total amount consumed [11, 17, 44]. Each type of alcoholic beverage (beer only, wine and beer, wine only or spirits) is associated with cancer risk, but the association is much stronger for consumption of spirits [11].

It is worth emphasising the importance of alcohol consumption patterns with special focus on the frequency and quantity over a predefined period of time. The patterns of drinking reflect drinking behaviours including frequency of drinking occasions, variations in drinking over periods of time and the number and characteristics of unsafe drinking occasions [45]. Other aspects to consider are the types of beverages consumed, discussed in this section, and the clusters of drinking norms and behaviours referred to as 'drinking cultures' [46]. The key measure to alcohol consumption patterns is to calculate the average number of alcoholic beverages consumed a day and the number of drinking days. The daily amount of alcohol consumption is increasingly important to ensure safe drinking limits. In the UK, the Chief Medical Officers' Alcohol Guidelines Review in 2016 proposed a new weekly guideline for people who drink frequently or regularly [47]. These guidelines state that it is safe to not drink regularly more than 14 units/week and that these units are best to be spread evenly over 3 days or more. These limits apply to men and women. The Australian Guidelines to reduce health risks from drinking alcohol cover four aspects in which the first two include recommendations to reduce the risk of alcohol-related harm over a lifetime and recommendations to reduce the risk of injury on a single occasion of drinking [45]. The former guideline states that for healthy men and women, no more than two standard alcoholic drinks a day reduced the lifetime risk of harm from alcohol-related disease or injury. The second guideline recommends that drinking no more than four standard alcoholic drinks on a single occasion reduced the risk of alcohol-related injury arising from that occasion. The third guideline accounts for children and young people under 18 years of age [45]. This directs particular attention to children under 15 years of age where the greatest risk of harm from drinking can occur and advises that young people aged 15–17 years should delay drinking for as long as possible. With that said, the relationship between age and drinking habits is affected by gender and culture. Alcohol intake is increasing in low- and middle-income countries and remains steadily high in high-income countries [48]. Drinking habits generally decrease with increasing age; however, some countries have different tendencies [49]. From another perspective, socioeconomic status reflects drinking habits where people with higher socioeconomic status are more likely to consume alcohol compared to people with lower socioeconomic status [50]. Additionally, women of higher socioeconomic status are found to be heavy drinkers and have heavy episodic drinking habits compared to men [51]. Educational status may also impact drinking patterns. Lower educational status is positively related to minimal alcohol consumption in the Netherlands [52]. In the German population, men of middle status had increased odds for heavy episodic drinking, and men of lower socioeconomic status had higher odds for symptoms of alcohol dependence [51]. The degree of employment has also been found to affect prevalence of alcoholic beverage consumption in the UK [53]. A UK study found that those with a higher employment degree were heavier drinkers and women who had a much higher rate of heavier drinking [53]. Kunst et al. found that men with a lower level of education in certain European countries consumed excessive amounts of alcohol (up to four glasses or more per day) [54]. In contrast, higher levels of education were consistently associated with higher rates of heavier drinking among both men and women in Brazil and Argentina [51, 55].

5.4 Topical Effects

Ethanol and its first metabolite, acetaldehyde, can act as risk factors, both locally and systemically in the development of oral cancer [56]. Alcohol may increase the penetration of carcinogens across the oral mucosa by either increasing their solubility or by increasing the permeability of the oral mucosa by dissolving the lipid component of the epithelium that normally acts as a protective barrier [56, 57]. In the context of mucosal permeability, one must note the differences in permeability between the oral tissues of certain oral cavity subsites. The buccal mucosa, the lateral border of the tongue and the floor of the mouth are non-keratinised tissues and therefore account for greater permeability than keratinised tissue such as the gingivae and the hard palate [58]. Changes in mucosal morphology have been found in human tongues, and these changes were characterised by the histopathological features of reduced epithelial thickness due to reduced maturation layer and cell shrinkage. Moreover, increased thickness of the basal cell layer due to hypertrophy was severe in human tongues of alcoholic patients [59]. This results in an atrophic oral mucosa and increased proliferative activity which leads to an increased susceptibility to carcinogens [60]. Further, tissue damage to rabbit oral mucosa by long-term exposure to alcohol has demonstrated dysplastic changes with keratosis, increased basal cell layer density and increased number of mitotic figures [61]. Acetaldehyde is a mutagenic and carcinogenic substance that exhibits many effects on human cells such as interference with the synthesis and repair of DNA, production of gene mutations and binding of cellular proteins and DNA resulting in morphological and cellular injury [56]. Acetaldehyde also induces exchanges between sister chromatids and inhibits enzyme *O*6-methylguanine transferase which is responsible for DNA injury repair [62]. It can also potentiate the genotoxicity of other mutagenic, clastogenic (ability to disrupt chromosomal material) or carcinogenic agents [25]. Further, chronic alcohol consumption leads to atrophy and lipomatous transformation of the parenchyma of the parotid and submandibular glands, resulting in impaired saliva flow and an increase in its viscosity. Due to the impaired salivary flow, the oral mucosa is therefore inadequately rinsed and is exposed to higher concentrations of locally acting carcinogens [63]. Hyposalivation and the resultant reduced salivary flow can therefore prolong the contact time of the carcinogens with the mucosa, increasing the risk of cancer development [56, 63].

Within the oral cavity, alcohol consumption has been found to be associated with an increased risk of oral epithelial dysplasia (OED) [64]. In particular, oral potentially malignant disorders and invasive OSCC development and alcohol drinking are associated in a frequency-response relationship [9, 64, 65]. In addition, the frequency-response relationship was found to have a stronger trend for beer and hard liquor than for wine [21, 66]. More importantly, heavy alcohol consumption was more strongly associated with oral cancer than OED among both current and never smokers [67].

Although the bulk of alcohol metabolism is carried out in the liver, extrahepatic metabolism of alcohol to acetaldehyde has been shown to occur elsewhere in the body including the oral cavity. An early study demonstrated considerable acetaldehyde production in saliva (up to 143 μM) after moderate consumption of alcohol (0.5 g/kg body weight) [68]. The level of acetaldehyde formed was well above endogenous AA level of 1 μM [69, 70] and was within the range that is capable of inducing mutagenic changes 50–150 μM [62, 71]. Furthermore, studies have also found that ingested alcohol may in fact be metabolised to acetaldehyde by commensal organisms in the oral cavity via microbial alcohol dehydrogenase. Microorganisms that have been documented to be significantly associated with higher acetaldehyde production include *Streptococcus* spp., particularly *S. salivarius*, *Neisseria* spp. and *Candida albicans* [62, 72, 73]. The known toxic effect of acetaldehyde as well as its local production in the mouth has led to increasing interest in the level of salivary AA formed after alcohol-containing mouthwash use and its association with oral cancer development.

5.5 Systemic Effects

The systemic effects of ethanol consumption may play a contributing role in carcinogenesis. Chronic alcohol consumption may affect the liver's ability to contend with toxic or potentially carcinogenic compounds [25]. Firstly, ethanol consumption results in reduced first-pass metabolism of nitrosamine by the liver, resulting in an increased metabolism in extrahepatic tissues, and this plays a contributing role in carcinogenesis [74]. Secondly, the impairment of both innate and acquired immune systems leads to an increased susceptibility to infection and certain neoplasms [74]. Chronic alcohol exposure may suppress natural killer (NK) cell activity which is involved in tumour cell surveillance [75]. Moreover, the recruitment of polymorphonuclear leukocytes during infection and inflammation can be impaired due to excessive alcohol consumption as well as impaired production of haemopoeitic stem cells [76–80]. Immunosuppression related to alcohol consumption can also be caused by vitamin deficiencies, hepatic cirrhosis and malnutrition [80]. Lastly, heavy alcohol consumers are more prone to nutritional deficiencies due to decreased consumption, or impaired absorption, utilisation or storage of nutrients, thus increasing the risk of cancer development [75]. The concept of malnutrition and oral cancer development can be supported by the evidence of the greater reported risk of oral cancer and high intake of meat and processed meat products [81]. In contrast, frequent consumptions of citrus fruit, vegetables, fish and vegetable oils are associated with a low risk of oral cavity cancer [82]. On the other hand, deficiencies of folate, zinc, iron and selenium have been associated with an increased risk of cancer development [83]

It has also been discovered that a poorer prognosis is associated with head and neck cancer alcoholic patients compared to non-alcoholic patients [84]. This finding is due to an increased risk for other alcohol-related diseases. Moreover, chronic alcohol consumption and a history of alcohol-related disease were found to be associated with an increased risk of death [84]. Interestingly, this was independent of age, site of tumour, tumour staging, histopathological grade, smoking habits or treatment modalities.

5.6 Synergistic Effects with Tobacco Use

Smoking and drinking are independently and synergistically associated with an increased risk of oral cancer, and the risks tend to increase with an increased frequency of exposure [11]. Moreover, oral epithelial dysplasia (OED) risk was positively associated with smoking and drinking in an independent, dose-dependent fashion, with evidence of a synergistic joint effect [64]. In 2009, the interaction between tobacco and alcohol and the risk of head and neck cancer were evaluated from a pooled analysis within INHANCE [16]. The aim of this evaluation was to test the multiplicative model of interaction between alcohol and tobacco use with a large sample size. Data was pooled from 18 individual case-control studies including 12,282 cases and 17,189 controls [15, 85–101]. Results have shown that the joint effect between alcohol and tobacco was larger than expected under the multiplicative model for head and neck cancer [16]. In addition, joint effects were found greater than multiplicative by subsite for oral cavity cancer and pharyngeal cancer. Other findings in the analysis included a higher proportion of head and neck cancers found in men who smoke and drink compared to women, with tobacco and alcohol combined accounting for a large proportion of cases. In contrast, tobacco and alcohol accounted for a smaller proportion of cases with head and neck cancers in a younger age group (<45 years). Evidence has shown that a simultaneous exposure to tobacco smoking and alcohol drinking increased oral cancer risk by approximately 13-fold compared to subjects never exposed to such habits [11]. A synergistic joint effect has been suggested due to the interaction between tobacco smoking status and alcohol drinking status being highly significant [11]. The risk of developing oral cancer was also assessed in the context of frequency of smoking and amount of alcohol consumption per day. Results have shown that there was a statistically significant fivefold increase in the risk of developing oral cancer and smoking 1–10 cigarettes coupled with 1–2 drinks/day [11]. That said, the same study has not shown statistically significant interactions between the type of tobacco smoked and the type of alcoholic beverage.

5.7 Alcohol-Related Oral Carcinogenesis

The main constituents of most alcoholic beverages are ethanol and water with some flavour compounds. The absorption of ethanol occurs rapidly through the gastric and duodenal mucosa and metabolised in the liver before being eliminated [25]. There are several steps involved in the hepatic metabolism of ethanol: firstly, oxidation of alcohol to acetaldehyde via the enzyme alcohol dehydrogenase (ADH). Acetaldehyde is a mutagenic and carcinogenic substance that exhibits many effects on human cells such as interference with the synthesis and repair of DNA, production of gene mutations and binding of cellular proteins and DNA resulting in morphological and cellular injury [56]. It can also potentiate the genotoxicity of other mutagenic, clastogenic or carcinogenic agents [25]. Secondly, conversion of acetaldehyde to acetate which is catalysed by the enzyme aldehyde dehydrogenase (ALDH). Acetate is then oxidised to produce carbon dioxide, fatty acids and water. It is important to note that extrahepatic metabolism of alcohol also occurs, and the involvement of ADH has been demonstrated in the oral mucosa [102, 103]. In addition, extrahepatic metabolism of acetaldehyde by ALDH has also been demonstrated in the oral mucosa [102]. The accumulation of acetaldehyde in oral tissues is thought to be due to the increased activity of ADH compared to ALDH activity [102].

Of concern is the role of genetic variation regarding the metabolism of alcohol and tobacco carcinogens. This belies the concept that genetic host factors influence the manner in which an individual would interact with environmental carcinogens [104, 105]. The different genetic polymorphism found in enzymes involved in alcohol and tobacco metabolism accounts for susceptibility of development of a particular type of cancer [105, 106]. An enzyme that is involved in the oxidation of acetaldehyde to acetate is the aldehyde dehydrogenase (ALDH) encoded by the *ALDH2* gene. This gene causes the accumulation of acetaldehyde after consumption of alcohol which has significant implications in the context of alcohol metabolism genes in head and neck cancer [107]. Bediaga et al. studied three *ALDH2* polymorphisms from the Basque Country and found that higher alcohol consumption was associated with heterozygous or homozygous carriers for any of *ALDH2* variant alleles. This leads to an increased predisposition to consuming alcohol and therefore an increased risk of developing head and neck squamous cell carcinoma [108]. This is also supported by the association between *ALDH2* and an increased risk of head and neck cancer in heavy drinkers [109]. Moreover, an increased risk of head and neck cancer has been found to be associated with *ALDH2* in Japanese populations [110, 111]. Tsai et al. found similar results where individuals with slow *ALDH2* genotypes were at an increased risk of developing head and neck cancer associated with alcohol consumption, mainly due to human acetaldehyde production. This study showed that the association between alcohol consumption and head and neck cancer risk may be modified by the interplay between genetic polymorphisms of *ALDH2* and *ADH1B* and oral hygiene [112]. One recent study evaluating the effects of *ADH1B* and *ALDH2* genetic polymorphisms in Japanese alcoholic men supports previously reported conclusions [113]. Results showed that salivary acetaldehyde levels were found to be higher and initially faster in carrier patients with either *ADH1B*2 or ALDH2*1/*2*. These findings suggest possible mechanistic explanations for *ALDH2*- and *ADH1B*-associated risk for alcohol consumption and upper aerodigestive tract cancer [113].

The gene that encodes the most important of the alcohol dehydrogenase enzymes, ADH1B, has two main functional allelic variants, ADH1B*2 and ADH1B*3. The homozygous genotype ADH1B*2/*2 encodes for an enzyme that has a maximum speed 40 times greater than the ADH1B*1/*1 genotype, and the ADH1B*3 allele encodes for an enzyme with a maximum speed 90 times higher than the wild-type allele [111]. It has been shown that individuals homozygous for ADH1B*1 with a normal catalytic speed bear alcohol consumption better, although in these subjects there is long-term damage, and this allele is known to be associated with an increased predisposition to head and neck cancer. The ADH1B*2 allele is presented in 93% of the Japanese population, while in Africans and Caucasians, it is present in only 20% of the population with the majority having ADH1B*1 allele [114].

ALDH2 is a mitochondrial enzyme whose wild-type allele is known as ALDH2*1, with a variant ALDH2*2 that is inactive, and individuals with ALDH2*1/*2 accumulate six times more acetaldehyde. ALDH2*2 allele is common among Asians being 30% of the population heterozygotes and 10% homozygotes, while virtually all European populations are homozygous for ALDH2*1. The presence of an ALDH2*1/*2 genotype plus alcohol consumption increases the risk of developing head and neck cancer, including oral cancer in the Japanese population. A recent case-control study of a Japanese population further reinforced the relationship between alcohol consumption and ALDH allele and extended these findings to include folate consumption. The majority of the cancers included in this study were oral cancers (257 of 409 patients), which were in turn matched with controls of the same age and gender at a ratio of 1–3 [111]. It was shown that not only was folate intake inversely associated with the risk of OPC, and alcohol consumption was positively associated, but there was a significant interaction of folate, alcohol and ALDH2 genotype in the risk of oropharyngeal cancer [111].

The role of alcohol in oral carcinogenesis has been studied repeatedly showing the capacity of alcohol to eliminate the lipid component of the oral cavity barrier surrounding epithelial spinous layer granules [115]. In one study, 15% ethanol significantly increased mucosal permeability suggesting that short-term exposure to ethanol caused the disruption of epithelial lipid molecules resulting in molecular rearrangement of the permeability barrier, in particular, the mucosa of the human ventral tongue [116]. As research moves forward, a close focus to the role of alcohol in dysplastic and malignant epithelial cells of precancerous lesions such as oral leukoplakia and cancerous lesions has been investigated [117]. One study assessed the generation and subcellular distribution of protein adducts with acetaldehyde, the first metabolite of ethanol and end products of lipid peroxidation. Results indicated that a number of distinct types of adducts may be found in precancerous and cancerous lesions of chronic alcohol consumers supporting the proposed mechanism of ethanol-induced carcinogenesis [117]. The formation of these adducts interferes with DNA synthesis and replication leading to disincorporation and mutations. The most abundant acetaldehyde adduct formed in DNA is N^2-ethyl-2′-deoxyguanosine (N^2-ethyl-dGTP) which was found to be only incorporated opposite the correct base [118]. Following alcohol exposure, significant increases in the number of adducts are seen in oral keratinocytes [119]. Another adduct that has been found to form from the interaction of croton aldehyde (CrA) and DNA is 1,N^2-propano-2′-deoxyguanosine (1,N^2-PdG) [118]. This adduct is more ominous than N^2-ethyl-dGTP due to its mutagenic, genotoxic and carcinogenic properties [120, 121]. Such properties can lead to chromosomal damage in humans which can be used as an early biomarker [122]. Chromosomal aberrations have been investigated with evidence postulating that acetaldehyde was responsible for changes in lymphocytes [123]. It is worth emphasising the role of cytochrome P450 enzyme (CYP2E1) induction in response to chronic alcohol consumption [124]. Consumption of 40 g/day, equivalent to three drinks, can induce CYP2E1, and the proportion of ethanol that is oxidised by CYP2E1 has been found to be up to 30% in chronic alcohol consumers [7, 125]. In oral and oesophageal epithelium, the induction of CYP2E1 has several implications regarding carcinogenesis. The activation of procarcinogens such as *N*-nitroso compounds and polycyclic aromatic hydrocarbons into their carcinogenic form is derived by CYP2E1 [7, 33, 126, 127]. This activation accounts for the mechanism in which synergistic effects of tobacco smoking and alcohol are associated with the development of OSCC.

The production of reactive oxygen species by the microsomal ethanol-oxidising system leads to DNA damage by single- and double-strand breaks, base oxidation and fragmentation and DNA-protein cross-links [128]. Examples of reactive oxygen species include hydrogen peroxide, hydroxyl radicals, peroxynitrate and superoxide [129]. In the context of oral carcinogenesis, high amounts of reactive oxygen species were found in OSCC samples [130]. In addition, 8-oxo-dG adducts were also found in greater amounts with a reduction in antioxidant compounds [131].

5.8 Alcohol-Containing Mouthwashes and Oral Cancer

Studies have investigated the potential risks of head and neck cancers in long-term and frequent users of mouthwash. Of particular importance is the evidence towards the role of alcohol-containing mouthwashes and its contribution to the increased risk of oral cancer development [132, 133]. Alcohol itself has long been established as a risk factor in the development of oral cancer, and this has been well demonstrated by the literature in the previous section. Ethanol is used in mouthwashes as a solvent for other ingredients and as a preservative for the preparations of the many different formulas available [134]. From the different available products, the concentrations of ethanol vary, reaching up to 26% v/v. The quantity of alcohol in mouthwashes and the prolonged exposure to the oral mucosa affect the mucosal permeability leading to many detrimental changes including epithelial detachment, keratosis, mucosal ulceration, hyperkeratotic lesions, mucosal ulcerations, periodontal diseases and petechiae, all of which have been proven in human oral mucosa and laboratory animals [134, 135]. The theory of a causal relationship between alcohol-containing mouthwashes and oral cancer has been studied since 1979 [112, 136–153]. Currie and Farah have modelled the pathways leading to oral mucosal carcinogenesis following alcohol-containing mouthwash use. This model was interpreted through the field of cancerisation concept under a unifying hypothesis [133]. They posited that regular topical exposure to alcohol-containing mouthwash leads to a dramatic rise in the level of salivary acetaldehyde to a point where there is the potential for mutagenic events to occur [69, 154]. Additionally, the use of alcohol-containing mouthwash increases the permeation of mucosa and induces cytochrome P450 2E1, which acts to enhance tobacco-related carcinogens evidenced by a greater than multiplicative increase in OSCC risk associated with concurrent smoking and drinking [33]. These combined effects would have a carcinogenic contribution especially to a sensitised field. With this in mind, it is also worth noting that alcohol containing mouthwash use is more likely to increase the risk of oral cancer development in patients diagnosed with oral epithelial dysplastic lesions as they tend to be smokers and alcohol consumers, but also tend to overuse alcohol-containing mouthwash causing further tissue damage [133].

Although evidence of the possible carcinogenicity of alcohol-containing mouthwashes exists arguably through the field of cancerisation theory [133], it is still considered to be controversial. Previous studies have shown conflicting results regarding an increasing risk of OSCC from the use of mouthwashes, and this is due to variations in study design [112, 136–153, 155]. Other reasons for the conflicting results are due to the variables tested, with some studies assessing the frequency of mouthwash use, others assessing the history of mouthwash use or the retention time in the mouth and others again assessing the rationale behind using mouthwashes. Further, the incidence of alcohol-containing mouthwash use in smokers and in patients who consume alcohol raises another difficulty in the context of effect quantification [139].

In 1983, a retrospective study found that mouthwash use increased the risk of oral cancer development in females only [152]. In addition, this excess risk is associated with non-drinking and nonsmoking women. However, the study concluded no causal significance to the association between daily mouthwash use and the development of oral cancer in women due to the absence of a dose-response relationship [137]. Following this study, another case-control study in North Carolina involving 206 women with oral and pharyngeal cancers and 352 controls evaluated the possibility of mouthwash use and its involvement in the aetiology of the development of oral cancer. Findings from this study showed nearly twofold increased risk associated with regular mouthwash use among women who abstained from tobacco. These results supported previous studies in which excess risk related to mouthwash use occurred in nonsmoking and non-drinking females [38, 149]. In contrast, Elmore and Horwitz evaluated the previous studies stating that mouthwash use and subsequent oropharyngeal cancer adhered to basic methodologic principles of case-control designs and that neither the data for the overall association nor the analysis in patients with no other clinical risk factors supported the association between mouthwash use and oral cancer [156]. Moreover, in 2004, a critical analysis of the literature found limited evidence to support the proposed causal relationship between the use of alcohol-containing mouthwashes and the development of oral cancer [134]. However, a suggestion was made to clarify the mechanisms of the role of alcohol-containing mouthwashes in oral carcinogenesis, due to the findings of an elevated, but not statistically significant, risk for oral cancer in nonsmokers and non-drinkers [151]. Results of two multicentric case-control studies assessing oral health and risk of squamous cell carcinoma of the head and neck and oesophagus showed that mouthwash use was a significant factor for all subsites with the exception for the eosophagus due to the unlikely contact with mouthwash [143]. More importantly, mouthwash use showed a strong association with cancer in the oral cavity in which mouthwash use twice daily increased the risk among current and past smokers and drinkers as well as among lifelong alcohol abstainers. The latter association supports the proposed mechanism of the role of alcohol in oral carcinogenesis with particular reference to alcohol-containing mouthwashes [132].

These results support findings from previous studies where the use of mouthwash increased the risk of oral cancer in smokers and drinkers [137, 144, 147, 148, 150–152] as well as tobacco and alcohol abstainers [137, 149, 151]. In addition, the first study investigating salivary acetaldehyde levels after use of alcohol-containing mouthwashes and mouthrinses found acetaldehyde contents in saliva which were significantly above endogenous levels and corresponding to concentrations found after alcohol consumption [69]. This systemic acetaldehyde exposure reached concentrations associated with DNA adduct formation and sister chromatid exchange in vitro suggesting a role of local oral carcinogenesis. An update on mouthwash use and the risk of oral cancer development was published in 2008 after the debate on this matter was reignited [132] with summarised findings of at least ten case-control studies over the last three decades [157]. The update concluded the proposed link between mouthwash use, in particular, alcohol-containing mouthwash, and oral cancer is not supported by epidemiological evidence. This conclusion is mainly due to studies not including specific information on alcohol-containing mouthwash [137, 143, 144, 149, 152, 153, 155] with only two studies including this information [150, 151]. Results of this update are supported by a recent quantitative meta-analysis of epidemiologic studies of mouthwash and oral cancer, specifically, mouthwash-containing alcohol content of more than 25% [158]. The meta-analysis included 18 studies and concluded that there was no statistically significant association found between regular mouthwash use and risk of oral cancer (RR = 1.3; 95% CI (0.95–1.35) and that there was no significant trend in risk of oral cancer associated with increased daily mouthwash use ($p = 0.11$). In addition, there was no association found between reported use of mouthwash, specifically alcohol-containing mouthwash, and risk of oral cancer (RR = 1.16; 95% CI (0.44, 3.08). The authors have noted that more epidemiologic studies with a greater focus on certain aspects of mouthwash use and the development of oral cancer are needed [158]. Following the latter meta-analysis, a very recent pooled analysis from the International Head and Neck Cancer Epidemiology Consortium (INHANCE) in 2015 proposed more definitive evidence on examining the association between mouthwash use and head and neck cancer by using individual-level data on a very large number of cases and controls [159]. The pooled analysis involved 8981 cases of head and neck cancer and 10,090 controls from 12 case-control studies with comparable information on mouthwash use in the INHANCE. An advantage of this pooled analysis is the use of standard methods to control for confounding, whereas meta-analyses may not adequately control for confounders due to their limitations to summary effect estimates reported in the original studies. Another advantage is that the data used from included studies originated from mouthwash use questionnaires in the INHANCE, whereas meta-analyses included published studies with a potential chance of bias [160]. Considerations were given to include data on regular mouthwash use, duration of use and daily frequency of use which indicates extent of exposure. However, these were only available in some studies. Results provided strong evidence for an association of long-term and high-dose use of mouthwash with the risk of head and neck cancer with a potential relation to the alcohol content in many of the products. However, some of the results do not support the proposed causal relationship in which no association was found between mouthwash use and never smokers or never drinkers suggesting no effect independent from that of these two habits. The authors concluded no overall increased risk of head and neck cancer development in individuals who ever used mouthwash, but an association in long-term frequent mouthwash users, stating that this analysis provides the most precise estimate of such association [159]. Further, prospective cohort studies on mouthwash use and oral cancer can avoid potential biases in case-control studies. Interestingly, mouthwash use was found to be a risk factor for head and neck squamous cell carcinomas in a study involving 513 cancer cases and 567 controls from a population-based study [142]. Results showed mouthwash use, regardless of alcohol content, is associated with an increased risk of head and neck squamous cell carcinomas. Alcohol-containing mouthwash was also found to be associated in the development of cancer in the same study, supporting the previously recognised proposition in 2008 [132].

5.9 Prevention

Oral cancer is a preventable disease and early detection can reduce cancerous transformation of oral premalignant disorders and hence potentially improve the survival rate. With increased understanding of this disease, the 5-year survival rate has remained at 50% for the past three decades [161]. Primary prevention of oral cancer is therefore paramount.

Primary prevention of oral cancer is the approach which focuses on the avoidance of the well-recognised risk factors implicated in the development of oral cancer with the intention of minimising the incidence of the disease. Avoidance of the many known aetiological factors for the development of OSCC including tobacco use, alcohol consumption, prolonged exposure to sunlight and alterations in lifestyle and behaviours may prevent OSCC development. Moderating alcohol intake and keeping consumption within recommended guidelines is an important primary prevention aspect that should be considered. Cessation of alcohol consumption has been associated with a 40% decreased risk of head and neck cancer after ≥20 years of cessation compared with current drinkers [162]. More importantly, there should be increased awareness of the synergistic effect between alcohol and smoking which holds a risk greater than that of alcohol alone or tobacco alone [163]. Regulations on alcoholic beverage consumption are available widely, and these aim for alcohol control and harm-reduction strategies. Alcohol control policy can be defined as any measure put in place to control the supply and/or affect the demand for alcoholic beverages, minimise alcohol-related harm and promote public health in a population. Such policies include education and treatment programmes to mitigate the burden of alcoholic beverages on societies by limiting and regulating alcohol beverage consumption and their distribution. Levels and patterns of alcohol consumption would be impacted, if alcohol policies were to be implemented with support and continuous enforcement. While the relationship between alcohol policies and levels of alcohol beverage consumption and alcohol-related harm continues to evolve, it is hoped that it will address social problems, prevent disability and promote health protection.

References

1. Ogden GR. Alcohol and oral cancer. Alcohol. 2005;35(3):169–73.
2. Ogden GR, Wight AJ. Aetiology of oral cancer: alcohol. Br J Oral Maxillofac Surg. 1998;36(4):247–51.
3. Ezzati M, Lopez AD, Rodgers A, Vander Hoorn S, Murray CJL. Selected major risk factors and global and regional burden of disease. Lancet. 2002;360(9343):1347–60.
4. Boffetta P, Hashibe M. Alcohol and cancer. Lancet Oncol. 2006;7(2):149–56.
5. Baan R, Straif K, Grosse Y, Secretan B, El Ghissassi F, Bouvard V, et al. Carcinogenicity of alcoholic beverages. Lancet Oncol. 2007;8(4):292–3.
6. Petti S. Lifestyle risk factors for oral cancer. Oral Oncol. 2009;45(4-5):340–50.
7. Seitz HK, Stickel F. Acetaldehyde as an underestimated risk factor for cancer development: role of genetics in ethanol metabolism. Genes Nutr. 2010;5(2):121–8.
8. Balaram P, Sridhar H, Rajkumar T, Vaccarella S, Herrero R, Nandakumar A, et al. Oral cancer in southern India: the influence of smoking, drinking, paan-chewing and oral hygiene. Int J Cancer. 2002;98(3):440–5.
9. Blot WJ, McLaughlin JK, Winn DM, Austin DF, Greenberg RS, Preston-Martin S, et al. Smoking and drinking in relation to oral and pharyngeal cancer. Cancer Res. 1988;48(11):3282–7.
10. Castellsague X, Munoz N, De Stefani E, Victora CG, Castelletto R, Rolon PA, et al. Independent and joint effects of tobacco smoking and alcohol drinking on the risk of esophageal cancer in men and women. Int J Cancer. 1999;82(5):657–64.
11. Castellsague X, Quintana MJ, Martinez MC, Nieto A, Sanchez MJ, Juan A, et al. The role of type of tobacco and type of alcoholic beverage in oral carcinogenesis. Int J Cancer. 2004;108(5):741–9.
12. Franceschi S, Levi F, Dal Maso L, Talamini R, Conti E, Negri E, et al. Cessation of alcohol drinking and risk of cancer of the oral cavity and pharynx. Int J Cancer. 2000;85(6):787–90.
13. Garrote LF, Herrero R, Reyes RMO, Vaccarella S, Anta JL, Ferbeye L, et al. Risk factors for cancer of the oral cavity and oro-pharynx in Cuba. Br J Cancer. 2001;85(1):46–54.
14. Gillison ML. Current topics in the epidemiology of oral cavity and oropharyngeal cancers. Head Neck. 2007;29(8):779–92.
15. Hashibe M, Brennan P, Benhamou S, Castellsague X, Chen C, Curado MP, et al. Alcohol drinking in never users of tobacco, cigarette smoking in never drinkers, and the risk of head and neck cancer: pooled analysis in the International Head and Neck Cancer Epidemiology Consortium. J Natl Cancer Inst. 2007;99(10):777–89.
16. Hashibe M, Brennan P, Chuang SC, Boccia S, Castellsague X, Chen C, et al. Interaction between tobacco and alcohol use and the risk of head and neck cancer: pooled analysis in the International Head and Neck Cancer Epidemiology Consortium. Cancer Epidemiol Biomarkers Prev. 2009;18(2):541–50.
17. Huang WY, Winn DM, Brown LM, Gridley G, Bravo-Otero E, Diehl SR, et al. Alcohol concentration and risk of oral cancer in Puerto Rico. Am J Epidemiol. 2003;157(10):881–7.
18. La Vecchia C, Tavani A, Franceschi S, Levi F, Corrao G, Negri E. Epidemiology and prevention of oral cancer. Oral Oncol. 1997;33(5):302–12.
19. Lissowska J, Pilarska A, Pilarski P, Samolczyk-Wanyura D, Piekarczyk J, Bardin-Mikollajczak A, et al. Smoking, alcohol, diet, dentition and sexual practices in the epidemiology of oral cancer in Poland. Eur J Cancer Prev. 2003;12(1):25–33.
20. Lubin JH, Purdue M, Kelsey K, Zhang ZF, Winn D, Wei Q, et al. Total exposure and exposure rate effects for alcohol and smoking and risk of head and neck cancer: a pooled analysis of case-control studies. Am J Epidemiol. 2009;170(8):937–47.
21. Maserejian NN, Joshipura KJ, Rosner BA, Giovannucci E, Zavras AI. Prospective study of alcohol consumption and risk of oral premalignant lesions in men. Cancer Epidemiol Biomarkers Prev. 2006;15(4):774–81.
22. Pelucchi C, Talamini R, Negri E, Levi F, Conti E, Franceschi S, et al. Folate intake and risk of oral and pharyngeal cancer. Ann Oncol. 2003;14(11):1677–81.

23. Philip M, Rowley DA, Schreiber H. Inflammation as a tumor promoter in cancer induction. Semin Cancer Biol. 2004;14(6):433–9.
24. Talamini R, Franceschi S, Barra S, La Vecchia C. The role of alcohol in oral and pharyngeal cancer in non-smokers, and of tobacco in non-drinkers. Int J Cancer. 1990;46(3):391–3.
25. Wight AJ, Ogden GR. Possible mechanisms by which alcohol may influence the development of oral cancer--a review. Oral Oncol. 1998;34(6):441–7.
26. Zavras AI, Douglass CW, Joshipura K, Wu T, Laskaris G, Petridou E, et al. Smoking and alcohol in the etiology of oral cancer: gender-specific risk profiles in the south of Greece. Oral Oncol. 2001;37(1):28–35.
27. Tramacere I, Negri E, Bagnardi V, Garavello W, Rota M, Scotti L, et al. A meta-analysis of alcohol drinking and oral and pharyngeal cancers. Part 1: overall results and dose-risk relation. Oral Oncol. 2010;46(7):497–503.
28. Bagnardi V, Rota M, Botteri E, Tramacere I, Islami F, Fedirko V, et al. Light alcohol drinking and cancer: a meta-analysis. Ann Oncol. 2013;24(2):301–8.
29. Li Y, Mao Y, Zhang Y, Cai S, Chen G, Ding Y, et al. Alcohol drinking and upper aerodigestive tract cancer mortality: a systematic review and meta-analysis. Oral Oncol. 2014;50(4):269–75.
30. Goldstein BY, Chang SC, Hashibe M, La Vecchia C, Zhang ZF. Alcohol consumption and cancers of the oral cavity and pharynx from 1988 to 2009: an update. Eur J Cancer Prev. 2010;19(6):431–65.
31. Jarl J, Gerdtham UG. Time pattern of reduction in risk of oesophageal cancer following alcohol cessation--a meta-analysis. Addiction. 2012;107(7):1234–43.
32. Turati F, Garavello W, Tramacere I, Pelucchi C, Galeone C, Bagnardi V, et al. A meta-analysis of alcohol drinking and oral and pharyngeal cancers: results from subgroup analyses. Alcohol Alcohol. 2013;48(1):107–18.
33. Seitz HK, Stickel F. Molecular mechanisms of alcohol-mediated carcinogenesis. Nat Rev Cancer. 2007;7(8):599–612.
34. Obot IS, Room R, editors. Alcohol, gender and drinking problems: perspectives from low and middle income countries. Geneva: World Health Organization; 2005.
35. IARC Working Group on the Evaluation of Carcinogenic Risks to Humans. Alcohol consumption and ethyl carbamate. IARC Monogr Eval Carcinog Risks Hum. 2010;96:3–1383.
36. Kabat GC, Wynder EL. Type of alcoholic beverage and oral cancer. Int J Cancer. 1989;43(2):190–4.
37. McCoy GD, Wynder EL. Etiological and preventive implications in alcohol carcinogenesis. Cancer Res. 1979;39(7 Pt 2):2844–50.
38. Wynder EL, Bross IJ, Feldman RM. A study of the etiological factors in cancer of the mouth. Cancer. 1957;10(6):1300–23.
39. Bamforth CW, editor. Beer: health and nutrition. Oxford: Blackwell Science; 2004.
40. Rogers MA, Vaughan TL, Davis S, Thomas DB. Consumption of nitrate, nitrite, and nitrosodimethylamine and the risk of upper aerodigestive tract cancer. Cancer Epidemiol Biomarkers Prev. 1995;4(1):29–36.
41. Franco EL, Kowalski LP, Oliveira BV, Curado MP, Pereira RN, Silva ME, et al. Risk factors for oral cancer in Brazil: a case-control study. Int J Cancer. 1989;43(6):992–1000.
42. Zambon P, Talamini R, La Vecchia C, Dal Maso L, Negri E, Tognazzo S, et al. Smoking, type of alcoholic beverage and squamous-cell oesophageal cancer in northern Italy. Int J Cancer. 2000;86(1):144–9.
43. La Vecchia C, Franceschi S, Favero A, Talamini R, Negri E. Alcohol intake and cancer of the upper digestive tract. Pattern of risk in Italy is different from that in Denmark. BMJ. 1999;318(7193):1289–90. author reply 91
44. Schlecht NF, Pintos J, Kowalski LP, Franco EL. Effect of type of alcoholic beverage on the risks of upper aerodigestive tract cancers in Brazil. Cancer Causes Control. 2001;12(7):579–87.
45. National Health and Medical Research Council AG. Australian Guidelines to Reduce Health Risks from Drinking Alcohol. Commonwealth of Australia; 2009.
46. Rehm J, Ashley MJ, Room R, Single E, Bondy S, Ferrence R, et al. On the emerging paradigm of drinking patterns and their social and health consequences. Addiction. 1996;91(11):1615–21.

47. Health Do. UK Chief Medical Officers' Alcohol Guidelines Review, Summary of the proposed new guidelines. London: 2016.
48. Roswall N, Weiderpass E. Alcohol as a risk factor for cancer: existing evidence in a global perspective. J Prev Med Public Health. 2015;48(1):1–9.
49. Makela P, Gmel G, Grittner U, Kuendig H, Kuntsche S, Bloomfield K, et al. Drinking patterns and their gender differences in Europe. Alcohol Alcohol Suppl. 2006;41(1):i8–18.
50. Keyes KM, Hasin DS. Socio-economic status and problem alcohol use: the positive relationship between income and the DSM-IV alcohol abuse diagnosis. Addiction. 2008;103(7):1120–30. doi:10.1111/j.360-0443.2008.02218.x.
51. Bloomfield K, Grittner U, Kramer S, Gmel G. Social inequalities in alcohol consumption and alcohol-related problems in the study countries of the EU concerted action 'Gender, Culture and Alcohol Problems: a Multi-national Study'. Alcohol Alcohol Suppl. 2006;41(1):i26–36.
52. van Oers JA, Bongers IM, van de Goor LA, Garretsen HF. Alcohol consumption, alcohol-related problems, problem drinking, and socioeconomic status. Alcohol Alcohol. 1999;34(1):78–88.
53. Marmot M. Inequality, deprivation and alcohol use. Addiction. 1997;92(Suppl 1):S13–20.
54. Kunst AE, Groenhof F, Mackenbach JP, Health EW. Occupational class and cause specific mortality in middle aged men in 11 European countries: comparison of population based studies. EU Working Group on Socioeconomic Inequalities in Health. BMJ. 1998;316(7145):1636–42.
55. Almeida-Filho N, Lessa I, Magalhaes L, Araujo MJ, Aquino E, James SA, et al. Social inequality and alcohol consumption-abuse in Bahia, Brazil--interactions of gender, ethnicity and social class. Soc Psychiatry Psychiatr Epidemiol. 2005;40(3):214–22.
56. Figuero Ruiz E, Carretero Pelaez MA, Cerero Lapiedra R, Esparza Gomez G, Moreno Lopez LA. Effects of the consumption of alcohol in the oral cavity: relationship with oral cancer. Med Oral. 2004;9(1):14–23.
57. Squier CA. The permeability of oral mucosa. Crit Rev Oral Biol Med. 1991;2(1):13–32.
58. Squier CA, Cox P, Wertz PW. Lipid content and water permeability of skin and oral mucosa. J Invest Dermatol. 1991;96(1):123–6.
59. Valentine JA, Scott J, West CR, St Hill CA. A histological analysis of the early effects of alcohol and tobacco usage on human lingual epithelium. J Oral Pathol. 1985;14(8):654–65.
60. Simanowski UA, Wright NA, Seitz HK. Mucosal cellular regeneration and colorectal carcinogenesis. In: Seitz HK, Simanowski UA, Wright NA, editors. Colorectal cancer: from pathogenesis to prevention? Berlin: Springer; 1989. p. 225–36.
61. Muller P, Hepke B, Meldau U, Raabe G. Tissue damage in the rabbit oral mucosa by acute and chronic direct toxic action of different alcohol concentrations. Exp Pathol. 1983;24(2-3):171–81.
62. Kurkivuori J, Salaspuro V, Kaihovaara P, Kari K, Rautemaa R, Gronroos L, et al. Acetaldehyde production from ethanol by oral streptococci. Oral Oncol. 2007;43(2):181–6.
63. Reidy J, McHugh E, Stassen LF. A review of the relationship between alcohol and oral cancer. Surgeon. 2011;9(5):278–83.
64. Morse DE, Katz RV, Pendrys DG, Holford TR, Krutchkoff DJ, Eisenberg E, et al. Smoking and drinking in relation to oral epithelial dysplasia. Cancer Epidemiol Biomarkers Prev. 1996;5(10):769–77.
65. Kabat GC, Chang CJ, Wynder EL. The role of tobacco, alcohol use, and body mass index in oral and pharyngeal cancer. Int J Epidemiol. 1994;23(6):1137–44.
66. Mashberg A, Garfinkel L, Harris S. Alcohol as a primary risk factor in oral squamous carcinoma. CA Cancer J Clin. 1981;31(3):146–55.
67. Morse DE, Psoter WJ, Cleveland D, Cohen D, Mohit-Tabatabai M, Kosis DL, et al. Smoking and drinking in relation to oral cancer and oral epithelial dysplasia. Cancer Causes Control. 2007;18(9):919–29.
68. Homann N, Karkkainen P, Koivisto T, Nosova T, Jokelainen K, Salaspuro M. Effects of acetaldehyde on cell regeneration and differentiation of the upper gastrointestinal tract mucosa. J Natl Cancer Inst. 1997;89(22):1692–7.

69. Lachenmeier DW, Gumbel-Mako S, Sohnius EM, Keck-Wilhelm A, Kratz E, Mildau G. Salivary acetaldehyde increase due to alcohol-containing mouthwash use: a risk factor for oral cancer. Int J Cancer. 2009;125(3):730–5.
70. Lachenmeier DW, Kanteres F, Rehm J. Carcinogenicity of acetaldehyde in alcoholic beverages: risk assessment outside ethanol metabolism. Addiction. 2009;104(4):533–50.
71. Salaspuro M. Interrelationship between alcohol, smoking, acetaldehyde and cancer. Novartis Found Symp. 2007;285:80–9; discussion 9–96, 198–9.
72. Muto M, Hitomi Y, Ohtsu A, Shimada H, Kashiwase Y, Sasaki H, et al. Acetaldehyde production by non-pathogenic Neisseria in human oral microflora: implications for carcinogenesis in upper aerodigestive tract. Int J Cancer. 2000;88(3):342–50.
73. Homann N, Tillonen J, Meurman JH, Rintamaki H, Lindqvist C, Rautio M, et al. Increased salivary acetaldehyde levels in heavy drinkers and smokers: a microbiological approach to oral cavity cancer. Carcinogenesis. 2000;21(4):663–8.
74. Swann PF, Coe AM, Mace R. Ethanol and dimethylnitrosamine and diethylnitrosamine metabolism and disposition in the rat. Possible relevance to the influence of ethanol on human cancer incidence. Carcinogenesis. 1984;5(10):1337–43.
75. Poschl G, Seitz HK. Alcohol and cancer. Alcohol Alcohol. 2004;39(3):155–65.
76. Ballard HS. Alcohol-associated pancytopenia with hypocellular bone marrow. Am J Clin Pathol. 1980;73(6):830–4.
77. Heermans EH. Booze and blood: the effects of acute and chronic alcohol abuse on the hematopoietic system. Clin Lab Sci. 1998;11(4):229–32.
78. Liu YK. Effects of alcohol on granulocytes and lymphocytes. Semin Hematol. 1980;17(2):130–6.
79. Michot F, Gut J. Alcohol-induced bone marrow damage. A bone marrow study in alcohol-dependent individuals. Acta Haematol. 1987;78(4):252–7.
80. Zhang P, Bagby GJ, Happel KI, Raasch CE, Nelson S. Alcohol abuse, immunosuppression, and pulmonary infection. Curr Drug Abuse Rev. 2008;1(1):56–67.
81. Warnakulasuriya S. Causes of oral cancer--an appraisal of controversies. Br Dent J. 2009;207(10):471–5.
82. Llewellyn CD, Linklater K, Bell J, Johnson NW, Warnakulasuriya S. An analysis of risk factors for oral cancer in young people: a case-control study. Oral Oncol. 2004;40(3):304–13.
83. Petti S, Scully C. Oral cancer: the association between nation-based alcohol-drinking profiles and oral cancer mortality. Oral Oncol. 2005;41(8):828–34.
84. Deleyiannis FW, Thomas DB, Vaughan TL, Davis S. Alcoholism: independent predictor of survival in patients with head and neck cancer. J Natl Cancer Inst. 1996;88(8):542–9.
85. Baron AE, Franceschi S, Barra S, Talamini R, La Vecchia C. A comparison of the joint effects of alcohol and smoking on the risk of cancer across sites in the upper aerodigestive tract. Cancer Epidemiol Biomarkers Prev. 1993;2(6):519–23.
86. Benhamou S, Tuimala J, Bouchardy C, Dayer P, Sarasin A, Hirvonen A. DNA repair gene XRCC2 and XRCC3 polymorphisms and susceptibility to cancers of the upper aerodigestive tract. Int J Cancer. 2004;112(5):901–4.
87. Boccia S, Cadoni G, Sayed-Tabatabaei FA, Volante M, Arzani D, De Lauretis A, et al. CYP1A1, CYP2E1, GSTM1, GSTT1, EPHX1 exons 3 and 4, and NAT2 polymorphisms, smoking, consumption of alcohol and fruit and vegetables and risk of head and neck cancer. J Cancer Res Clin Oncol. 2008;134(1):93–100.
88. Bosetti C, Gallus S, Trichopoulou A, Talamini R, Franceschi S, Negri E, et al. Influence of the Mediterranean diet on the risk of cancers of the upper aerodigestive tract. Cancer Epidemiol Biomarkers Prev. 2003;12(10):1091–4.
89. Cui Y, Morgenstern H, Greenland S, Tashkin DP, Mao J, Cao W, et al. Polymorphism of Xeroderma Pigmentosum group G and the risk of lung cancer and squamous cell carcinomas of the oropharynx, larynx and esophagus. Int J Cancer. 2006;118(3):714–20.
90. Elahi A, Zheng Z, Park J, Eyring K, McCaffrey T, Lazarus P. The human OGG1 DNA repair enzyme and its association with orolaryngeal cancer risk. Carcinogenesis. 2002;23(7):1229–34.

91. Franceschi S, Talamini R, Barra S, Baron AE, Negri E, Bidoli E, et al. Smoking and drinking in relation to cancers of the oral cavity, pharynx, larynx, and esophagus in northern Italy. Cancer Res. 1990;50(20):6502–7.
92. Hashibe M, Boffetta P, Zaridze D, Shangina O, Szeszenia-Dabrowska N, Mates D, et al. Evidence for an important role of alcohol- and aldehyde-metabolizing genes in cancers of the upper aerodigestive tract. Cancer Epidemiol Biomarkers Prev. 2006;15(4):696–703.
93. Hayes RB, Bravo-Otero E, Kleinman DV, Brown LM, Fraumeni JF Jr, Harty LC, et al. Tobacco and alcohol use and oral cancer in Puerto Rico. Cancer Causes Control. 1999;10(1):27–33.
94. Herrero R, Castellsague X, Pawlita M, Lissowska J, Kee F, Balaram P, et al. Human papillomavirus and oral cancer: the International Agency for Research on Cancer multicenter study. J Natl Cancer Inst. 2003;95(23):1772–83.
95. Levi F, Pasche C, La Vecchia C, Lucchini F, Franceschi S, Monnier P. Food groups and risk of oral and pharyngeal cancer. Int J Cancer. 1998;77(5):705–9.
96. Muscat JE, Richie JP Jr, Thompson S, Wynder EL. Gender differences in smoking and risk for oral cancer. Cancer Res. 1996;56(22):5192–7.
97. Olshan AF, Weissler MC, Watson MA, Bell DA. GSTM1, GSTT1, GSTP1, CYP1A1, and NAT1 polymorphisms, tobacco use, and the risk of head and neck cancer. Cancer Epidemiol Biomarkers Prev. 2000;9(2):185–91.
98. Peters ES, McClean MD, Liu M, Eisen EA, Mueller N, Kelsey KT. The ADH1C polymorphism modifies the risk of squamous cell carcinoma of the head and neck associated with alcohol and tobacco use. Cancer Epidemiol Biomarkers Prev. 2005;14(2):476–82.
99. Rosenblatt KA, Daling JR, Chen C, Sherman KJ, Schwartz SM. Marijuana use and risk of oral squamous cell carcinoma. Cancer Res. 2004;64(11):4049–54.
100. Wang D, Ritchie JM, Smith EM, Zhang Z, Turek LP, Haugen TH. Alcohol dehydrogenase 3 and risk of squamous cell carcinomas of the head and neck. Cancer Epidemiol Biomarkers Prev. 2005;14(3):626–32.
101. Zhang Z, Shi Q, Liu Z, Sturgis EM, Spitz MR, Wei Q. Polymorphisms of methionine synthase and methionine synthase reductase and risk of squamous cell carcinoma of the head and neck: a case-control analysis. Cancer Epidemiol Biomarkers Prev. 2005;14(5):1188–93.
102. Dong YJ, Peng TK, Yin SJ. Expression and activities of class IV alcohol dehydrogenase and class III aldehyde dehydrogenase in human mouth. Alcohol. 1996;13(3):257–62.
103. Moreno A, Pares A, Ortiz J, Enriquez J, Pares X. Alcohol dehydrogenase from human stomach: variability in normal mucosa and effect of age, gender, ADH3 phenotype and gastric region. Alcohol Alcohol. 1994;29(6):663–71.
104. Raunio H, Husgafvel-Pursiainen K, Anttila S, Hietanen E, Hirvonen A, Pelkonen O. Diagnosis of polymorphisms in carcinogen-activating and inactivating enzymes and cancer susceptibility--a review. Gene. 1995;159(1):113–21.
105. Eriksson CJP. Genetic-epidemiological evidence for the role of acetaldehyde in cancers related to alcohol drinking. Adv Exp Med Biol. 2015;815:41–58.
106. Marichalar-Mendia X, Acha-Sagredo A, Rodriguez-Tojo MJ, Rey-Barja N, Hernando-Rodriguez M, Aguirregaviria JI, et al. Alcohol-dehydrogenase (ADH1B) Arg48His polymorphism in Basque Country patients with oral and laryngeal cancer: preliminary study. Anticancer Res. 2011;31(2):677–80.
107. Yoshida A, Huang IY, Ikawa M. Molecular abnormality of an inactive aldehyde dehydrogenase variant commonly found in orientals. Proc Natl Acad Sci U S A. 1984;81(1):258–61.
108. Bediaga NG, Marichalar-Mendia X, Rey-Barja N, Setien-Olarra A, Gonzalez-Garcia JA, de Pancorbo MM, et al. Polymorphisms in alcohol and tobacco metabolism genes in head and neck cancer in the Basque Country. J Oral Pathol Med. 2015;44(10):769–75.
109. Boccia S, Hashibe M, Galli P, De Feo E, Asakage T, Hashimoto T, et al. Aldehyde dehydrogenase 2 and head and neck cancer: a meta-analysis implementing a Mendelian randomization approach. Cancer Epidemiol Biomarkers Prev. 2009;18(1):248–54.
110. Oze I, Matsuo K, Hosono S, Ito H, Kawase T, Watanabe M, et al. Comparison between self-reported facial flushing after alcohol consumption and ALDH2 Glu504Lys polymorphism for risk of upper aerodigestive tract cancer in a Japanese population. Cancer Sci. 2010;101(8):1875–80.

111. Matsuo K, Rossi M, Negri E, Oze I, Hosono S, Ito H, et al. Folate, alcohol, and aldehyde dehydrogenase 2 polymorphism and the risk of oral and pharyngeal cancer in Japanese. Eur J Cancer Prev. 2012;21(2):193–8.
112. Tsai S-T, Wong T-Y, Ou C-Y, Fang S-Y, Chen K-C, Hsiao J-R, et al. The interplay between alcohol consumption, oral hygiene, ALDH2 and ADH1B in the risk of head and neck cancer. Int J Cancer. 2014;135(10):2424–36.
113. Yokoyama A, Kamada Y, Imazeki H, Hayashi E, Murata S, Kinoshita K, et al. Effects of ADH1B and ALDH2 genetic polymorphisms on alcohol elimination rates and salivary acetaldehyde levels in intoxicated Japanese alcoholic men. Alcohol Clin Exp Res. 2016;40(6):1241–50.
114. Marichalar-Mendia X, Rodriguez-Tojo MJ, Acha-Sagredo A, Rey-Barja N, Aguirre-Urizar JM. Oral cancer and polymorphism of ethanol metabolising genes. Oral Oncol. 2010;46(1):9–13.
115. Squier CA, Cox P, Hall BK. Enhanced penetration of nitrosonornicotine across oral mucosa in the presence of ethanol. J Oral Pathol. 1986;15(5):276–9.
116. Howie NM, Trigkas TK, Cruchley AT, Wertz PW, Squier CA, Williams DM. Short-term exposure to alcohol increases the permeability of human oral mucosa. Oral Dis. 2001;7(6):349–54.
117. Warnakulasuriya S, Parkkila S, Nagao T, Preedy VR, Pasanen M, Koivisto H, et al. Demonstration of ethanol-induced protein adducts in oral leukoplakia (pre-cancer) and cancer. J Oral Pathol Med. 2008;37(3):157–65.
118. Matsuda T, Terashima I, Matsumoto Y, Yabushita H, Matsui S, Shibutani S. Effective utilization of N2-ethyl-2′-deoxyguanosine triphosphate during DNA synthesis catalyzed by mammalian replicative DNA polymerases. Biochemistry. 1999;38(3):929–35.
119. Balbo S, Meng L, Bliss RL, Jensen JA, Hatsukami DK, Hecht SS. Kinetics of DNA adduct formation in the oral cavity after drinking alcohol. Cancer Epidemiol Biomarkers Prev. 2012;21(4):601–8.
120. Brooks PJ, Theruvathu JA. DNA adducts from acetaldehyde: implications for alcohol-related carcinogenesis. Alcohol. 2005;35(3):187–93.
121. Fernandes PH, Kanuri M, Nechev LV, Harris TM, Lloyd RS. Mammalian cell mutagenesis of the DNA adducts of vinyl chloride and crotonaldehyde. Environ Mol Mutagen. 2005;45(5):455–9.
122. Maffei F, Forti GC, Castelli E, Stefanini GF, Mattioli S, Hrelia P. Biomarkers to assess the genetic damage induced by alcohol abuse in human lymphocytes. Mutat Res. 2002;514(1-2):49–58.
123. Obe G, Ristow H. Acetaldehyde, but not ethanol, induces sister chromatid exchanges in Chinese hamster cells in vitro. Mutat Res. 1977;56(2):211–3.
124. Brooks PJ. DNA damage, DNA repair, and alcohol toxicity--a review. Alcohol Clin Exp Res. 1997;21(6):1073–82.
125. Albano E, Clot P, Morimoto M, Tomasi A, Ingelman-Sundberg M, French SW. Role of cytochrome P4502E1-dependent formation of hydroxyethyl free radical in the development of liver damage in rats intragastrically fed with ethanol. Hepatology. 1996;23(1):155–63.
126. Farin FM, Bigler LG, Oda D, McDougall JK, Omiecinski CJ. Expression of cytochrome P450 and microsomal epoxide hydrolase in cervical and oral epithelial cells immortalized by human papillomavirus type 16 E6/E7 genes. Carcinogenesis. 1995;16(6):1391–401.
127. Scully C, Bagan J. Oral squamous cell carcinoma: overview of current understanding of aetiopathogenesis and clinical implications. Oral Dis. 2009;15(6):388–99.
128. Rulten SL, Hodder E, Ripley TL, Stephens DN, Mayne LV. Alcohol induces DNA damage and the Fanconi anemia D2 protein implicating FANCD2 in the DNA damage response pathways in brain. Alcohol Clin Exp Res. 2008;32(7):1186–96.
129. Marnett LJ. Oxyradicals and DNA damage. Carcinogenesis. 2000;21(3):361–70.
130. Korde SD, Basak A, Chaudhary M, Goyal M, Vagga A. Enhanced nitrosative and oxidative stress with decreased total antioxidant capacity in patients with oral precancer and oral squamous cell carcinoma. Oncology. 2011;80(5-6):382–9.

131. Agha-Hosseini F, Mirzaii-Dizgah I, Farmanbar N, Abdollahi M. Oxidative stress status and DNA damage in saliva of human subjects with oral lichen planus and oral squamous cell carcinoma. J Oral Pathol Med. 2012;41(10):736–40.
132. McCullough MJ, Farah CS. The role of alcohol in oral carcinogenesis with particular reference to alcohol-containing mouthwashes. Aust Dent J. 2008;53(4):302–5.
133. Currie S, Farah C. Alcohol-containing mouthwash and oral cancer risk: a review of current evidence. OA Alcohol. 2014;2(1):4.
134. Carretero Pelaez MA, Esparza Gomez GC, Figuero Ruiz E, Cerero Lapiedra R. Alcohol-containing mouthwashes and oral cancer. Critical analysis of literature. Med Oral. 2004;9(2):120–3. 16-20
135. Bolanowski SJ, Gescheider GA, Sutton SV. Relationship between oral pain and ethanol concentration in mouthrinses. J Periodontal Res. 1995;30(3):192–7.
136. Ahrens W, Pohlabeln H, Foraita R, Nelis M, Lagiou P, Lagiou A, et al. Oral health, dental care and mouthwash associated with upper aerodigestive tract cancer risk in Europe: the ARCAGE study. Oral Oncol. 2014;50(6):616–25.
137. Blot WJ, Winn DM, Fraumeni JF Jr. Oral cancer and mouthwash. J Natl Cancer Inst. 1983;70(2):251–3.
138. Chang JS, Lo HI, Wong TY, Huang CC, Lee WT, Tsai ST, et al. Investigating the association between oral hygiene and head and neck cancer. Oral Oncol. 2013;49(10):1010–7.
139. Cole P, Rodu B, Mathisen A. Alcohol-containing mouthwash and oropharyngeal cancer: a review of the epidemiology. J Am Dent Assoc. 2003;134(8):1079–87.
140. Divaris K, Olshan AF, Smith J, Bell ME, Weissler MC, Funkhouser WK, et al. Oral health and risk for head and neck squamous cell carcinoma: the Carolina Head and Neck Cancer Study. Cancer Causes Control. 2010;21(4):567–75.
141. D'Souza G, Kreimer AR, Viscidi R, Pawlita M, Fakhry C, Koch WM, et al. Case-control study of human papillomavirus and oropharyngeal cancer. N Engl J Med. 2007;356(19):1944–56.
142. Eliot MN, Michaud DS, Langevin SM, McClean MD, Kelsey KT. Periodontal disease and mouthwash use are risk factors for head and neck squamous cell carcinoma. Cancer Causes Control. 2013;24(7):1315–22.
143. Guha N, Boffetta P, Wunsch Filho V, Eluf Neto J, Shangina O, Zaridze D, et al. Oral health and risk of squamous cell carcinoma of the head and neck and esophagus: results of two multicentric case-control studies. Am J Epidemiol. 2007;166(10):1159–73.
144. Kabat GC, Hebert JR, Wynder EL. Risk factors for oral cancer in women. Cancer Res. 1989;49(10):2803–6.
145. Macfarlane TV, Macfarlane GJ, Oliver RJ, Benhamou S, Bouchardy C, Ahrens W, et al. The aetiology of upper aerodigestive tract cancers among young adults in Europe: the ARCAGE study. Cancer Causes Control. 2010;21(12):2213–21.
146. Marques LA, Eluf-Neto J, Figueiredo RA, Gois-Filho JF, Kowalski LP, Carvalho MB, et al. Oral health, hygiene practices and oral cancer. Rev Saude Publica. 2008;42(3):471–9.
147. Marshall JR, Graham S, Haughey BP, Shedd D, O'Shea R, Brasure J, et al. Smoking, alcohol, dentition and diet in the epidemiology of oral cancer. Eur J Cancer B Oral Oncol. 1992;28B(1):9–15.
148. Talamini R, Vaccarella S, Barbone F, Tavani A, La Vecchia C, Herrero R, et al. Oral hygiene, dentition, sexual habits and risk of oral cancer. Br J Cancer. 2000;83(9):1238–42.
149. Weaver A, Fleming SM, Smith DB. Mouthwash and oral cancer: carcinogen or coincidence? J Oral Surg. 1979;37(4):250–3.
150. Winn DM, Blot WJ, McLaughlin JK, Austin DF, Greenberg RS, Preston-Martin S, et al. Mouthwash use and oral conditions in the risk of oral and pharyngeal cancer. Cancer Res. 1991;51(11):3044–7.
151. Winn DM, Diehl SR, Brown LM, Harty LC, Bravo-Otero E, Fraumeni JF Jr, et al. Mouthwash in the etiology of oral cancer in Puerto Rico. Cancer Causes Control. 2001;12(5):419–29.
152. Wynder EL, Kabat G, Rosenberg S, Levenstein M. Oral cancer and mouthwash use. J Natl Cancer Inst. 1983;70(2):255–60.

153. Young TB, Ford CN, Brandenburg JH. An epidemiologic study of oral cancer in a statewide network. Am J Otolaryngol. 1986;7(3):200–8.
154. McCullough MJ, Prasad G, Zhao S, Farah CS. The changing aetiology of oral cancer and the role of novel biomarkers to aid in early diagnosis. 2012. In: Oral cancer [Internet]. Rijeka: InTech; [130-48].
155. Mashberg A, Barsa P, Grossman ML. A study of the relationship between mouthwash use and oral and pharyngeal cancer. J Am Dent Assoc. 1985;110(5):731–4.
156. Elmore JG, Horwitz RI. Oral cancer and mouthwash use: evaluation of the epidemiologic evidence. Otolaryngol Head Neck Surg. 1995;113(3):253–61.
157. La Vecchia C. Mouthwash and oral cancer risk: an update. Oral Oncol. 2009;45(3):198–200.
158. Gandini S, Negri E, Boffetta P, La Vecchia C, Boyle P. Mouthwash and oral cancer risk quantitative meta-analysis of epidemiologic studies. Ann Agric Environ Med. 2012;19(2):173–80.
159. Boffetta P, Hayes RB, Sartori S, Lee YA, Muscat J, Olshan A, et al. Mouthwash use and cancer of the head and neck: a pooled analysis from the International Head and Neck Cancer Epidemiology Consortium. Eur J Cancer Prev. 2015;25(4):344–8.
160. Conway DI, Hashibe M, Boffetta P, INHANCE consortium, Wunsch-Filho V, Muscat J, et al. Enhancing epidemiologic research on head and neck cancer: INHANCE – The International Head and Neck Cancer Epidemiology Consortium. Oral Oncol. 2009;45(9):743–6.
161. Warnakulasuriya S. Global epidemiology of oral and oropharyngeal cancer. Oral Oncol. 2009;45(4–5):309–16.
162. Marron M, Boffetta P, Zhang ZF, Zaridze D, Wunsch-Filho V, Winn DM, et al. Cessation of alcohol drinking, tobacco smoking and the reversal of head and neck cancer risk. Int J Epidemiol. 2010;39(1):182–96.
163. Ogden GR, Macluskey M. An overview of the prevention of oral cancer and diagnostic markers of malignant change: 1. Prevention. Dent Update. 2000;27(2):95–9.

6 High-Risk Human Papillomaviruses and Epstein-Barr Virus Presence and Crosstalk in Human Oral Carcinogenesis

Ala-Eddin Al Moustafa, Farhan S. Cyprian, Noor Al-Antary, and Amber Yasmeen

6.1 Introduction

Human oral cancer refers to a subgroup of head and neck (HN) malignancies that develop at the lips, tongue, salivary glands, gingiva, floor of the mouth, oropharynx, buccal surfaces, and other intraoral locations, based on the International Classification of Diseases of the World Health Organization (WHO). This cancer is considered one of the most frequent types of malignancies in the head and neck (38%) with an incidence of 75% in male patients over the age of 60 years; about 95% of these cancer cases are squamous cell carcinomas (SCCs), which are of epithelial origin [1, 2]. "Oral carcinomas" is the term used for cancers that form in tissues of the oral cavity and the oropharynx [2, 3]. Oral squamous cell carcinomas are invasive lesions with the presence of perineural growth. It has a significant recurrence rate and frequently metastasizes to cervical lymph nodes [4]. Lymph node metastatic tumors occur in about 40% of patients with oral cancer. Clinically, their manifestations are hidden in rates of 15–34% [5, 6]. In general, tobacco, betel quid chewing, alcohol and virus infection including human papillomaviruses (HPVs) as well as Epstein-Barr virus (EBV) are regarded as major risk factors for oral cancer initiation and progression [3, 7, 8].

A.-E. Al Moustafa (✉)
College of Medicine & Biomedical Research Centre, Qatar University, Doha, Qatar

Oncology Department, McGill University, Montreal, QC, Canada

Syrian Research Cancer Centre of the Syrian Society Against Cancer, Aleppo, Syria
e-mail: aalmoustafa@qu.edu.qa; ala-eddin.almoustafa@mcgill.ca

F.S. Cyprian • N. Al-Antary
College of Medicine & Biomedical Research Centre, Qatar University, Doha, Qatar

A. Yasmeen
Oncology Department, McGill University, Montreal, QC, Canada

A.-E. Al Moustafa (ed.), *Development of Oral Cancer*,
DOI 10.1007/978-3-319-48054-1_6

High-risk human HPVs and EBV are considered as important etiological factors in the development and progression of human oral cancer, as more than 35 and 55% of these cancer cases are positive for high-risk HPVs and EBV, respectively [3, 9–12]. However, it is important to mention that high-risk HPVs or EBV infection alone is not sufficient to induce neoplastic transformation of normal epithelial cells; the infected cells must undergo additional genetic changes to reach full transformation and consequently tumor formation. Thus, we have demonstrated that E6/E7 oncoproteins of HPV type 16 cooperate with ErbB-2 receptor to induce cell transformation of human normal oral epithelial (NOE) cells [13]. On the other hand, several recent investigations revealed that high-risk HPVs and EBV can be copresent in human oral cancer where they could cooperate to induce cellular transformation of the coinfected cells, leading to cancer development; consequently, HPVs and EBV coinfection can enhance the progression of this malignancy. In this chapter, we will overview the presence and outcome of high-risk HPVs and EBV in human oral cancer; in addition, we will discuss the cooperative effect of these viruses in the initiation and progression of this malignancy.

6.2 High-Risk Human Papillomaviruses (HPVs) in Human Cancer

Currently, it is well established that infections with high-risk HPVs (types 16, 18, 31, 33, 35, 39, 45, 51, 52, 55, 56, 58, 59, 68, 73, 82, and 83) are associated with the development of cervical cancers where more than 96% of these cancers are positive for high-risk HPVs worldwide [14, 15]; thus, HPV prophylactic vaccines against the most frequent high-risk HPV types have been recently developed to prevent infection with the most frequent type of these viruses (HPV types 16 and 18) [16–18]. On the other hand, it was pointed out that high-risk HPVs have carcinogenic effects at several other anatomical sites in both men and women such as HN and colorectal [19–23]. Earlier studies revealed that approximately 35% of human oral cancers are positive for high-risk HPVs [24–26]. It is well known that high-risk HPV oncoproteins, E5, E6, and E7, provoke cellular alteration, and in cooperation with other oncogenes, this modification can lead to cellular transformation and consequently tumor development [27–29]. For instance, previous investigations demonstrated that the E5 oncoprotein could play an important role in cell alteration through its interaction with EGF-R1 signaling pathways (MAP kinase and PI3K-Akt) and proapoptotic proteins [30, 31]. E6 and E7 are assumed to work together in HPV-infected cells [32]. Both E6 and E7 have functions that deregulate cell cycle, apoptosis, and cell adhesion, through their interaction with p53, pRb, and other members of the pocket protein family [27, 33]. Nevertheless, it is important to emphasize that most HPV studies were performed on human cervical cancers.

On the other hand, and in order to address the role of E6/E7 genes in high-risk HPV-associated carcinogenesis in vivo, transgenic mice have been developed expressing E6/E7 of HPV type 16 individually and together under the human K14 promoter [34, 35]. These transgenic mice developed skin tumors, in general, and cervical cancer with chronic estrogen administration [35, 36]. In parallel, and to examine the oncogenic properties of E5 in vivo, K14-E5 transgenic mice were generated in which the expression of E5 was directed to the basal layer of the stratified squamous epithelia [37]; these mice exhibited epidermal hyperplasia, aberrant differentiation of the epithelium, and were susceptible to spontaneous skin tumors. Moreover, it was reported that K14-E6/E7 transgenic mice have susceptibility to colorectal cancers and precancerous lesions after dimethylbenz[a]anthracene treatment, which is a chemical carcinogen that is known to induce squamous cell carcinomas in other sites [38]. These studies show clearly that high-risk HPVs play an important role in cancer initiation and progression of several tissues composed of squamous epithelia, including the oral cavity, through their E5, E6, and E7 oncoproteins. Thus, we believe that high-risk HPVs can cooperate with other oncogenes in addition to certain human viruses such as EBV in order to initiate and/or enhance human cancer especially in the oral cavity since this part of the human body can be considered as the main site of EBV infection.

6.3 Epstein-Barr Virus (EBV) in Human Cancer

EBV is a human gammaherpesvirus that infects more than 90% of the human adult population [39]. Acute infection with EBV can cause infectious mononucleosis, and its latent state can evolve to yield several B-cell lymphomas, oral carcinomas (especially nasopharyngeal), gastric cancer, and other malignancies [40, 41]. EBV-infected cells express the latency III program of gene products, including six EBV nuclear antigens (EBNA1, EBNA2, EBNA3A, EBNA3B, EBNA3C, and EBNA-LP) as well as three latent membrane proteins (LMP1, LMP2A, and LMP2B) and multiple noncoding RNAs (EBERs and miRNAs) [42–44].

The differential expression patterns of these latent genes define the distinct latency programs linked with the types of cancers associated with EBV [40, 41]. For example, type II latency is characterized by a more restricted latent gene expression pattern (EBNA1, LMP1, and LMP2) and is associated with Hodgkin's lymphoma and nasopharyngeal as well as other carcinomas including gastric and probably breast [45–48]. While, LMP1 is considered the major EBV-encoded oncogenic protein as it is frequently expressed in EBV-associated human oral carcinomas; this oncoprotein induces a multitude of effects such as promoting cell growth, protecting cells from apoptosis, enhancing cell motility, and stimulating angiogenesis [47, 49]. In addition, it has been reported that EBV is present in more than 95% of nasopharyngeal carcinomas worldwide [50–54].

Certain investigations have shown, in vivo, that LMP1 expressed under the control of the polyomavirus early promoter resulted in hyper-proliferation of the basal epithelium [55, 56]. More specifically, transgenic mice expressing LMP1 under the ED-L2 EBV early lytic promoter induce corrosive lesions that could progress to invasive carcinomas [57, 58]. Recently, transgenic mice that express LMP1 and LMP2 of EVB using the K14 promoter were generated to assess the role of these two genes in cancer initiation and progression in vivo [59]. It was reported that

K14-LMP1 transgenic mice developed papillomas and SCCs after dimethyl benzanthracene (DMBA) and TPA treatment. Although, K14-LMP2 mice were similar to non-transgenic controls; however, double transgenic mice (LMP1 and LMP2) developed papillomas comparable to the single transgenic K14-LMP1 mice, indicating the lack of LMP2 effect on LMP1-enhanced papilloma formation. However, the development of SCCs was significantly increased in double transgenic animals. Identification of pathways known to be activated by LMP1 and/or LMP2 revealed that all tumors have high levels of activated ERK and Stat3, with the highest levels in double transgenic carcinomas. This was the first analysis of jointly expressed LMP1 and LMP2 genes in epithelial cells in transgenic mice. This study indicates clearly that the expression of LMP1 and LMP2 increases susceptibility to tumor development.

Overall, these findings demonstrate that EBV is present and plays an important role in several human carcinomas including oral. Based on this fact, EBV vaccines are presently under clinical trials in several institutions; thus, it is important to identify the real role of EBV infection in human oral cancer initiation and progression; based on which, EBV vaccines can be used as important tools to prevent oral cancer. Meanwhile, we believe that the association between EBV and other human viruses particularly high-risk HPVs in human oral carcinogenesis needs more investigation mainly with regard to cancer progression and phenotypes. Thus, available data regarding the presence and role of HPVs and EBV in human oral carcinogenesis will be reviewed.

6.4 High Risk of HPVs and EBV in Human Oral Cancer

Today, it is well known that high-risk HPVs are considered important etiological factors for human HN carcinogenesis including oral cancer development, as roughly 30% of HN and 40% of oral cancers are positive for high-risk HPVs, especially HPV types (16, 18, 31, 33, and 35) [60, 61]. However, it is important to emphasize that high-risk HPV infection alone is not sufficient to induce neoplastic transformation of normal epithelial cells; the infected cells must undergo additional genetic changes to reach full transformation. Therefore, and based on this fact, we have developed a new model to study the cooperation effect between high-risk HPVs and ErbB-2 receptor in HN carcinogenesis, as ErbB-2 is overexpressed in 25% of human HN cancers [13]. In our model, we used human normal oral epithelial (NOE) cells [62]. Using this model, we established that E6/E7 oncoproteins of high-risk HPV type 16 cooperate with the ErbB-2 receptor to induce cellular transformation of human NOE cells (Fig. 6.1); this was accompanied by a delocalization of beta-catenin from the undercoat membrane to the nucleus in NOE cells. Furthermore, we reported that cyclin D1 is the downstream target of E6/E7/ErbB-2 cooperation [63]. In parallel, we revealed that D-type cyclins (D1, D2, and D3) are essential for cell transformation induced by E6/E7/ErbB-2 cooperation in human NOE and mouse

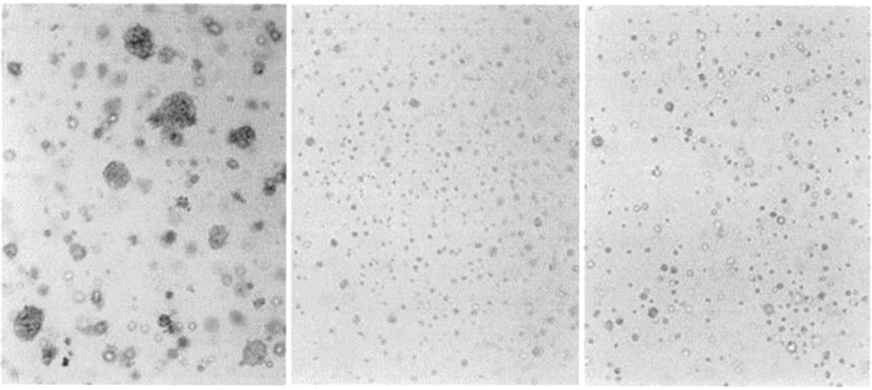

Fig. 6.1 Cellular transformation of human normal oral epithelial (NOE) cells induced by E6/E7 of HPV type 16 and ErbB-2 cooperation. We note that NOE-E6/E7-ErbB-2 cells form colonies in soft agar but not NOE-E6/E7 and NOE-ErbB-2 cells; thus, NOE cells expressing E6/E7 and ErbB-2 form tumor in nude mice but not those expressing E6/E7 alone or ErbB-2 alone [13, 63]

normal embryonic fibroblast (NEF) cells [63, 64]. Finally, we were able to show that the cooperation effect of E6/E7 with ErbB-2, in human NOE and cancer cells, occurs via the conversion of beta-catenin's role from a cell-cell adhesion molecule to a transcriptional regulator through beta-catenin tyrosine phosphorylation by pp60 (c-Src) kinase activation [65]. On the other hand, and in order to investigate the incidence of high-risk HPVs in human HN cancers including oral cancer in the Syrian population, we examined the presence of these viruses in a cohort of 80 oral cancer tissue samples from Syria by immunohistochemistry and tissue microarray methodologies. Our data revealed that 43% of these cancers are positives for high-risk HPVs [61, 66]. Genotyping investigation of high-risk HPVs showed that HPV types 16, 18, 31, 33, and 35 are the most frequent HPV types in HN cancers in Syria.

While, it has been revealed that HPV-positive oral SCC is an emerging clinical entity with features that distinguish it from HPV-negative oral SCC, which is strongly correlated to smoking and alcohol consumption, as we mentioned earlier. HPV-positive oral SCC exhibits a more rapid onset development in younger adults [20, 67]. Patients with HPV-positive oral SCC frequently present with disseminated metastatic disease; however, HPV-positive oral SCC exhibits a better prognosis compared to HPV-negative oral SCC [68, 69]. In addition, HPV-positive oral SCCs display features of poorly or undifferentiated epithelial cells [20, 70].

Although, it has been well documented that EBV is present in more than 95% of nasopharyngeal carcinomas (NPC) especially in Asian countries [50, 51, 53, 54]. A few studies have correlated the presence of EBV with HPV in human oral cancer. In oropharyngeal cancer, the presence of EBV and HPV viruses together is approximately 15–20% of oral SCC [11, 71]. Meanwhile, Jiang et al. [12] found that 75%

of tonsillar SCC and 90% of base of tongue SCC were HPV-positive. However, EBV alone was found in 42 and 80% of tonsillar and tongue SCCs, respectively. In parallel, EBV and HPV coinfection was observed in 25% of tonsillar and 70% of tongue SCC [12].

Further support for interactions between EBV and HPV has also been noted in NPC. The NPC is a rare cancer in Caucasians but is common in Asia accounting for up to 20% of all cancers in endemic regions. A high incidence of NPC is also observed in Mediterranean Africa and among the Inuit population [72]. The WHO has categorized NPC into three types that describe the tumor's differentiation and keratin states. Type 1 NPC is a rare keratinizing, differentiated squamous cell carcinoma, accounting for 20–25% of all NPC. Type 2 NPC is a nonkeratinizing, differentiated squamous cell carcinoma, whereas type 3 NPC is nonkeratinizing, undifferentiated squamous cell carcinoma. EBV is an established etiological factor in the development of NPC and is associated with nearly all type 2 and 3 NPC from endemic regions. Elevated IgA antibody titer to EBV capsid and early antigens is predictive of NPC development within a window of about 3 years [73, 74]. Despite the nearly complete association of EBV in types 2 and 3 endemic NPC, HPV has been detected at frequencies ranging from 10 to 47% in endemic NPC cohorts from Japan, Iran, Morocco, and China [75–78]. Although both low-risk and high-risk HPVs (6, 11, 16, and 18) were detected, HPV types 16 and 18 were more prevalent, accounting for 66.7% of HPV-positive NPC tumors in a Chinese cohort [78]. In contrast, coinfections were rarely detected in NPC from non-endemic areas [79], and several studies have suggested that HPV and EBV appear to be mutually exclusive in NPC with oncogenic HPV types 16, 18, 39, 45, and 59 only detected in EBV-negative NPC [80–84]. The presence of EBV or HPV in NPC correlated with an overall improved survival compared to virally negative NPC, a similarity noted for HPV-positive oral SCC [69, 79, 80]. In our lab and in collaboration with Dr. Sabrina da Silva from McGill University, we explored the copresence of high-risk HPVs and EBV in oral cancer tissue samples in the Canadian population. We noted that around 20% of our Canadian samples are positive for both high-risk HPVs and EBV (Da Silva et al., in preparation).

Collectively, it is evident that high-risk HPVs and EBV are present together and can cooperate in human oral cancer. Regarding the molecular pathways of HPVs and EBV interaction in human oral carcinogenesis, we believe that high-risk HPVs or EBV alone can immortalize (precancer) human normal oral epithelial (NOE) cells which can subsequently transform into cancer cells under the effect of another oncogene or infection with both viruses, high-risk HPVs and EBV. On the other hand, noninvasive cancer cells could be converted into invasive cells under the effect of one of these viruses or both via the initiation of the epithelial-mesenchymal transition (Fig. 6.2), which is a major event of cancer progression into metastasis [85]. Thus, more investigations, using cells and animal models, are necessary to identify the molecular machineries of HPVs/EBV cooperation.

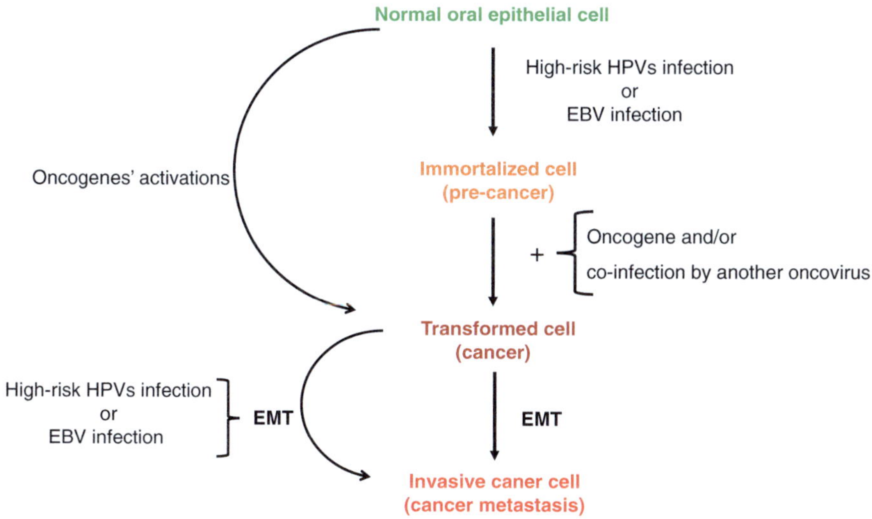

Fig. 6.2 High-risk HPVs and EBV cooperation in human normal oral epithelial (NOE) cells. High-risk HPV or EBV alone can immortalize (precancer) NOE cells which can subsequently transform into cancer cells under the effect of another oncogene or infection with more than one oncovirus (e.g., HPVs and EBV together). Meanwhile, noninvasive cancer cells (induced by oncogene activation) could be converted into invasive cells under the effect of one of these viruses or both together via the initiation of the epithelial-mesenchymal transition (EMT), which is a major event of cancer progression into metastasis [85]

6.5 Conclusion and Perspectives

This chapter presented substantial evidence that oncoviruses especially high-risk HPVs and EBV are important factors in human oral cancer, thereby enhancing the progression of this cancer via the activation of several oncogenes related to cancer progression in HPV-/EBV-infected cells. However, we believe that further studies are required to elucidate the high-risk HPVs/EBV signaling pathways and their association in human oral cancer initiation and/or progression. In parallel, we assume that developing new in vitro and in vivo models such as cell lines and animal models, double transgenic mice, are necessary to identify the exact role of high-risk HPVs and EBV separately and together, in order to discern their role in the initiation and progression of human oral carcinomas which can lead to generate new targets to manage this cancer and other human carcinomas where these oncoviruses are present and/or copresent.

Alternatively and with regard to the prevention of oral malignancy as well as other human cancers, we assume that the elimination of a number of known risk factors especially tobacco, betel quid chewing, and alcohol and oncovirus infections such as high-risk HPVs and EBV could diminish the development of these malignancies and reduce their metastases, since it was clearly demonstrated that these viruses could convert noninvasive and nonmetastatic cancer into invasive and metastatic forms [60, 61, 85]. Therefore, we firmly believe that prevention of high-risk HPV and EBV infection by using the presently available and/or upcoming vaccines, respectively, could greatly reduce high-risk HPV and EBV-associated cancers, including oral, and their progression into invasive form, which is responsible for the majority of cancer-related deaths.

Acknowledgments We are grateful to Mrs. A. Kassab for her critical reading of the chapter. Our research works are supported by Qatar University and its College of Medicine Grant #: GCC-2017-002 QU/KU.

References

1. Bagan J, Sarrion G, Jimenez Y. Oral cancer: clinical features. Oral Oncol. 2010;46:414–7.
2. Noguti J, De Moura CF, De Jesus GP, Da Silva VH, Hossaka TA, Oshima CT, Ribeiro DA. Metastasis from oral cancer: an overview. Cancer Genomics Proteomics. 2012;9: 329–35.
3. Al Moustafa AE, Chen D, Ghabreau L, Akil N. Association between human papillomavirus and Epstein-Barr virus infections in human oral carcinogenesis. Med Hypotheses. 2009;73:184–6.
4. Okura M, Aikawa T, Sawai NY, Iida S, Kogo M. Decision analysis and treatment threshold in a management for the N0 neck of the oral cavity carcinoma. Oral Oncol. 2009;45:908–11.
5. Fan S, Tang QL, Lin YJ, Chen WL, Li JS, Huang ZQ, Yang ZH, Wang YY, Zhang DM, Wang HJ, et al. A review of clinical and histological parameters associated with contralateral neck metastases in oral squamous cell carcinoma. Int J Oral Sci. 2011;3:180–91.
6. Lea J, Bachar G, Sawka AM, Lakra DC, Gilbert RW, Irish JC, Brown DH, Gullane PJ, Goldstein DP. Metastases to level IIb in squamous cell carcinoma of the oral cavity: a systematic review and meta-analysis. Head Neck. 2010;32:184–90.
7. Farris C, Petitte DM. Head, neck, and oral cancer update. Home Healthc Nurse. 2013;31:322–8; quiz 328-330
8. Lambert R, Sauvaget C, de Camargo Cancela M, Sankaranarayanan R. Epidemiology of cancer from the oral cavity and oropharynx. Eur J Gastroenterol Hepatol. 2011;23:633–41.
9. Higa M, Kinjo T, Kamiyama K, Chinen K, Iwamasa T, Arasaki A, Sunakawa H. Epstein-Barr virus (EBV)-related oral squamous cell carcinoma in Okinawa, a subtropical island, in southern Japan—simultaneously infected with human papillomavirus (HPV). Oral Oncol. 2003;39:405–14.
10. Jalouli J, Ibrahim SO, Sapkota D, Jalouli MM, Vasstrand EN, Hirsch JM, Larsson PA. Presence of human papilloma virus, herpes simplex virus and Epstein-Barr virus DNA in oral biopsies from Sudanese patients with regard to toombak use. J Oral Pathol Med. 2010;39:599–604.
11. Jalouli J, Jalouli MM, Sapkota D, Ibrahim SO, Larsson PA, Sand L. Human papilloma virus, herpes simplex virus and Epstein Barr virus in oral squamous cell carcinoma from eight different countries. Anticancer Res. 2012;32:571–80.
12. Jiang R, Ekshyyan O, Moore-Medlin T, Rong X, Nathan S, Gu X, Abreo F, Rosenthal EL, Shi M, Guidry JT, et al. Association between human papilloma virus/Epstein-Barr virus coinfection and oral carcinogenesis. J Oral Pathol Med. 2015;44:28–36.
13. Al Moustafa AE, Foulkes WD, Benlimame N, Wong A, Yen L, Bergeron J, Batist G, Alpert L, Alaoui-Jamali MA. E6/E7 proteins of HPV type 16 and ErbB-2 cooperate to induce neoplastic transformation of primary normal oral epithelial cells. Oncogene. 2004;23:350–8.
14. Castellsague X, Diaz M, de Sanjose S, Munoz N, Herrero R, Franceschi S, Peeling RW, Ashley R, Smith JS, Snijders PJ, et al. Worldwide human papillomavirus etiology of cervical adenocarcinoma and its cofactors: implications for screening and prevention. J Natl Cancer Inst. 2006;98:303–15.

15. Smith JS, Lindsay L, Hoots B, Keys J, Franceschi S, Winer R, Clifford GM. Human papillomavirus type distribution in invasive cervical cancer and high-grade cervical lesions: a meta-analysis update. Int J Cancer. 2007;121:621–32.
16. Brown DR, Kjaer SK, Sigurdsson K, Iversen OE, Hernandez-Avila M, Wheeler CM, Perez G, Koutsky LA, Tay EH, Garcia P, et al. The impact of quadrivalent human papillomavirus (HPV; types 6, 11, 16, and 18) L1 virus-like particle vaccine on infection and disease due to oncogenic nonvaccine HPV types in generally HPV-naive women aged 16–26 years. J Infect Dis. 2009;199:926–35.
17. Darus CJ, Mueller JJ. Development and impact of human papillomavirus vaccines. Clin Obstet Gynecol. 2013;56:10–6.
18. Paavonen J, Naud P, Salmeron J, Wheeler CM, Chow SN, Apter D, Kitchener H, Castellsague X, Teixeira JC, Skinner SR, et al. Efficacy of human papillomavirus (HPV)-16/18 AS04-adjuvanted vaccine against cervical infection and precancer caused by oncogenic HPV types (PATRICIA): final analysis of a double-blind, randomised study in young women. Lancet. 2009;374:301–14.
19. Abramowitz L, Jacquard AC, Jaroud F, Haesebaert J, Siproudhis L, Pradat P, Aynaud O, Leocmach Y, Soubeyrand B, Dachez R, et al. Human papillomavirus genotype distribution in anal cancer in France: the EDiTH V study. Int J Cancer. 2011;129:433–9.
20. Gillison ML, Koch WM, Capone RB, Spafford M, Westra WH, Wu L, Zahurak ML, Daniel RW, Viglione M, Symer DE, et al. Evidence for a causal association between human papillomavirus and a subset of head and neck cancers. J Natl Cancer Inst. 2000;92:709–20.
21. Shukla S, Bharti AC, Mahata S, Hussain S, Kumar R, Hedau S, Das BC. Infection of human papillomaviruses in cancers of different human organ sites. Indian J Med Res. 2009;130:222–33.
22. Umudum H, Rezanko T, Dag F, Dogruluk T. Human papillomavirus genome detection by in situ hybridization in fine needle aspirates of metastatic lesions from head and neck squamous cell carcinomas. Cancer. 2005;105:171–7.
23. Varnai AD, Bollmann M, Griefingholt H, Speich N, Schmitt C, Bollmann R, Decker D. HPV in anal squamous cell carcinoma and anal intraepithelial neoplasia (AIN). Impact of HPV analysis of anal lesions on diagnosis and prognosis. Int J Color Dis. 2006;21:135–42.
24. Ragin CC, Taioli E. Survival of squamous cell carcinoma of the head and neck in relation to human papillomavirus infection: review and meta-analysis. Int J Cancer. 2007;121:1813–20.
25. Termine N, Panzarella V, Falaschini S, Russo A, Matranga D, Lo Muzio L, Campisi G. HPV in oral squamous cell carcinoma vs head and neck squamous cell carcinoma biopsies: a meta-analysis (1988–2007). Ann Oncol. 2008;19:1681–90.
26. Venuti A, Badaracco G, Rizzo C, Mafera B, Rahimi S, Vigili M. Presence of HPV in head and neck tumours: high prevalence in tonsillar localization. J Exp Clin Cancer Res. 2004;23:561–6.
27. Doorbar J. The papillomavirus life cycle. J Clin Virol. 2005;32(Suppl 1):S7–15.
28. Grm HS, Massimi P, Gammoh N, Banks L. Crosstalk between the human papillomavirus E2 transcriptional activator and the E6 oncoprotein. Oncogene. 2005;24:5149–64.
29. Moody CA, Laimins LA. Human papillomavirus oncoproteins: pathways to transformation. Nat Rev Cancer. 2010;10:550–60.
30. Kim SH, Juhnn YS, Kang S, Park SW, Sung MW, Bang YJ, Song YS. Human papillomavirus 16 E5 up-regulates the expression of vascular endothelial growth factor through the activation of epidermal growth factor receptor, MEK/ERK1,2 and PI3K/Akt. Cell Mol Life Sci. 2006;63:930–8.
31. Suprynowicz FA, Disbrow GL, Krawczyk E, Simic V, Lantzky K, Schlegel R. HPV-16 E5 oncoprotein upregulates lipid raft components caveolin-1 and ganglioside GM1 at the plasma membrane of cervical cells. Oncogene. 2008;27:1071–8.
32. Stacey SN, Jordan D, Williamson AJ, Brown M, Coote JH, Arrand JR. Leaky scanning is the predominant mechanism for translation of human papillomavirus type 16 E7 oncoprotein from E6/E7 bicistronic mRNA. J Virol. 2000;74:7284–97.
33. Ghittoni R, Accardi R, Hasan U, Gheit T, Sylla B, Tommasino M. The biological properties of E6 and E7 oncoproteins from human papillomaviruses. Virus Genes. 2010;40:1–13.

34. Herber R, Liem A, Pitot H, Lambert PF. Squamous epithelial hyperplasia and carcinoma in mice transgenic for the human papillomavirus type 16 E7 oncogene. J Virol. 1996;70: 1873–81.
35. Song S, Pitot HC, Lambert PF. The human papillomavirus type 16 E6 gene alone is sufficient to induce carcinomas in transgenic animals. J Virol. 1999;73:5887–93.
36. Riley RR, Duensing S, Brake T, Munger K, Lambert PF, Arbeit JM. Dissection of human papillomavirus E6 and E7 function in transgenic mouse models of cervical carcinogenesis. Cancer Res. 2003;63:4862–71.
37. Genther Williams SM, Disbrow GL, Schlegel R, Lee D, Threadgill DW, Lambert PF. Requirement of epidermal growth factor receptor for hyperplasia induced by E5, a high-risk human papillomavirus oncogene. Cancer Res. 2005;65:6534–42.
38. Stelzer MK, Pitot HC, Liem A, Schweizer J, Mahoney C, Lambert PF. A mouse model for human anal cancer. Cancer Prev Res (Phila). 2010;3:1534–41.
39. Niedobitek G, Meru N, Delecluse HJ. Epstein-Barr virus infection and human malignancies. Int J Exp Pathol. 2001;82:149–70.
40. Munz C, Moormann A. Immune escape by Epstein-Barr virus associated malignancies. Semin Cancer Biol. 2008;18:381–7.
41. Thompson MP, Kurzrock R. Epstein-Barr virus and cancer. Clin Cancer Res. 2004;10: 803–21.
42. Kulwichit W, Edwards RH, Davenport EM, Baskar JF, Godfrey V, Raab-Traub N. Expression of the Epstein-Barr virus latent membrane protein 1 induces B cell lymphoma in transgenic mice. Proc Natl Acad Sci U S A. 1998;95:11963–8.
43. Murata T, Tsurumi T. Switching of EBV cycles between latent and lytic states. Rev Med Virol. 2014;24:142–53.
44. Young LS, Rickinson AB. Epstein-Barr virus: 40 years on. Nat Rev Cancer. 2004;4:757–68.
45. Aboulkassim T, Yasmeen A, Akil N, Batist G, Al Moustafa AE. Incidence of Epstein-Barr virus in Syrian women with breast cancer: a tissue microarray study. Hum Vaccin Immunother. 2015;11:951–5.
46. Amarante MK, Watanabe MA. The possible involvement of virus in breast cancer. J Cancer Res Clin Oncol. 2009;135:329–37.
47. Dawson CW, Port RJ, Young LS. The role of the EBV-encoded latent membrane proteins LMP1 and LMP2 in the pathogenesis of nasopharyngeal carcinoma (NPC). Semin Cancer Biol. 2012;22:144–53.
48. Michelow P, Wright C, Pantanowitz L. A review of the cytomorphology of Epstein-Barr virus-associated malignancies. Acta Cytol. 2012;56:1–14.
49. Morris MA, Dawson CW, Young LS. Role of the Epstein-Barr virus-encoded latent membrane protein-1, LMP1, in the pathogenesis of nasopharyngeal carcinoma. Future Oncol. 2009;5: 811–25.
50. Babu KG. Oral cancers in India. Semin Oncol. 2001;28:169–73.
51. Ng RH, Ngan R, Wei WI, Gullane PJ, Phillips J. Trans-oral brush biopsies and quantitative PCR for EBV DNA detection and screening of nasopharyngeal carcinoma. Otolaryngol Head Neck Surg. 2014;150:602–9.
52. Popat SR, Liavaag PG, Morton R, McIvor N, Irish JC, Freeman JL. Epstein Barr virus genome in nasopharyngeal carcinomas from New Zealand. Head Neck. 2000;22:505–8.
53. Whitney BM, Chan AT, Rickinson AB, Lee SP, Lin CK, Johnson PJ. Frequency of Epstein-Barr virus-specific cytotoxic T lymphocytes in the blood of Southern Chinese blood donors and nasopharyngeal carcinoma patients. J Med Virol. 2002;67:359–63.
54. Yip KW, Shi W, Pintilie M, Martin JD, Mocanu JD, Wong D, MacMillan C, Gullane P, O'Sullivan B, Bastianutto C, et al. Prognostic significance of the Epstein-Barr virus, p53, Bcl-2, and survivin in nasopharyngeal cancer. Clin Cancer Res. 2006;12:5726–32.
55. Curran JA, Laverty FS, Campbell D, Macdiarmid J, Wilson JB. Epstein-Barr virus encoded latent membrane protein-1 induces epithelial cell proliferation and sensitizes transgenic mice to chemical carcinogenesis. Cancer Res. 2001;61:6730–8.

56. Wilson JB, Weinberg W, Johnson R, Yuspa S, Levine AJ. Expression of the BNLF-1 oncogene of Epstein-Barr virus in the skin of transgenic mice induces hyperplasia and aberrant expression of keratin 6. Cell. 1990;61:1315–27.
57. Charalambous CT, Hannigan A, Tsimbouri P, McPhee GM, Wilson JB. Latent membrane protein 1-induced EGFR signalling is negatively regulated by TGF alpha prior to neoplasia. Carcinogenesis. 2007;28:1839–48.
58. Stevenson D, Charalambous C, Wilson JB. Epstein-Barr virus latent membrane protein 1 (CAO) up-regulates VEGF and TGF alpha concomitant with hyperlasia, with subsequent up-regulation of p16 and MMP9. Cancer Res. 2005;65:8826–35.
59. Shair KH, Raab-Traub N. Transcriptome changes induced by Epstein-Barr virus LMP1 and LMP2A in transgenic lymphocytes and lymphoma. MBio. 2012;3:e00288–12.
60. Al Moustafa AE, Al-Awadhi R, Missaoui N, Adam I, Durusoy R, Ghabreau L, Akil N, Ahmed HG, Yasmeen A, Alsbeih G. Human papillomaviruses-related cancers. Presence and prevention strategies in the Middle East and North African regions. Hum Vaccin Immunother. 2014;10:1812–21.
61. Al Moustafa AE, Ghabreau L, Akil N, Rastam S, Alachkar A, Yasmeen A. High-risk HPVs and human carcinomas in the Syrian population. Front Oncol. 2014;4:68.
62. Al Moustafa AE, Alaoui-Jamali MA, Batist G, Hernandez-Perez M, Serruya C, Alpert L, Black MJ, Sladek R, Foulkes WD. Identification of genes associated with head and neck carcinogenesis by cDNA microarray comparison between matched primary normal epithelial and squamous carcinoma cells. Oncogene. 2002;21:2634–40.
63. Al Moustafa AE, Foulkes WD, Wong A, Jallal H, Batist G, Yu Q, Herlyn M, Sicinski P, Alaoui-Jamali MA. Cyclin D1 is essential for neoplastic transformation induced by both E6/E7 and E6/E7/ErbB-2 cooperation in normal cells. Oncogene. 2004;23:5252–6.
64. Yasmeen A, Bismar TA, Kandouz M, Foulkes WD, Desprez PY, Al Moustafa AE. E6/E7 of HPV type 16 promotes cell invasion and metastasis of human breast cancer cells. Cell Cycle. 2007;6:2038–42.
65. Al Moustafa AE, Kassab A, Darnel A, Yasmeen A. High-risk HPV/ErbB-2 interaction on E-cadherin/catenin regulation in human carcinogenesis. Curr Pharm Des. 2008;14:2159–72.
66. Al Moustafa AE, Yasmeen A, Ghabreau L, Akil N. Does the Syrian population have to wait for the new generation of human papillomaviruses vaccine? Hum Vaccin Immunother. 2012;8:1867–8.
67. Mellin H, Friesland S, Lewensohn R, Dalianis T, Munck-Wikland E. Human papillomavirus (HPV) DNA in tonsillar cancer: clinical correlates, risk of relapse, and survival. Int J Cancer. 2000;89:300–4.
68. Benson E, Li R, Eisele D, Fakhry C. The clinical impact of HPV tumor status upon head and neck squamous cell carcinomas. Oral Oncol. 2014;50:565–74.
69. Guidry JT, Scott RS. The interaction between human papillomavirus and other viruses. Virus Res. 2016;231:139–47.
70. Dahlstrom KR, Adler-Storthz K, Etzel CJ, Liu Z, Dillon L, El-Naggar AK, Spitz MR, Schiller JT, Wei Q, Sturgis EM. Human papillomavirus type 16 infection and squamous cell carcinoma of the head and neck in never-smokers: a matched pair analysis. Clin Cancer Res. 2003;9:2620–6.
71. Polz-Gruszka D, Morshed K, Stec A, Polz-Dacewicz M. Prevalence of human papillomavirus (HPV) and Epstein-Barr virus (EBV) in oral and oropharyngeal squamous cell carcinoma in South-Eastern Poland. Infect Agent Cancer. 2015;10:37.
72. Nielsen NH, Mikkelsen F, Hansen JP. Nasopharyngeal cancer in Greenland. The incidence in an Arctic Eskimo population. Acta Pathol Microbiol Scand A. 1977;85:850–8.
73. Henle W, Henle G, Zajac BA, Pearson G, Waubke R, Scriba M. Differential reactivity of human serums with early antigens induced by Epstein-Barr virus. Science. 1970;169:188–90.
74. Ji MF, Wang DK, Yu YL, Guo YQ, Liang JS, Cheng WM, Zong YS, Chan KH, Ng SP, Wei WI, et al. Sustained elevation of Epstein-Barr virus antibody levels preceding clinical onset of nasopharyngeal carcinoma. Br J Cancer. 2007;96:623–30.

75. Deng Z, Uehara T, Maeda H, Hasegawa M, Matayoshi S, Kiyuna A, Agena S, Pan X, Zhang C, Yamashita Y, et al. Epstein-Barr virus and human papillomavirus infections and genotype distribution in head and neck cancers. PLoS One. 2014;9:e113702.
76. Laantri N, Attaleb M, Kandil M, Naji F, Mouttaki T, Dardari R, Belghmi K, Benchakroun N, El Mzibri M, Khyatti M. Human papillomavirus detection in Moroccan patients with nasopharyngeal carcinoma. Infect Agent Cancer. 2011;6:3.
77. Mirzamani N, Salehian P, Farhadi M, Tehran EA. Detection of EBV and HPV in nasopharyngeal carcinoma by in situ hybridization. Exp Mol Pathol. 2006;81:231–4.
78. Tung YC, Lin KH, Chu PY, Hsu CC, Kuo WR. Detection of human papilloma virus and Epstein-Barr virus DNA in nasopharyngeal carcinoma by polymerase chain reaction. Kaohsiung J Med Sci. 1999;15:256–62.
79. Stenmark MH, McHugh JB, Schipper M, Walline HM, Komarck C, Feng FY, Worden FP, Wolf GT, Chepeha DB, Prince ME, et al. Nonendemic HPV-positive nasopharyngeal carcinoma: association with poor prognosis. Int J Radiat Oncol Biol Phys. 2014;88:580–8.
80. Dogan S, Hedberg ML, Ferris RL, Rath TJ, Assaad AM, Chiosea SI. Human papillomavirus and Epstein-Barr virus in nasopharyngeal carcinoma in a low-incidence population. Head Neck. 2014;36:511–6.
81. Lin Z, Khong B, Kwok S, Cao H, West RB, Le QT, Kong CS. Human papillomavirus 16 detected in nasopharyngeal carcinomas in white Americans but not in endemic Southern Chinese patients. Head Neck. 2014;36:709–14.
82. Lo EJ, Bell D, Woo J, Li G, Hanna EY, El-Naggar AK, Sturgis EM. Human papillomavirus & WHO type I nasopharyngeal carcinoma. Laryngoscope. 2010;120(Suppl 4):S185.
83. Maxwell JH, Kumar B, Feng FY, Worden FP, Lee JS, Eisbruch A, Wolf GT, Prince ME, Moyer JS, Teknos TN, et al. Tobacco use in human papillomavirus-positive advanced oropharynx cancer patients related to increased risk of distant metastases and tumor recurrence. Clin Cancer Res. 2010;16:1226–35.
84. Robinson M, Suh YE, Paleri V, Devlin D, Ayaz B, Pertl L, Thavaraj S. Oncogenic human papillomavirus-associated nasopharyngeal carcinoma: an observational study of correlation with ethnicity, histological subtype and outcome in a UK population. Infect Agent Cancer. 2013;8:30.
85. Al Moustafa AE, Achkhar A, Yasmeen A. EGF-receptor signaling and epithelial-mesenchymal transition in human carcinomas. Front Biosci (Schol Ed). 2012;4:671–84.

Oral Cancer: Epidemiology and Infections (Bacterial and Fungal) Global Incidence

7

Mohammed Jaloudi, Maria Aamir,
Mohammad Ahmad Lahej Alfelasi, and Jihad Kanbar

7.1 Introduction

Cancer is amongst the most common causes of morbidity and mortality today with more than ten million new cases and more than six million deaths each year worldwide [1]. Globally more than 20 million persons are diagnosed with cancer, and more than half of all cancer cases occur in the developing countries. Cancer is responsible for about 20% of all deaths in high-income countries and 10% in low-income countries. It is projected that by 2020, there will be every year 15 million new cancer cases and 10 million cancer deaths. This alarming increase in numbers may well be caused by the ageing of populations worldwide and enhanced cancer registry. The cancer epidemic in high-income countries, and increasing numbers in low- and middle-income countries, is also caused by the prevalence of cancer risk factors such as tobacco use, unhealthy diets, alcohol consumption, inactive lifestyles and infections.

Oral cancer is an emerging problem in many countries. According to WHO, it is amongst the most prevalent cancers worldwide. It is the sixth most common cancer in the world [2]. In 2002, two-thirds of the new cases and deaths occurring in the world due to oral cancer were observed in less-resourced countries [3].

There is a huge geographical variation in the incidence of oral cancer worldwide. Variances in the incidence rates across different countries are particularly due to

M. Jaloudi • J. Kanbar (✉)
Oncology Department, Tawam Hospital, Al-Ain, UAE
e-mail: jkanbar@seha.ae

M. Aamir
Cancer Registry Department, Tawam Hospital, Al-Ain, UAE

M.A.L. Alfelasi
ENT/Maxillo Facial Department, Tawam Hospital, Al-Ain, UAE

A.-E. Al Moustafa (ed.), *Development of Oral Cancer*,
DOI 10.1007/978-3-319-48054-1_7

distinct risk factors and availability as well as accessibility of health services. In developed countries, oral cancer is relatively less common; however the incidence rates vary a great deal.

The worldwide estimated annual incidence of oral cancer is approximately 275,000 which is mainly reported from developing countries [4]. The world incidence rate on oral cancer significantly increased during 1983–2002 predominantly in economically developed countries [5]. There has been sharp increase reported in several parts of the world, for instance, Denmark, France, Germany, Scotland, Central and Eastern Europe and to a lesser extent Australia, Japan, New Zealand and the USA [6]. The highest crude rates in the world have been reported from Melanesia, Hungary, France, Sri Lanka and Croatia [7].

Incidence rates increased in many countries mainly due to tobacco epidemics. In some countries the incidence of oral cancer has been declined; however rates of oropharyngeal cancer have been risen presumably due to human papillomavirus infection [8].

In the **USA**, it accounts for 3% of all cancer. Each year 30,000 new cases of oral cavity and pharynx are diagnosed in the USA [9]. According to 2004 National Cancer Institute Survey, oral cancer rates have increased approximately 15% from the mid-1970s until the latest. Studies in the USA have found increased incidence of oral cancer among minorities mainly in black males [10].

In **Canada**, there were 3400 new cases of oral cancer in 2008. According to Canadian cancer society, there were 4350 new cases diagnosed in 2015.

Although the incidence rates of mouth cancer reported a decline in some countries, a large increase is observed in **southern South America** [11]. In **South America and the Caribbean**, oral cancer together with pharynx ranks fifth in male and sixth in female. It is the seventh most common cancer in Brazil with 13,470 new cases with the highest incidence in males [12]. The highest incidence was reported in Latin America with huge regional variation across the country. Puerto Rico reported the highest incidence of oral cancer in the Caribbean region with the incidence more than 15 per 100,000 [11].

In the **UK**, oral cancer incidence is relatively low. It was reported as the 14th most common cancer in 2013 accounted for 2% of all cases [13]. There were 7591 new cases of oral cancer registered in the UK in 2013. In England and Wales, the incidence of oral cancer decreased from 1970s to mid-1980s but increased later on. According to the National Cancer Intelligence Report 2010, the incidence of oral cavity has risen more than 30% mainly due to immigrants from the Indian subcontinents. In Scotland, studies have shown a significant increase in male incidence since the 1980s [14].

Within **European Union**, France has the highest incidence rates reporting 15,500 cancers of lip, oral cavity and pharynx annually [15]. Data from these countries revealed that the oral and pharyngeal cancer ranks the seventh position in the European Union countries registering 67,000 in 2004 [16]. France and Eastern Europe including Hungary, Slovakia and Slovenia have been marked as regions with higher incidence of oral cancer on the globe [15]. The lowest incidence rates have been recorded from Greece, Finland and Sweden within Europe [16]. Continuing upward trends have also been reported for Belgium, Denmark, Greece, Portugal and Scotland [15].

Countries with the highest incidence of oral cancer in the world are mainly from the **Asia.** It is the sixth most common cancer in the region with 274,300 new cases reported with poor survival prospects [7, 17].

There are striking differences in incidence rates within Asian subcontinent. The highest incidence rates are reported from **south central and southeast** regions mainly Sri Lanka, India, Pakistan, Bangladesh and Taiwan where oral cancer is ranked as the top most common cancer [18].

Among the 23 counties, Changhua (Taiwan) has ranked top in oral cancer incidence in recent years [19]. According to Sri Lankan Centre of Research in oral cancer (2015), a total of 16,511 new cases of oral cancer were reported with the incidence rate of 81.6 per 100,000.

In India one-third of the total cancer burden is attributed to oral cancer [18]. In India, it is most common in men whereas in women, these rates are three to seven times higher than in other developed countries [20]. The highest rates were reported as 15.7 per 100,000. The increased rates in Indian subcontinent are mainly due to poor hygiene, tobacco use, use of chewing tobacco leave and smoking whereas in Pakistan, the higher incidence is mainly attributed to the local custom of chewing tobacco products such as paan, gutka and naswar [21].

Other Asian countries including Hong Kong, the Philippines, Singapore, Vietnam, China and Israel have comparatively low incidence rates of less than 6 per 100,000 in both males and females [17]. In China, the estimate of new cases diagnosed with oral cancer was 39,450 including 26,160 males and 13,290 females [22]. In Vietnam, 19.80% of all malignant neoplasms are diagnosed as oral cancer [3]. In Japan the rates of oral cancer are relatively low which is 0.2 per 100,000 [20]; however the rates were previously reported from Osaka Cancer Registry with a dramatic increase for both males and females between 1965 and 1999 [7].

Reported rates from **Africa** do not reveal the higher incidence; this could be due to limited data available from cancer registries in that region.

7.2 Worldwide Incidence of Oral Cancer by Gender, Age and Primary Site

Oral cancer is the eighth most common cancer globally, accounting for an estimated 300,000 new cases and 145,000 deaths in 2012 and 702,000 prevalent cases over a period of 5 years (Tables 7.1, 7.2 and 7.3).

Incidence and mortality as a result of oral cancer are higher in developing countries when compared to developed countries [23]. According to the latest World Health Organization (WHO) data recorded in 2010, the death rate due to oral cancer in the Middle East is reported to be approximately 2 in 100,000, which is much lower than that in other parts of the world [24] (Table 7.4).

Table 7.1 Oral cancer in men (all ages): global incidence, mortality and prevalence, World Health Organization geographic classification, 2012

	Incidence		Mortality		Prevalence	
Population	Number	ASR (W)	Number	ASR (W)	Number	5-year
World	198,975	5.5	97,919	2.7	198,267	467,157
More developed regions	68,042	7	23,380	2.3	67,978	195,233
Less developed regions	130,933	5	74,539	2.8	130,289	271,924
WHO Africa region	8009	3.4	5026	2.2	7763	18,446
WHO Americas region	31,898	5.9	8532	1.5	31,805	94,953
WHO East Mediterranean region	11,601	5.1	6185	2.8	11,533	27,236
WHO Europe region	45,567	7.1	18,621	2.8	45,499	118,151
WHO Southeast Asia region	70,816	8.9	45,247	5.7	70,667	122,976
WHO Western Pacific region	31,013	2.7	14,292	1.2	30,929	85,233
Africa	10,230	3.3	6083	2.1	9961	23,560
Latin America and Caribbean	12,988	4.6	5244	1.9	12,918	32,424
Asia	111,994	5.2	65,045	3	111,683	230,389
Europe	42,573	7.5	17,598	3	42,539	111,347
Oceania	2280	9.6	661	2.7	2279	6908

Source: Incidence/mortality data: Ferlay et al. (2013). Prevalence data: (Bray et al. 2013; Ferlay et al. 2013)
Note: ASR (W) = age-standardized incidence rate per 100,000 population, for the world population structure; WHO = World Health Organization

Oral cancer might be considered as the most common cancer in head-neck region affecting predominantly male with 75% of diagnosed cases around 60-year-old among which 90% are oral squamous cell carcinoma [10].

Although the oral cancer is mostly found in middle-aged and older persons, recent studies has shown that 4–6% of oral cancers now occur at ages younger than 40 years [7]. Surprisingly it could also occur in children as early as 10 years of age in the absence of any known risk factors [25].

There has been a significant age shift in the past few decades presenting quite a heterogeneous figure of oral cancer around the globe [26]. Latest studies have also revealed an alarming increase in the incidence among younger people from many parts of the world [27]. In the past few decades, there has been a 60% increase in oral cancer in adults under age 40 [28]. The mean age reported from different countries is around 56–62 years [7].

The current male-to-female worldwide ratio is about 2:1. These gender differences in oral cancer incidence are very much associated with heavier indulgence in tobacco and alcohol habits in males [7, 26].

More than 90% of oral malignancies are squamous cell carcinoma [26], whereas 'tongue cancer' is the most common type of oral cancer reported among

Table 7.2 Oral cancer in women (all ages): global incidence, mortality and prevalence, World Health Organization geographic classification, 2012

	Incidence		Mortality		Prevalence	
Population	Number	ASR (W)	Number	ASR (W)	Number	5-year
World	101,398	2.5	47,409	1.2	100,784	234,992
More developed regions	32,781	2.6	9908	0.6	32,683	93,180
Less developed regions	68,617	2.5	37,501	1.4	68,101	141,812
WHO Africa region	5475	2	3504	1.4	5349	12,766
WHO Americas region	17,302	2.6	4271	0.6	17,204	48,526
WHO East Mediterranean region	9080	4.1	4812	2.2	8993	21,570
WHO Europe region	20,366	2.4	6556	0.7	20,305	51,933
WHO Southeast Asia region	32,648	3.9	20,487	2.5	32,482	58,034
WHO Western Pacific region	16,511	1.3	7776	0.6	16,435	42,123
Africa	7046	2	4258	1.3	6892	16,409
Latin America and Caribbean	7645	2.2	2381	0.7	7586	17,813
Asia	56,856	2.5	32,363	1.4	56,549	117,362
Europe	18,843	2.5	6033	0.7	18,789	48,653
Oceania	1351	5.3	484	1.9	1350	4042

Sources: Incidence/mortality data: Ferlay et al. (2013). Prevalence data. Bray et al. (2013)
Note: ASR (W) = age-standardized incidence rate per 100,000 population, for the world population structure; WHO = World Health Organization

every ethnicity which accounts for around 40% of all cases in the oral cavity proper [7, 29]. Rao et al. [17] reported that the young adults of age 45 or below suffer more from tongue cancer whereas older people have tendency to develop cancer of buccal mucosa of which 60% of cancer occur in tongues followed by buccal mucosa and other sites. A study conducted in Spain discovered that 3% of malignant tumours originate in the oral cavity of which majority are squamous cell carcinoma [30].

According to Surveillance, Epidemiology, and End Results (SEER) Program by the National Cancer Institute, cancer rates are significantly higher in males than in females in the **USA**. Data shows that the median age at diagnosis for oral cancer in the USA was 62 years [7]. The age-adjusted incidence rates in the country were 15.6 per 100,000 for men and 6.1 per 100,000 for women. These rates were predominantly higher in black males particularly for oropharynx [15]. A significant increase was reported in cancer of the tongue and tonsils in population under 40 in the USA between 1973 and 2001 [7].

In **Canada,** the oral cancer contributes to approximately 2.6% of all cancer in males and 1.4% in females [3] where the highest rates of lip cancer are reported in white population.

Table 7.3 Worldwide cancer deaths in 2012 at ages 0–69 by cancer site and country income grouping and 5-year survival rates in low-, middle- and high-income countries

Cancer, by site (ICD-10 C00-99)	Annual deaths, age 0–69 years (thousands) by World Bank country income group					5-year survival (%), cancer registry data	
	Low	Lower	Upper	High	World	Low or	High
Lung, mouth and oesophagus	70	260	560	300	1200	10	20
Liver	30	90	270	60	440	10	20
Breast	30	140	110	80	360	75	90
Stomach	20	80	210	50	360	20	40
Colon or rectum	20	80	120	100	310	50	60
Cervix	40	90	60	20	200	55	65
Ovary	8	30	30	30	100	25	40
Leukaemia, age 0–14 years	3	10	10	2	30	65	90
age 15–69 years	10	40	60	30	140	30	50
Prostate	4	10	20	20	60	70	90
Other/unknown site	110	330	470	310	1220	–	–
All cancers (% of all causes)	350 (6%)	1170 (6%)	1920 (22%)	1000 (37%)	4400 (14%)	–	–
All noncommunicable diseases	1660	6300	5950	2200	16,070	–	–
Communicable/external causes	4100	7380	2650	500	14,660	–	–
All causes	5760	13,680	8600	2700	30,730	–	–

Sources: Population and mortality based on data from the UN Population Division and WHO Global Health Estimates (WHO 2012). Estimated 5-year survival based on Allemani et al. (2015)
Note: A number of deaths above 10,000 are rounded to the nearest 10,000, so totals may differ. Estimated 5-year survival rounded to the nearest 5%. – = Not applicable

The rising of oropharyngeal cancer incidence has been noticed in both USA and Canada which is presumed to be associated with HPV infection; however the reason for rising incidence of oral tongue cancer is currently unclear in that region [31].

The incidence rates in Australia have also been reported mounting overtime both in males and females as well as in **New Zealand** predominantly in non-Maori population [7]. In Australia, 50% of oral cancers are located on the lip [32] which is quite rare in non-white population.

An increased risk also has been observed in 19 out of 24 **European countries** [30]. In **France**, the incidence of both oral and oropharyngeal cancer among males is extremely high in the northern region with a rate of almost 42.3 per 100,000 [15]. **Hungary** has the highest incident of oral and pharyngeal cancer in both genders [33] and the lowest among females in Cyprus and Greece (1.5 and 2.0 per 100,000, respectively) [7]. Other countries including Spain, Portugal, Germany, Switzerland

Table 7.4 World Health Organization, 2012

	Rank	Deaths	Rank	Deaths
Coronary heart disease	1	7,356,061	1	1658
Stroke	2	6,670,934	3	666
Lung disease	3	3,104,330	18	135
Lung cancers	5	1,599,557	15	153
HIV/AIDS	6	1,533,760	73	0
Diarrhoeal diseases	7	1,497,724	42	23
Diabetes mellitus	8	1,497,371	7	296
Road traffic accidents	9	1,254,526	2	908
Liver cancer	18	740,373	29	66
Stomach cancer	19	733,499	27	78
Colon-rectum cancers	20	723,913	21	117
Breast cancer	25	536,521	20	123
Oesophagus cancer	30	405,803	36	39
Pancreas cancer	35	331,918	32	52
Prostate cancer	36	321,728	40	27
Lymphomas	37	312,302	19	124
Oral cancer	**38**	**298,027**	**34**	**46**
Leukaemia	40	276,097	25	90
Cervical cancer	42	264,225	39	28
Other neoplasms	46	193,025	52	9
Bladder cancer	47	172,813	44	19
Ovary cancer	48	151,039	35	42

and northern regions of Italy have reported intermediate rates compared with other countries of Europe [15].

In **South America and the Caribbean**, oral cancer including mouth and pharynx ranks fifth in men and sixth in women. Several population-based cancer registries in **Brazil, Sao Paulo and Puerto Alegre** have registered highest rates for tongue and mouth cancer rates [15]. **Brazil** has the highest risk in the world for cancer of mouth in males. In Brazilian males, the primary site of oral cancer is found to be the first one-third anterior portion of tongue, lower lip, mouth floor and hard palate [10].

According to Cancer Research **UK** [13], oral cancer is the 11th most common cancer in male (3% of all male cases), whereas in females, it is the 16th most common cancer (1% of all new cases). The male-to-female incidence rate ratio is around 21:10 in the UK.

There are 16 new oral cancer cases for every 100,000 males in the UK and 8 for every 100,000 females. In the **UK**, the oral cancer is increasing in young adults. It is more common in migrants mainly in South Asians due to predisposing social and cultural habits acquired in the home countries [3]. Rates in Scotland are higher than in other parts of the UK for both men and women. UK cancer registries currently show that 6% of all oral cancers occur in people under the age of 45 years [34].

Between 1990 and 1999, an increase in incidence rates was reported In UK in both in males of all ages (18%) and in females (30%) whereas in **Scotland**, the incidence rates increased dramatically in younger males between 1980s and 1990s [7].

There is very high incidence of oral cancer in **Southern Asia** whereas in **Southeast Asia**, oral and nasopharyngeal cancer ranks on the top and accounts for 40% of all malignancies (Johnson et al. [7]). The common anatomic sites of oral cancer in Southeast Asia are the buccal mucosa, gingiva and tongue.

In Asia, most cases of oral cancer occur between age 50 and 70 years. Data from high-risk countries including Sri Lanka, India, Pakistan and Bangladesh, shows that the oral cancer is most common in men which and may contribute up to 25% of all new cases of cancer [15].

In **India,** oral cancer is the most common in men and third most common in women after cervical and breast amongst women (Khan [20]). In India, 8–10% of all cancers occur in the oral cavity [35] whereas the tongue cancer constitutes about 36.5% [36]. Johnson et al. [7] reported a decline in incidence rates between 1982 and 2000 in mouth and tongue in females and for males in tongue cancer rates likely associated with the economic growth and change in habits from betel quid to other forms of tobacco (smoking).

Rao et al. [17] reported that cheek and buccal mucosa cancer exceed all other oral cancers in Pakistan. Few reports from Pakistan and India have shown equal male-to-female ratio of oral cancer. However institutional studies from India reported two to four times increase rates in men than women [17]. Franceschia et al. [37] reported the highest incidence of oral cancer in women in India and the Philippines with clear predominance of cancer in the oral cavity. He also indicated that the incidence rate of oral cancer in Indian women exceeds that of males.

Taiwan had an alarming 5.3-fold increase in the incidence of male oral cancer from 1982 to 2001, and in Changhua, the incidence of oral cancer in male was among the highest in the world in 2001 and predominantly occurs in the buccal mucosa [19]. The highest male-to-female ratio was also reported from Taiwan which is 10.5 [38]. According to the World Health Organization, the incidence of oral cancer in men has been triple folded since 1980s in China and Taiwan mainly due to chewing of betel quid [3, 39], whereas global cancer forum has reported a significant decline in Hong Kong in the incidence of oral cancer in recent years.

In Sri Lanka, it is the most common cancer in males with 15.5% of all cancers reported in the mouth. In Bangladesh, oral cancer is equally common in both genders. There are about 200,000 patients diagnosed each year with oral cancer in Bangladesh among which around 7000 cases are of lip, oral cavity and pharynx [40].

In **Africa**, the data on cancer is quite limited; however some regional studies had shown that the incidence is higher in males [15] which are mainly associated with oral snuff of toombak intake [41]. According to global cancer forum, a wide variability in oral cancer incidence has been observed in the regional burden of lip and oral cavity cancers with highest incidence reported in Djibouti, Somalia, Sudan, Madagascar, Botswana, Mauritius and Mozambique. In Central Africa the cancer of the oral mucosa is common, whereas in East, West and South Africa, the frequent anatomic sites of oral cancer are alveolar ridge and tongue cancers.

7.3 Oral Cancer Mortality and Survival

Oral cancer is responsible for more deaths in the world than melanoma, Hodgkin's disease or cervical cancer [3]. Most of these deaths occurred in the poor-resourced countries.

Mortality rates due to oral cancer do vary across the globe. Variation in outcome and survival are associated with the access to healthcare; studies in the USA have shown that black patients with oral cancer have poorer overall and disease survival than whites mainly due to the lack of access to healthcare [42]. Improved survival has also been observed in affluent group and younger than older patient.

Oral cancer is one of the few cancers whose survival rate has not improved over 30 years [3]. There is a little evidence of improved survival rates globally [7]. Five-year survival rate has improved only marginally over the past few decades, and it remains at about 50–55% [29]. Another US study showed that there will be approximately 60% of people diagnosed with oral cancer that will survive in the USA only up to 5 years [43].

Since 5-year survival is directly related to stage at diagnosis, the survival rates for stage I disease is 80% and for stage IV is 15% [44]. Most oral cancer patients are elderly with a life expectancy less than 5 years. The overall 5-year survival for tongue and oral cavity cancer ranges from 45 to 72% worldwide.

For most countries, the age-adjusted death rates from oral cancer have been estimated at 3–4 per 100,000 in males and 1.5–2 per 100,000 in females for the period of 2005–2009 [26].

According to Globocan 2012 [45], the highest mortality from oral cancer is found in **Melanesia** which was 16.6 per 100,000 in males and 6.2 per 100,000 in females. These rates are the highest among both genders across the globe.

There has been a steady increase in oral cancer mortality in young population mainly from the oropharynx in the USA [26]. It is estimated that approximately 8000 Americans die of oral cancer each year [46]. In 2008, there were 7590 deaths reported due to oral cancer in the **USA** representing 1.64% of all deaths due to oral cancer in the country [7]. In 2005, the mortality rate in the **USA** due to oral and pharyngeal cancer in males was 3.9 and 1.4 per 100,000 in females which was reported relatively much higher in 1975 (male, 6.9, and female, 2.3). Surveillance epidemiology and end results data show better 5-year 62.2% survival rate in white males and 37.5% in black men during the period of 1999–2006.

There were 1150 deaths that occurred in **Canada** due to oral cancer [3]. According to Canadian cancer society (2015), the mortality rates due to oral cancer have declined by 2.4% per year for males between 2001 and 2010; however, in females these rates are stable during the same period which are more likely reflect patterns of smoking prevalence. The observed survival in both males and females has been reported as 57% in Canada.

In **France** about 5000 deaths are reported per year [15] due to oral cancer. Oral cancer mortality reflects the different patterns in tobacco smoking and alcohol drinking, including drinking patterns and type of alcohol in central Europe [47].

In the **European Union** (EU), male mortality rates rose by 2.1% per year between 1975 and 1984, by 1.0% between 1984 and 1993 and declined by 1.3% between 1993 and 2004. There was a steady increase in oral cancer mortality in men during early decades in France, Hungary, Slovakia, Slovenia and Russia which decreased in past decade; however these rates are increasing steadily in females as well in that region [7].

Exceedingly high rates have been reported **in Hungary and Slovakia**. A study showed almost tenfold increase within one generation in mortality from oral cancer in men aged 35–44 in Germany, Czechoslovakia and Hungary [7]. Between 1984 and 1994, the Hungarian mortality rates for oral cancers increased by 84% in males and 72% in females whereas these rates peaked in the 1980s and decreased after 1990 among Italian and French males [47].

A study conducted in the **UK** to compare the mortality risk in persons born in the Indian subcontinent who migrated to England and Wales with native population showed significant raised risks in Indian ethnic migrants for cancers of the mouth and pharynx [16].

In **Scotland**, oropharyngeal cancer accounted for more male death than any other cancer. A study from Canniesburn hospital, Glasgow, in 2000 suggested no improvement in survival in the last 16 years despite the advances in cancer diagnosis and treatment, indicating a 5-year survival rate of 44% [30].

India is the country that has the highest mortality of oral cancer in Southeast Asia. In India, oral cancer is the most fatal in men and accounts as the fourth most cause of death in women in age group 30–69 years [48].

In **China,** there were 16,933 deaths that occurred in 2011 due to oral cancer accounting for 0.80% of all cancer deaths. Mortality rates in China were mainly reported higher in urban than rural areas as well as predominantly in males than females [22].

According to Su et al. [19], it is the fourth leading cause of death in **Taiwan** with an overall survival rate of 61% [49].

In **Bangladesh**, the mortality rate due to oral cancer has been reported 8.3% in males and 4.3% in females. Access to healthcare in rural health has been considered the major barrier as people in those areas are not warned about health issues as well as they have not been educated to visit dentists for their oral health problems [40].

Sargeran et al. [50] emphasized the planning of prevention campaigns, awareness programmes, population literacy rate and efficiency of healthcare system are pivotal to control oral cancer mortality. A Canadian study reported higher incidence rates among people with lower median income, less than eighth grade education and visiting dentists less than once a year. Continued surveillance is a prerequisite to establish informed global policies as well as to develop prevention and care strategies. There is a huge variability of oral cancer incidence and mortality rate around the world.

7.4 Bacteria and Cancer

Primary tumours of the oral cavity may arise from the surface epithelium, minor salivary glands or submucosal soft tissues. The oral cavity is continuously exposed to inhale and consume carcinogens, and thus it is the most common site for the origin of malignant epithelial neoplasms in the head and neck region. Known carcinogens in the oral cavity include those present in tobacco, alcohol, radiation, ultraviolet radiation exposure (lip cancer), Plummer-Vinson syndrome, poor oral hygiene and betel nuts. It has been clearly proven that HPV is related to oropharyngeal cancer; no evidence shows clear-cut relation between bacteria and fungus to be an aetiology to oral cancer.

An overwhelming body of evidence has determined that relationships among certain bacteria and cancers exist. The bacterial mechanisms involved are as yet unclear. These knowledge gaps make it impossible to state the exact progression of events by which specific bacteria may cause, colonize or cure cancer [51].

7.4.1 Anatomy

The various anatomic sites within the oral cavity are described by the American Joint Committee on Cancer/International Union Against Cancer staging system.

The oral cavity is the space located between the lips and cheeks on the external surface to the palatoglossal fold on the internal surface. It is lined by squamous epithelium with interspersed minor salivary glands. The oral cavity also contains the dento-alveolar structures with the upper and lower dentition.

7.4.2 Clinical Presentation

Patients present with a non-healing ulcer or oral pain, loosening of teeth, ill-fitting dentures, dysphagia, odynophagia, weight loss, bleeding or referred otalgia. Risk increase to have cervical lymph node involvement is substantially dependent on the size of the primary cancer and depth of invasion.

Oral cancer may grow as an ulcerative and/or infiltrative and/or exophytic lesion. The presenting symptom is often pain, with or without dysarthria. Dysarthria implies deep muscle invasion of advanced tumour stage. There may be a history of longstanding leukoplakia or erythroplakia.

7.4.3 Pathology

More than 90% of malignant tumours in the oral cavity are squamous cell carcinomas, they can be classified as well differentiated, moderately differentiated and poorly differentiated tumours. SCC of the head and neck cancers often develop through a series of changes from premalignant entities which includes leukoplakia, erythroplakia and dysplasia. The remainder are minor salivary gland carcinomas and other rare tumours. The TNM staging system of the American Joint Committee on Cancer (AJCC) and the International Union for Cancer Control (UICC) is used to classify cancers of the head and neck.

Diagnosis and staging evaluation will depend on initial assessment of the primary tumour based on a thorough history and examination of the nasal cavity, oral cavity, pharynx and larynx. A direct biopsy of the lesion is required in the clinic setting; if patients present with metastatic cervical lymph node, a fine needle aspiration is required. Furthermore, depending on the lesion site and lymph node, different modality imagings are recommended including CT scan, MRI and PET scan.

The main causes of oral cancer as mentioned earlier are smoking and alcohol consumption; in addition there are other known factors such as:

- Human Papilloma virus 'HPV'
- Tobacco chewing
- Poor diet
- Previous cancers
- AIDS & HIV
- Family history
- Excessive exposure to the sun or sunbeds
- Genetic conditions like fanconi anaemia or dyskeratosis congenita
- Oral phenomenon like leukoplakia or erythroplakia
- Medication drugs like antihypertensive drug 'hydrochlorothiazide'

An overwhelming body of evidence has also been determined that relationships among certain bacteria and cancers exist, yet our knowledge in its relation to oral cancers remains inadequate. The bacterial mechanism involved is still unclear. These gaps in knowledge make it impossible to state the exact progression of events by which specific bacteria may cause, colonize or cure cancer. It is estimated that over 15% of malignancies worldwide can be attributed to infections or about 1.2 million cases per year [52].

Convincing evidence has linked *Helicobacter pylori* with both gastric cancer and mucosa-associated lymphoid tissue (MALT) lymphoma [53]; other species associated with cancers include: *Salmonella typhi* and gallbladder cancer [54], *Streptococcus bovis* and colon cancer [55] and *Chlamydia pneumoniae* with lung cancer [56–58].

The complex relationship between bacteria and humans is demonstrated by *Helicobacter pylori* and *Salmonella typhi* infections; (Table 7.5) [59]. Research has shown that *H. pylori* can cause gastric cancer or MALT lymphoma in some individuals. In contrast, exposure to *H. pylori* appears to reduce the risk of oesophageal cancer in others. *Salmonella typhi* infection has been associated with the development of gallbladder cancer; chronic hyperplastic candidosis, a rare oral fungal infection, is associated with the invasion of candidal hyphae into the oral epithelium and known to cause oral cancers [60].

Table 7.5 Various evidence-based cancers associated with specific bacterial aetiology

Carcinomas of various regions	Associated pathogen
Gastric carcinoma	*Helicobacter pylori*
Gall bladder carcinoma	*Salmonella typhi*
Cervical carcinoma	*Chlamydia trachomatis*
Lung cancer	*Chlamydia pneumonia*
Intestinal cancer	*Streptococcus bovis*

It has been shown that several bacteria can cause chronic infections or produce toxins that disturb the cell cycle resulting in altered cell growth and the resulting damage to DNA is similar to that caused by carcinogenic agents as the genes that are altered control normal cell division and apoptosis. Processes that encourage the loss of cellular control may be tumour initiators (directly causing mutations) or promoters (facilitating mutations). Tumorigenesis is initiated when cells are freed from growth restraints, later promotion results when the immune system is evaded favouring further mutations and increased loss of cell control. As the tumour proliferates, an increased blood supply is needed resulting in the organization of blood vessels or angiogenesis. Subsequent invasion occurs if the tumour breaks down surrounding tissues. The worst outcome is metastasis which results when cells break away from the tumour and seed tumours at distant sites [56–58, 61].

7.4.4 Virus

7.4.4.1 HPV

Oral HPV infection is strongly associated with oropharyngeal SCC among those with or without established risk factors of alcohol and tobacco use [62]; HPV is a mucosotropic virus that has been closely associated with cervical carcinoma in women, such that HPV 16 and 18 are considered carcinogenic. In oral cavity specimens, variable detection has been reported with rates ranging from 19 to 78% [63].

Findings of HPV 16 within normal tissue at the margins of tumour specimens have suggested that infection is not a sole event preceding malignant transformation. Rather, it has been postulated that HPV may play a role in the early events of carcinogenesis. HPV oncoproteins E6 and E7 have the ability to bind and degrade tumour suppressor gene products of p53 and pRB, respectively. This binding can impair the capacity of the cell cycle to arrest for the repair of DNA damage and results in an accumulation of genetic changes assisting transformation [64].

Smith and colleagues detected a significant increase in the presence of HPV DNA within oral cavity carcinoma samples (15%) compared with controls (5%). In addition, they noted that HPV (odds ratio [OR] = 3.7) was a risk factor for carcinoma, independent of tobacco (OR = 2.63) and alcohol use (OR = 2.57); [65]. Maden and co-workers noted an increased risk for oral cavity carcinoma with the presence of HPV 6 and HPV 16. Similar to Smith and colleagues, they also demonstrated HPV infection to be a risk factor, independent of age and tobacco and alcohol use; [66].

7.4.4.2 Human Immunodeficiency Virus

Human immunodeficiency virus (HIV) has shown an emerging association with head and neck squamous cell carcinoma. In a recent study from New York, HIV infection was present in almost 5% of patients with head and neck cancer [67].

Patients with HIV were younger than non-HIV patients, and HIV infection was present in over 20% of head and neck cancer patients who were under 45 year of age. The site of tumour presentation did not vary with respect to HIV status, but tumours were larger and more advanced in the HIV group. As in most cases of head and neck squamous cell carcinoma, a history of tobacco and alcohol use is prevalent in the HIV population [68].

7.4.4.3 Herpes Simplex Virus

Herpes simplex virus (HSV) has been associated with cancer of the oral cavity. In a study utilizing patient questionnaires for data collection, a history of proven HSV-1 infections was associated with oral cancer (OR = 1.9). A stronger association was seen with a history of a suspected HSV-1 infection (OR = 3.3); [69]. While this study raises concerns about reporting bias, support for this association is provided by a finding of HSV type 1 protein in 42% of patients with oral cancer and no positive results in control patients [70].

7.4.5 Dental Considerations

7.4.5.1 Hygiene

Poor oral hygiene is associated with oral cancer, but no causal relationship has been established. A case control study of patients with upper aerodigestive tract squamous cell carcinoma matched 100 patients with 214 age- and sex-matched controls and found significantly worse oral hygiene and dental status in the tumour patients. Chronic inflammation of the gingiva was more often seen in the cancer patients. [71]. Similarly, oral cancers have been significantly associated with a history of chronic oral infections (OR = 3.8); [69].

Other studies have also supported the relationship between poor oral hygiene and increased risk of oral cancer. Less-than-daily brushing has been associated with an approximate twofold increased risk of tongue and other oral cancers in a Brazilian population [72], but no association was seen in a US study [73].

The frequent use of mouthwash has been discouraged due to the fact that several preparations contain ethanol. The association between mouthwash use and risk of oral or pharyngeal cancer has been the subject of previous studies with mixed results [74].

7.4.5.2 Dentures

A large Brazilian case-control study has demonstrated an association between oral sores from loosefitting dentures and risk of oral cancer. Brazilian study above these results and those relating hygiene to oral cancer may describe the role of chronic inflammation as a risk for oral cancer [75].

7.4.5.3 Oral Cancer in the UAE

A multicentre, retrospective study of oral biopsies was conducted in four hospitals in the UAE. Oral biopsy reports were retrieved from Tawam Hospital in Al Ain and Al Mafraq Hospital in Abu Dhabi. Data were taken from Tawam Hospital and Al Mafraq Hospital, and data from the Iranian and Al Baraha Hospitals in Dubai were also reviewed. Data recorded included age, sex, site of the lesion, clinical presentation, histological grade and information pertaining to neck dissections, if any. The distribution of the cases is shown in Table 7.6. A more detailed analysis was

Table 7.6 The distribution of the cases among various hospitals

Hospitals	Study years	Total no. of oral biopsies retrieved	Malignant lesions	OSCC
Tawam	2008–2011	223	74	60
Mafraq	2009–2012	248	21	17
Baraha	2005–2011	133	44	3
Iranian	2007–2010	388	8	23

Note: OSCC, oral squamous cell carcinoma [76]

Table 7.7 Distribution of the various histopathological diagnoses of malignant lesions in the UAE for the studied time periods

Diagnosis	Frequency	Percentage of malignant tumours (%)
Malignant neoplasms of epithelial origin		
Squamous cell carcinoma	103	70
Papillary carcinoma (variant)	8	5.4
Spindle cell carcinoma (variant)	2	1.4
Malignant melanoma	2	1.4
Total: 115		78.2
Malignant neoplasms of glandular origin		
Mucoepidermoid carcinoma	8	5.4
Adenoid cystic carcinoma	4	2.7
Adenocarcinoma	4	2.7
Malignant salivary gland tumour (type unspecified)	2	1.4
Clear cell carcinoma	1	0.7
Salivary duct carcinoma	1	0.7
Total: 20		13.6
Malignant neoplasms of mesenchymal origin		
Rhabdomyosarcoma	4	2.7
Ewing's sarcoma	2	1.4
B-cell lymphoma	2	1.4
Burkitt's lymphoma	2	1.4
Plasma cell tumour	2	1.4
Total: 12		8.3
Total	147	100

conducted for cases of OSCC diagnosed at the Mafraq and Tawam Hospitals. Cases of OSCC included all cancers of the oral cavity (i.e. those found on the lips, tongue, buccal mucosa, palate and other areas of the oral cavity).

Analysis of the records showed that the most prevalent malignant lesion was OSCC, followed by mucoepidermoid carcinoma of the salivary glands (Table 7.7). A total of 113 cases of OSCC were diagnosed, which makes up 77% of the total malignancies biopsied. Of the 77 cases of OSCC diagnosed at the Tawam and Mafraq Hospitals, 62 were found in males and 15 in females, which corresponds to a male-to-female (M:F) ratio of 4.13. The average age at diagnosis of OSCC was 54.9 years. The commonest site of diagnosis of OSCC was the tongue, followed by the buccal mucosa and lip. Of the lesions diagnosed as SCCs, 31.17% presented clinically as ulcers, followed by lumps (18.18%) and white lesions (3.9%). Well-differentiated OSCC is followed by moderately differentiated (20.8%) and poorly differentiated OSCC (6.5%) [76].

According to the World Health Organization, 2 in 100,000 people in the Middle East died of oral cancer in 2010. The number of cases was, however, lower than those reported in India and in the USA. People who are most vulnerable to the oral disease are heavy smokers and those that don't follow a healthy diet. Frequent exposure of the lip to direct sunlight is another contributing factor. The high prevalence of smoking, less than healthy diet and the lack of health awareness and promotion are all contributing factors that put people in the Middle East at great risk of oral cancer.

In the UAE oral cancer is not an uncommon disease. This could prove the need for more awareness campaigns, including screening procedures for early detection of cancerous lesions and other potentially malignant oral diseases.

The great challenge is the early detection of OC, which improves prognosis and quality of life. OC screening of high-risk population is needed to decrease the severity of disease at diagnosis or diagnose potentially malignant lesions before malignant transition occurs.

References

1. World Health Organization. The world cancer report 2013; 2013.
2. Parkin DM, Bray FI, Devesa SS. Cancer burden in the year 2000: the global picture. Eur J Cancer 2001;37:54–66.
3. Priebe LS, Aleksejuniene J, Dharamsi S, Zed C. Oral cancer and cultural factors in Asia. Evidence for practice. Can J Dent Hyg. 2008;42(6):291–5.
4. Ferlay J, Pisani P, Parkin DM. GLOBOCAN 2002: Cancer incidence, mortality and prevalence worldwide. IARC Cancer Base (2002 estimates). Lyon: IARC Press; 2004.
5. Chaturvedi KA, et al. Worldwide trends in incidence rates for oral cavity and oropharyngeal cancers. J Clin Oncol. 2013. doi:10.1200/JCO.2013.50.3870.
6. WHO. Strengthening the prevention of oral cancer: the WHO perspective. Community Dent Oral Epidemiol. 2005;33:397–9.
7. Johnson WN, Jayasekara P, Amarasinghe KH. Squamous cell carcinoma and precursor lesions of the oral cavity: epidemiology and aetiology. Periodontol. 2011. doi:10.1111/j.1600-0757.2011.00401.x.
8. Simmard PE, Torre AL, Jemal A. International trends in head and neck cancer incidence rates: differences by country, sex and anatomic site. Oral Oncol. 2014. doi:10.1016/j.oraloncology.2014.01.016.
9. CDC. Division of oral health, National Center for Chronic Disease Prevention and Health Promotion; 2013.
10. Bittar OT, Raranhos RL, Fornazari HD, Pereira CA. Epidemiological features of oral cancer – a world public health matter. RFO UPF. 2010;15(1):87–93.
11. Wunsch-Fiho V, De-Camargo A. The burden of mouth cancer in Latin America and the Caribbean: epidemiologic issues. Semin Oncol. 2001;28:158–68.

12. Losi-Guembarovski R, Paes de Menezes R, Polisel F, Chaves NV, Kuasne H, Leichsenring A, Maciel EM, Guembarovski LA, Oliveira WB, Ramos G, Mizuno TL, Cavalli JI, Riberiro MFE, Colus MSI. Oral carcinoma epidemiology in Paraná State, Southern Brazil. Cad Saúde Pública. 2009;25(2):393–400.
13. Cancer Research UK. Oral cancer incidence statistics; 2016.
14. Møller H, Brewster D. Lip, mouth and pharynx. In: Cancer atlas of the United Kingdom and Ireland; 2005. p. 129–38.
15. Bosetti C, Bertuccio P, Levi F, Lucchini F, Negri E, La-Vecchia C. Cancer mortality in the European Union, 1970–2003, with a joinpoint analysis. Ann Oncol. 2008;19:631–40.
16. Warnakulasuriya S. Global epidemiology of oral and oropharyngeal cancer. Oral Oncol. 2009;45:309–16.
17. Rao VKS, Mejia G, Roberts-Thomson K, Logan R. Epidemiology of oral cancer in Asia in the past decade – an update (2000–2012). Asian Pac J Cancer Prev. 2013;14(10):5567–77.
18. Parkin DM, Bray F, Ferlay J, Pisani P. Global cancer statistics, 2002. CA Cancer J Clin. 2005;55(2):74–108.
19. Su C-C, Yang H-F, Huang S-J, Lian I-B. Distinctive features of oral cancer in Changhua County: high incidence, buccal mucosa preponderance, a close relation to betel quid chewing habit. J Formos Med Assoc. 2007;106:225–33. doi:10.1016/S0929-6646(09)60244-8.
20. Khan UZ. An overview of oral cancer in Indian subcontinent and recommendations to decrease its incidence. WebmedCentral Cancer. 2012;3(8):WMC003626. doi:10.9754/journal.wmc.2012.003626.
21. Siddiqui QRP. Oral cancer: a new epidemic can be foreseen in Pakistan. Pakistan J Med Dent. 2013;2(01):1–2.
22. Zhang S-K, Zheng R, Chen Q, Zhang S, Sun X, Chen W. Oral cancer incidence and mortality in China, 2011. Chin J Cancer Res. 2015;27(1):44–51.
23. Boyle P, Levin B. World cancer report. Geneva: World Health Organization & International Agency for Research on cancer; 2008.
24. Cancer Research UK. CancerStats report – lip and oral cavity cancer. London: Cancer Research UK; 2008.
25. Khan MH, Naushad QN. Oral squamous cell carcinoma in a 10 year old boy. Mymensingh Med J. 2011;20:145–50.
26. Warnakulsuriya S, Tilakaratne MW. Oral medicine and pathology: a guide to diagnosis and management. Published by Jaypee Brothers Medical Publisher (P) Ltd.; 2014. ISBN: 978-93-5025-221-5.
27. Annertz K, Anderson H, Biorklund A, Moller T, Kantola S, Mork J, Olsen JH, Wennerberg J. Incidence and survival of squamous cell carcinoma of the tongue in Scandinavia, with special reference to young adults. Int J Cancer. 2002;101:95–9.
28. Myers JN, Elkins T, Roberts D, Byers RM. Squamous cell carcinoma of the tongue in young adults: increasing incidence and factors that predict treatment outcomes. Otolaryngol Head Neck Surg. 2000;122(1):44–51.
29. Neville WB, Day AT. Oral cancer and precancerous lesions. CA Cancer J Clin. 2002;52(4):195–215.
30. Vallecillo-Capilla M, Romero-Olid MN, Olmedo-Gaya MV, Reyes-Botella C, Bustos-Ruíz V. Factors related to survival from oral cancer in an Andalusian population sample (Spain). Med Oral Patol Oral Cir Bucal. 2007;12(7):E518–23.
31. Global Cancer Forum, White Papers. Group 1: Global burden of oral cavity and pharyngeal cancers.
32. Sugerman PB, Savage NW. Oral cancer in Australia: 1983–1996. Aust Dent J. 2002;47:45–56.
33. Ferlay J, Parkin DM, Steliarova-Foucher E. Estimates of cancer incidence and mortality in Europe in 2008. Eur J Cancer. 2010;46:765–81.
34. Warnakulasuriya S, Sutherland G, Scully C. Tobacco, oral cancer, and treatment of dependence. Oral Oncol. 2005;41:244–60.

35. Bhurgri Y. Cancer of the oral cavity – trends in Karachi south (1995–2002). Asian Pac J Cancer Prev. 2005;6:22–6.
36. Iype EM, Pandey M, Mathew A, Thomas G, Sebastian P, Nair MK. Squamous cell carcinoma of the tongue among young Indian adults. Neoplasia. 2001;3(4):273–7.
37. Franceschia S, Bidolia E, Herrerob E, Muñozb N. Comparison of cancers of the oral cavity and pharynx worldwide: etiological clues. Oral Oncol. 2000. doi:10.1016/S1368-8375(99)00070-6.
38. Chiang C-T, Hwang Y-H, Su C-C, Tsai KY, Lian IB, Yuan TH, Chang TK. Elucidating the underlying causes of oral cancer through spatial clustering in high-risk areas of Taiwan with a distinct gender ratio of incidence. Geospat Health. 2010;4(2):230–42.
39. Ho P-S, Ko Y-C, Yang Y-H, Shieh TY, Tsai CC. The incidence of oropharyngeal cancer in Taiwan: an endemic betel quid chewing area. J Oral Pathol Med. 2002;31:213–9. doi:10.1034/j.1600-0714.2002.310404.x.
40. Sultana N, Malik M. The overview of oral cancer and risk factors in Bangladesh. Int J Dent Sci Res. 2014;2(5A):8–10.
41. Idris AM, Ahmed HM, Mukthar BI, Gander AF, El-Beshir EI. Descriptive epidemiology of oral neoplasms in Sudan 1970–1985 and the role of toombak. Int J Cancer. 1995;61:155–8.
42. Gourin CG, Podolsky RH. Racial disparities in patients with head and neck squamous cell carcinoma. Laryngoscope. 2006;116:1093–106.
43. Jemal A, Tiwari RC, Murray T, Ghafoor A, Samuels A, Ward E. Cancer statistics, 2004. CA Cancer J Clin. 2004;54(1):8–29.
44. Rubin PH. Clinical oncology. A multidisciplinary approach to physicians and students. 7th ed. Philadelphia: Saunders; 1993.
45. Globocan 2012: Estimated cancer incidence, mortality and prevalence worldwide in 2012.
46. NIH Fact sheet (2013).
47. Garavello W, Bertuccio P, Levi F, Lucchini F, Bosetti C, Malvezzi M, Negri E, La-Vecchia C. The oral cancer epidemic in central and eastern Europe. Int J Cancer. 2009;127:160–71.
48. Dikshit R, Gupta PC, Ramasundarahettige C. Cancer mortality in India: a nationally representative survey. Lancet. 2012;379:1807–16.
49. Liu S-Y, Lu C-L, Chiou C-T, Yen C-Y, Liaw G-A, Chen Y-C, Liu Y-C, Chaing W-F. Surgical outcomes, prognostic factors of oral cancer associated with betel quid chewing, tobacco smoking in Taiwan. Oral Oncol. 2010;46:276–82. doi:10.1016/j.oraloncology.2010.01.008.
50. Sargeran K, Murtomaa H, Safavi SM, Vehkhalahti MM, Teronen O. Survival after diagnosis of cancer of the oral cavity. Br J Oral Maxillofac Surg. 2008;46:187–91. doi:10.1016/j.bjoms.2007.11.004.
51. Mager DL. Bacteria and cancer: cause, coincidence or cure? A review. J Transl Med. 2006;4:14. doi:10.1186/1479-5876-4-14.
52. Pisani P, Parkin DM, Munoz N, Ferlay J. Cancer and infection: estimates of the attributable fraction in 1990. Cancer Epidemiol Biomark Prev. 1997;6:387–400.
53. Crowe SE. Helicobacter infection, chronic inflammation, and the development of malignancy. Curr Opin Gastroenterol. 2005;1:32–8.
54. Vaishnavi C, Kochhar R, Singh G, Kumar S, Singh S, Singh K. Epidemiology of typhoid carriers among blood donors and patients with biliary, gastrointestinal and other related diseases. Microbiol Immunol. 2005;49:107–12.
55. Biarc J, Nguyen IS, Pini A, Gosse F, Richert S, Thierse D, Van DA, Leize-Wagner E, Raul F, Klein JP, Scholler-Guinard M. Carcinogenic properties of proteins with pro-inflammatory activity from *Streptococcus infantarius* (formerly *S. bovis*). Carcinogenesis. 2004;25:1477–84. doi:10.1093/carcin/bgh091.
56. Littman AJ, White E, Jackson LA, Thornquist MD, Gaydos CA, Goodman GE, Vaughan TL. Chlamydia pneumoniae infection and risk of lung cancer. Cancer Epidemiol Biomark Prev. 2004;13:1624–30.
57. Koyi H, Branden E, Gnarpe J, Gnarpe H, Steen B. An association between chronic infection with Chlamydia pneumoniae and lung cancer. A prospective 2-year study. APMIS. 2001;109:572–80. doi:10.1034/j.1600-0463.2001.d01-177.x.

58. Anttila T, Koskela P, Leinonen M, Laukkanen P, Hakulinen T, Lehtinen M, Pukkala E, Paavonen J, Saikku P. Chlamydia pneumoniae infection and the risk of female early-onset lung cancer. Int J Cancer. 2003;107:681–2. doi:10.1002/ijc.11353.
59. Noureen C, Pankaj C, Rushikesh D. The role of bacteria in oral cancer. Ind J Med Paediatr Oncol. 2010;31(4):126–31. doi:10.4103/0971-5851.76195.
60. Cawson RA. Leukoplakia and oral cancer. Proc R Soc Med. 1969;62:610–4.
61. Kuper H, Adami HO, Trichopoulos D. Infections as a major preventable cause of human cancer. J Intern Med. 2000;248:171–83. doi:10.1046/j.1365-2796.2000.00742.x.
62. Mork J, Lie AK, Glattre E, et al. Human papillomavirus infection as a risk factor for squamous-cell carcinoma of the head and neck. N Engl J Med. 2001;244:1125–31.
63. Holladay EB, Gerald WL. Viral gene detection in oral neoplasms using the polymerase chain reaction. Am J Clin Pathol. 1993;100:36–40.
64. Snijders PJF, Scholes AGM, Hart CA, et al. Prevalence of mucosa tropic human papillomaviruses in squamous cell carcinomas of the head and neck. Int J Cancer. 1996;66:464–9.
65. Smith EM, Hoffman H, Summersgill KS, et al. Human papillomavirus and risk of oral cancer. Laryngoscope. 1998;108:1098–103.
66. Maden C, Beckmann AM, Thomas DB. Human papillomaviruses, herpes simplex viruses, and the risk of oral cancer in men. Am J Epidemiol. 1992;135:1093–102.
67. Singh B, Balwally AN, Shaha AR, et al. Aerodigestive tract squamous cell carcinoma. The human immunodeficiency virus connection [published erratum appears in Arch Otolaryngol Head Neck Surg 1996;122(9):944]. Arch Otolaryngol Head Neck Surg. 1996;122:639–43.
68. Spitz MR, McPherson RS, Jiang H, et al. Correlates of mutagen sensitivity in patients with upper aerodigestive tract cancer. Cancer Epidemiol Biomark Prev. 1997;6:687–92.
69. Schildt EB, Eriksson M, Hardell L, Magnuson A. Oral infections and dental factors in relation to oral cancer: a Swedish case-control study. Eur J Cancer Prev. 1998;7:201–6.
70. Kassim KH, Daley TD. Herpes simplex virus type proteins in human oral squamous cell carcinoma. Oral Surg Oral Med Oral Pathol Oral Radiol Endod. 1988;65:445–8.
71. Maier H, Zoller J, Herrmann A, et al. Dental status and oral hygiene in patients with head and neck cancer. Otolaryngol Head Neck Surg. 1993;108:655–61.
72. Velly AM, Franco EL, Schlecht N, et al. Relationship between dental factors and risk of upper aerodigestive tract cancer. Oral Oncol. 1998;34:284–91.
73. Young TB, Ford CN, Brandenburg JH. An epidemiologic study of oral cancer in a statewide network. Am J Otolaryngol. 1986;7:200–8.
74. Mashberg A, Barsa P, Grossman ML. A study of the relationship between mouthwash use and oral and pharyngeal cancer. J Am Dent Assoc. 1985;110:731–4.
75. Marur S, D'Souza G, Westra WH, et al. HPV-associated head and neck cancer. A virus-related cancer epidemic. Lancet Oncol. 2010;11:781–9.
76. Anis R, Gaballah K. Oral cancer in the UAE: a multicenter, retrospective study. Libyan J Med. 2013;8. doi:10.3402/Ljm.V8i0.21782.

Oral Cancer and Chewing Habits

8

Shahid Pervez and Brooj Abro

8.1 Introduction

Oral cancer (OC) is becoming a growing concern worldwide, and its prevalence in the subcontinent and Southeast Asia is reaching epidemic proportions. It ranks as the 11th most common cancer worldwide, with an incidence of about 300,000 and mortality close to 145,000 in 2012 [1, 2]. Great majority of malignant neoplasms in the oral cavity are oral squamous cell carcinomas (OSCC). Other uncommon malignant tumors include tumors of minor salivary gland origin [3].

OC is often preceded by precursor and premalignant lesions in the oral cavity, which includes proliferative verrucous leukoplakia, dysplasia, oral submucous fibrosis (OSF), and lichen planus, among others [4]. The established risk factors shown by several studies are alcohol, cigarette smoking, and chewing of smokeless tobacco, betel quid, and other alternative chewing substances such as gutka, pan masala, and naswar (a mixture of sun-dried powdered tobacco, ash oil, lime, and flavoring agents).

In this chapter we will discuss the factors responsible for such a high risk of OC with particular reference to betel quid and alterative chewing substances which are widely prevalent in the Asian population.

8.2 Oral Cancer Statistics: Global Incidence, Prevalence, Mortality, and Survival

The incidence of OC is variable in different parts of the world due to unique lifestyles. The incidence is closely related to the trends of alcohol, tobacco, and betel nut use. According to data from Globocan 2012, the estimated age-standardized

S. Pervez (✉) • B. Abro
Section of Histopathology, Department of Pathology & Laboratory Medicine, Aga Khan University Hospital, Karachi, Pakistan
e-mail: shahid.pervez@aku.edu

A.-E. Al Moustafa (ed.), *Development of Oral Cancer*,
DOI 10.1007/978-3-319-48054-1_8

incidence rate (per 100,000) was 2.1% worldwide with mortality and 5-year prevalence rates of 1.8% and 2.2%, respectively.

Survival after diagnosis of OC depends on stage at diagnosis and availability of treatment. In the USA and UK, the overall 5-year survival is about 65% and 50%, respectively [5, 6]. In India, Pakistan, and China, the survival is between 35 and 55% [7, 8].

8.3 Epidemiology in Asia: A Region with High Burden of Oral Cancer

In WHO Southeast Asia Region (SEARO), oral cavity and lip cancer has the highest incidence and prevalence when compared to other regions. It is the third most common cancer among men and sixth most common among women. Overall, in this region it is the fifth most common cancer, with an estimated age-standardized incidence rate of 6%, mortality rate of 5.6%, and 5-year prevalence rate of 5.5% (Globocan 2012).

The highest incidence rates have been seen in Papua New Guinea, Maldives, Sri Lanka, Bangladesh, Pakistan, and India, with incidence rates ranging from 7.2 per 100,000 per annum in India to 25.0 per 100,000 reported in Papua New Guinea [1]. A study from Karachi, Pakistan, reported a rising incidence of OC. The study showed an exponential increase in OC cases in the last two decades, i.e., from 15.6 per 100,000 cases in 1995–2007 to 27.8 per 100,000 in 2003–2007 in males surpassing lung cancer as the most common cancer. Similar trend was observed in females where it progressed from 14.9 per 100,000 to 25.3 per 100,000 as the second most common cancer after breast cancer [9].

8.4 Risk Factors

To reduce the burden of this devastating disease, it is important to understand the contributing risk factors. Depending on the geographic location, risk factors may vary. The most common in Europe, North America, and Latin America are smoking and alcohol. Many studies conducted in Asia have demonstrated other factors to play a more important role in this region, such as chewing of smokeless tobacco and/or betel quid [10]. OC predominantly seems to occur in populations with lower socioeconomic status [11]. Other risk factors include infection with human papillomavirus (HPV), diet, and oral hygiene, among others.

8.4.1 Betel Quid and Tobacco Chewing

Betel quid is a compound of several substances, including betel leaf (*Piper betle*), fruit/nut of the areca palm (*Areca catechu*), and lime (calcium hydroxide). Areca nut is however the most important component and is known to be the fourth most widely used stimulant, after nicotine, ethanol, and caffeine [12].

Around the world, estimates show about 600 million people use betel quid in some form [4]. These users are predominantly concentrated in the Indo-Pakistan subcontinent, South and Southeast Asian countries, islands in the Pacific, and immigrant population in Africa, Europe, and North America [13].

The contents and preparations of betel quid may vary in different parts of the world. It may be chewed with and without tobacco. Other substances added to it are usually for flavor such as saffron, cloves, cardamom, sweeteners, turmeric, mustard, and other spices. In 1996, a workshop for consensus was held in Malaysia and defined the term "quid" as "a substance, or mixture of substances, placed in the mouth or chewed and remaining in contact with the mucosa, usually containing one or both of the two basic ingredients, tobacco and/or areca nut, in raw or any manufactured or processed form" [14].

The origin of betel quid usage may be traced back to Southeast Asia, most likely Malaysia, which has a province named Penang, meaning "island of the areca nut palm" [15]. Practices related to betel usage have been described in China and India (subcontinent) since more than two millennia ago. From ancient times, it has also been a part of India's traditional medicine, Ayurveda [16].

8.4.1.1 Preparations of Chewing Products and Geographic Prevalence of Usage

According to *IARC Monographs on the Evaluation of Carcinogenic Risks to Humans* (2004), volume 85, a chewing substance may primarily consist of:

1. Areca nut alone
2. Smokeless tobacco, chewed without areca nut
3. Areca combined with components of betel vine and other ingredients except tobacco
4. Areca combined with components of betel vine and other ingredients including tobacco

Betel quid is known to be used in various forms in several countries including Pakistan, India, Sri Lanka, Bangladesh, Malaysia, Thailand, Cambodia, China, Indonesia, Papua New Guinea, Pacific Islands, and migrant populations in South Africa and Eastern Africa, the UK, North America, and Australia [17]. About 20–40% of the population in India, Pakistan, and Nepal are betel quid chewers since the past 2–3 decades.

In India, betel quid is commonly prepared by crushing the areca nut, shredding it, and then garnishing with lime and certain spices and finally wrapped in the betel leaf [18]. In Papua New Guinea, the lime is applied separately at the commissure of the mouth by betel quid chewers [19]. Figure 8.1 shows a preparation of betel quid known as "paan" in Karachi, Pakistan, and the crushed form or areca nut used in commercial packaged products of betel. In South Central Asia (India, Pakistan, and Bangladesh), tobacco is commonly added to betel quid, whereas in some other countries such as Papua New Guinea, China, and Taiwan, betel is chewed without tobacco.

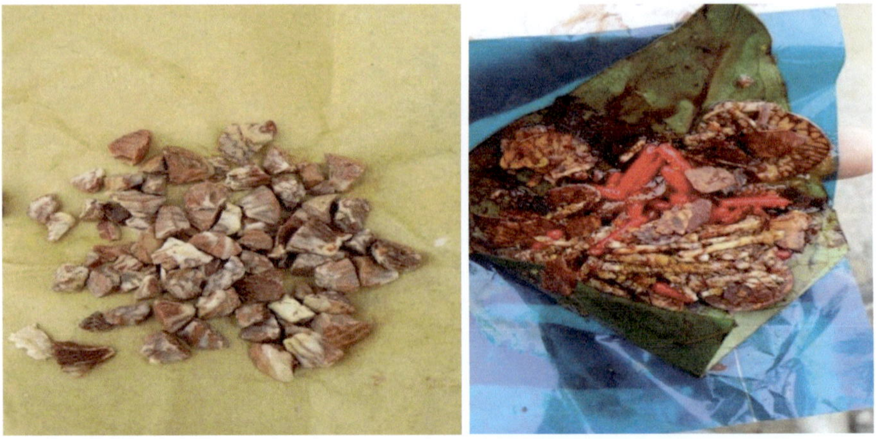

Fig. 8.1 *Right image*: a preparation of betel nut made in Karachi, Pakistan. It is placed on betel leaf combined with sweeteners and other spices, known as "paan" by the local population. *Left*: crushed areca nut used in several betel quid products in Southeast Asia (pictures taken at a local pan shop in Karachi, Pakistan)

A large Asian betel quid consortium study was conducted in 2009 [20] which revealed significant cultural and demographic differences in practice and patterns of betel quid use in six Asian countries: Nepal, Sri Lanka, Malaysia, Mainland China, Taiwan, and Indonesia. The results of the study showed higher lifetime chewing rates in men (16–44%) compared to women (2–35%) in population from Taiwan, Mainland China, Nepal, and Sri Lanka, whereas in Malaysia and Indonesia, the prevalence in women (32–48%) was much higher than in men (15–31%). In the latter, betel quid was also more common among older women (about 50% chewers were women >40 years old), and conversely in China, chewing was more prevalent in the younger male population (32% were <41 years old). The highest daily betel quid quantity used by both men and women was found in Taiwan (16–20 quids per day). People who chewed tobacco-added quid were found to chew more frequently compared to ones who used tobacco-free quid.

In regard to spitting out betel juice after chewing, population from Taiwan, Malaysia, Indonesia, and Sri Lanka were more inclined to follow this practice, whereas in Mainland China and Nepal the juice was swallowed instead.

8.4.1.2 Cultural Significance: Accounting for Widespread Use

In about 20% of the human population, betel chewing is an integral part of the cultural practices in their society [16]. Habitual users can chew betel throughout the day, and some mothers may even give their infants pre-masticated quids [21]. Betel is also known for its ceremonial significance. It is commonly given to guests at joyous occasions such as weddings. Since the practice of quid chewing is culturally well accepted, its use is common among all strata of society.

Unlike cigarette smoking and alcohol drinking, people usually do not associate betel quid with serious health consequences [22, 23]. This lack of awareness opens the gateway for tobacco manufacturers to sell tobacco in this form without any regulations.

8.4.1.3 Pan Masala and Gutka: Betel Quid Alternative Products

Pan masala and gutka are mixtures of the components of betel quid but do not contain betel leaf. They are packaged and marketed as betel quid alternatives [24]. The betel leaf itself is known to have anticarcinogenic activity [25]. A study identified the specific effects of betel leaf extract against tobacco carcinogens using mice subjects [26]. The absence of betel leaf in these products possibly enhances the genotoxic effect of areca nut and tobacco components.

These preparations are packaged in forms that are long lasting and easy to store. Gutka contains areca nut, catechu, slaked lime, condiments, and powdered tobacco in a dry form. Pan masala is similar to gutka except that it does not contain tobacco. Figure 8.2 shows gutka prepared at a local shop in Karachi, Pakistan. Both these products have been aggressively advertised since their arrival in market in the 1960s and 1970s. With their emergence, the Indian market for areca nut experienced a massive growth with increased sale of products worldwide [24].

Specific epidemiologic data pertaining to their use is not yet available; however the prevalent use of these products can be assessed by the value of the Indian market for pan and gutka which was estimated to be several hundred million US dollars [27]. Gutka is marketed through many different brands and exported to about 22 countries worldwide [28]. In Southeast Asia, studies show that gutka has an increasing demand and is frequently sold to even minors in this region [29, 30].

The packaged forms are colorful, with added sweeteners to enhance the taste. These forms have attracted children's attention over the years. Surveys conducted in India have shown that about 13–50% students chew pan masala and gutka regularly [31]. Two studies conducted in Karachi, Pakistan, showed widespread use of gutka.

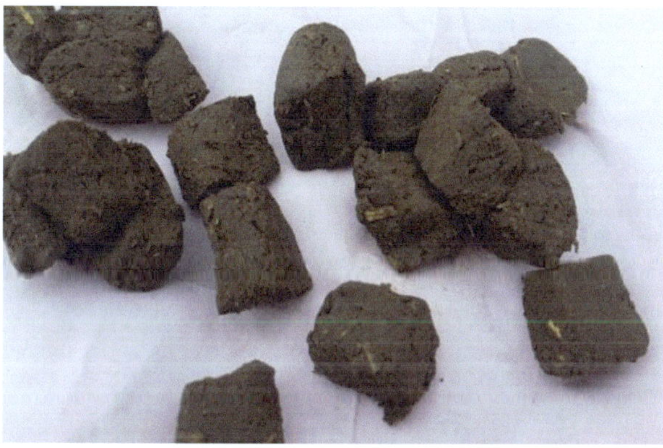

Fig. 8.2 The image is showing a dry powdered form of areca nut and tobacco mixed together with other ingredients to make gutka (picture taken from a local shop in Karachi, Pakistan)

One reported that 46% of the population of a community in Karachi were habitually using gutka [32]. The second study investigated its use in patients visiting a local health-care center, and the results showed 35% of patients were using gutka [33]. In 2010, a report was published which reviewed literature between 1956 and 2009 on gutka usage and associated oral disorders [34]. Three studies included in this review reported a significant association of habitual gutka usage with periodontal inflammation which included conditions like gingivitis, gingival recession, and periodontal pockets. Seven studies supported the evidence that OSF was more common in gutka chewers when compared to those who did not chew tobacco, and one reported that OC was more prevalent in gutka users when compared to nonusers [35].

8.4.1.4 Carcinogenesis

There is significant evidence that supports the carcinogenic potential of the areca nut and smokeless tobacco. The IARC monographs have classified betel quid both with and without tobacco as carcinogenic to humans [4]. A recent meta-analysis that reviewed 50 reports published between 1933 and 2013 further supports the evidence that betel quid is a significant independent risk factor for cancers of the oral cavity and oropharynx [36]. This study also identified the dose-response relationship, showing an increasing risk of OC with an increasing duration and frequency of betel quid chewing.

The precise biochemical pathways that lead to the development of precancerous and cancerous lesions due to betel quid chewing have not yet been well understood. Figure 8.3 is illustrating the role of different contents of betel in carcinogenesis. The

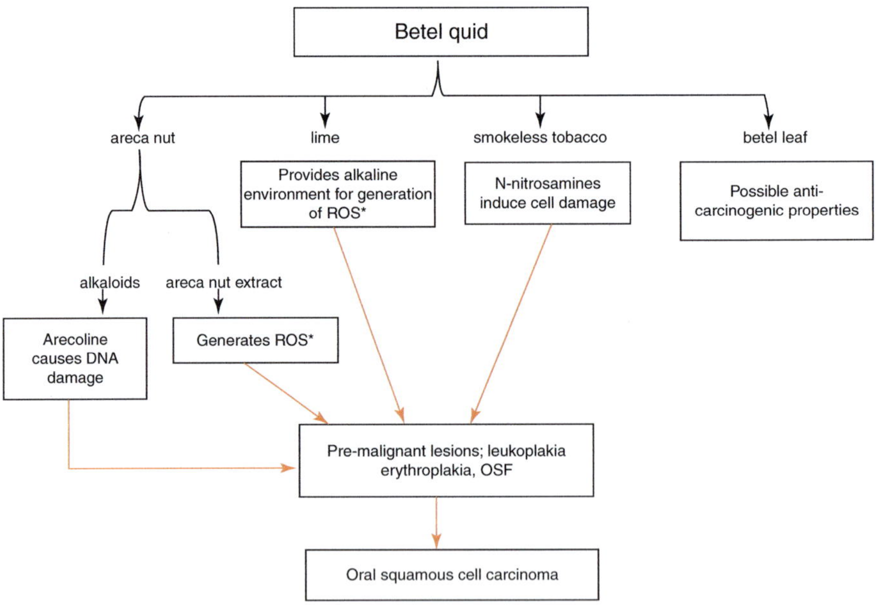

Fig. 8.3 This figure is illustrating the potential pathways for pathogenesis of OC caused by betel quid contents. *ROS = reactive oxygen species

carcinogenicity of chemicals in betel quid has been demonstrated by several animal studies [37–39] and experiments on cultured human cells [40, 41]. Areca nut extract (ANE) exposure to cultured human oral mucosal epithelial cells and fibroblasts has shown that it is cytotoxic and genotoxic to living cells with long-term exposure [42]. This study also showed that exposure to ANE results in generation of reactive oxygen species, genetic damage, and micronuclei formation. Arecoline, the major alkaloid in areca nut, is considered an important carcinogen [43]. It can induce certain changes in different types of cells; these changes observed in experimental studies include structural chromosomal aberrations, micronuclei formation, and sister chromatid exchanges [44, 45].

8.4.1.5 Oral Manifestations

Discoloration of teeth and mucosa: The betel quid juice produced after chewing is bright red in color and can cause staining of teeth and mucosa after prolonged exposure. The staining may range from red-yellow to black depending on years of exposure. The darkening effect is known to be caused by polymers of orthoquinones [46, 47].

Mechanical trauma: The hard consistency of areca nut can cause tooth abrasions, fractures, and damage to oral mucosa. Teeth frequently lose their enamel exposing the dentine which may increase sensitivity [48]. Root fractures have been observed in long-term areca nut chewers [48].

Oral mucosal lesions: It has been shown by various epidemiologic studies that quid chewing containing areca nut and/or tobacco is a significant risk factor for developing oral lesions such as leukoplakia [49], erythroplakia [50], OSF [51], and OSCC [43].

8.4.1.6 Betel Chewer's Mucosa

Studies have demonstrated the presence of this condition in long-term chewers of quid [52]. The area in direct contact with the quid shows certain changes, tendency of the mucosa to desquamate, and the incorporation of betel quid ingredients in the mucosa. The underlying tissue may be observed in the form of yellow or reddish-brown encrusted areas [53].

8.4.1.7 Betel Quid Lichenoid Lesion

This condition has similarities to oral lichen planus and has been identified exclusively in betel quid chewers [54]. It is characterized by the presence of white, wavy lines that are parallel to each other, that may radiate from a central erythematous lesion and appear flat on the mucosal surface [55]. This condition should be recognized as a separate entity since the course of betel quid lichenoid lesion is different from that of lichen planus as identified by interventional studies. This lesion may regress and even completely resolve on cessation of betel chewing [14].

8.4.1.8 Potentially Premalignant Disorders (PMDs): Leukoplakia, Erythroplakia, and OSF

Leukoplakia is a white patch or plaque on the oral mucosa which cannot be defined by any other disease or condition and is usually associated with tobacco and betel nut chewing [56, 57]. Leukoplakia can be homogenous or nonhomogenous. The extent of epithelial dysplasia indicates its malignant potential. There is an increased potential for the nonhomogenous types, speckled, verrucous, and nodular to transform into malignancy [58]. A 10-year prospective cohort study in India reported that about 70% cases of OC were preceded by leukoplakia [53].

Erythroplakia has been defined by WHO as "any lesion of the oral mucosa that presents as bright red velvety plaques which cannot be clinically or pathologically classified as any other recognizable condition." It has been considered the most severe premalignant lesion due to its high potential to transform into malignancy [59]. It may co-occur with leukoplakia, a condition known as erythroleukoplakia. A case-control study suggested that tobacco chewing and alcohol drinking combined with low intake of fruits and vegetables are strong risk factors for erythroplakia [50].

Oral submucous fibrosis (OSF) is a chronic progressive condition of the oral cavity which leads to stiffness, ulceration, and in later stages inability to open the mouth due to fibrotic changes. This condition was first described by Pindborg and Sirsat [60] in 1996 as a gradual, chronic premalignant disease of the oral cavity that may extend into the pharynx [61]. The 10-year cohort study in India reported a 7.6% transformation rate of OSF to malignancy [53]. Betel nut and tobacco chewing is proven to be an important risk factor in the development of OSF [62–64]. The areca nut component, arecoline, has been implicated in the pathogenesis of OSF. It has been postulated that arecoline stimulates fibroblast proliferation and also decreases breakdown of collagen, playing an important role in fibrous tissue formation [65].

8.4.1.9 Oral Squamous Cell Carcinoma (OSCC)

OSCC is the most common among cancers of the head and neck. In India and other parts of Southeast Asia, it is the fifth most common malignancy [66]. Ample data is available since historic times that shows the potential of betel quid and tobacco chewing in the development of OSCC [67–69]. A recent meta-analysis reported increasing risk of OC with increasing duration and frequency of quid chewing. The buccal mucosa and cheek were identified as the most common involved sites for development of OSCC in populations that chewed quid with added tobacco [70]. Figure 8.4 is showing two patients with extensive OSCC involving the cheek and tongue.

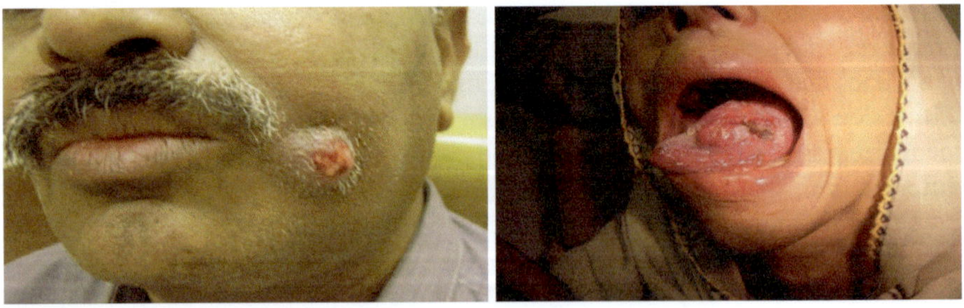

Fig. 8.4 *Right*: photo of SCC affecting the left lateral border of the tongue. *Left*: extensive SCC T4 lesion of the cheek involving the deep as well as superficial tissue (photos taken with patients' consent)

8.4.1.10 Systemic Effects and Addictive Potential

"They are always chewing Arecca, a certain Fruit like a Pear, cut in quarters and rolled up in leaves of a Tree called Bettre (or Vettele), like Bay leaves; which having chewed they spit forth. It makes the mouth red. A meta-analysis published in 2013, reviewed 17 Asian studies, that were published between 1951 and 2013 with data relevant to systemic effects of betel quid [71].

Above is an ancient writing about the practice of betel quid chewing. The last line highlights the addictive potential of areca nut. Betel nut chewing has been known to cause addiction in frequent users, and discontinuation can lead to withdrawal symptoms [72]. This association was also reported by a study that used DSM IV and ICD-10 criteria to show evidence of dependence in betel quid chewers even when used without tobacco [73]. Nicotine has already been proven to have significant addictive potential, and when combined with areca nut, the chances of dependence are much higher. This is one of the reasons it is quite challenging to convince chewers to discontinue its use despite the harmful effects.

The hazards of betel quid are not limited to the oral cavity. A meta-analysis published in 2013 reviewed 17 Asian studies (between 1951 and 2013) relevant to systemic effects of betel quid. The review concluded that betel consumption was associated with diverse health consequences including obesity, diabetes, metabolic syndrome, cardiovascular disease, and increase in all-cause mortality [74].

8.4.2 Tobacco Smoking and Alcohol Consumption

Both tobacco smoking and alcohol drinking have been independently associated with increased risk of cancer [75, 76]. Tobacco smoking in any form can increase the risk of OC by twofold to tenfold [75]. Alcohol was found to increase the risk of OC twofold to sixfold with the risk directly proportional to the quantity and duration of consumption [76]. Use of both tobacco and alcohol has a synergistic effect and substantially increases the risk of cancer [77].

The carcinogenic potential of tobacco has been identified, and there are several chemical constituents in it that play a role. The most important of them are tobacco-specific N-nitrosamines, N-nitrosonornicotine, and 4-(methylnitrosamino)-1-(3-pyridyl)-1-butanone [78].

Alcohol exerts its carcinogenic effects by both direct damage to individual cells and systemic effects. The chemicals in it are directly toxic to cell membranes and can alter membrane permeability and damage cell organelles. Systemic effects include nutritional deficiency, immunological deficiency, and, with chronic use, altered liver function [77].

8.4.3 Human Papillomavirus (HPV)

HPV is a small, non-envelope, epitheliotropic DNA virus which belongs to the Papovaviridae family of viruses. There are several different strains of this virus, some of them have been identified as having low malignant potential (HPV 6, 11,

42, 43, and 44) and others having moderate to high malignant potential (HPV 16, 18, 31, 33, 35, 39, 45, 51, 52, 56, 58, 65, 66) [79]. The IARC classified the high-risk types 16 and 18 as carcinogenic to humans [80]. These high-risk types are known to alter tumor suppressor genes including the p53 and retinoblastoma gene [81]. 30 to 65% of all head and neck cancers and 50–80% of all cancers arising in the oropharynx are HPV positive [82, 83]. The first evidence of HPV's contribution in OSCC was presented in 1977 [84], and since then numerous studies including reviews and meta-analyses have documented its prevalence in head and neck cancer including OSCC [85–87]. It has been suggested that most of the population with HPV-positive cancer are younger than those with tobacco- or alcohol-associated head and neck cancers, and also these younger patients may not have any other identifiable risk factors [88].

In reports from India, HPV 16 was identified in 27% of OC cases in the northern part of the country and about 25–31% of OC cases in Western India [89]. The presence of this high-risk HPV subtype in cases of HPV-positive OSCC supports the role of HPV in the multifactor pathogenesis of this cancer. A study conducted in Karachi, Pakistan, at our institute also showed an association of high-risk HPV, particularly HPV 16 in OSCC [79]. A systemic review evaluated the prevalence of HPV and its subtypes in different anatomical subsites of head and neck. It revealed that HPV prevalence was highest in oropharyngeal cancer (35.6%, 95% CI 32.6–38.7) followed by laryngeal cancers (24%, 95% CI 21.8–26.3) and lower in oral cavity malignant lesions (23.5%, 95% CI 21.9–25.1). Type 16 was detected in 86.7% of HPV-positive oropharyngeal cancers and 68.2% of HPV-positive OC. The prevalence of HPV was found to be almost equal in Asia (46.3%) and North America (47.0%) and lower in Europe (28.2%) [86]. The presence of high-risk HPV in head and neck cancer, particularly oropharyngeal cancer, is a double-edged sword. On one hand it is implicated in carcinogenesis, while on the other hand, HPV-positive cancers show good prognosis and increased survival. A recent review stated that HPV-positive head and neck cancer had a better 2-year and 5-year survival when compared to HPV-negative cancers, the reason being an overall better response of HPV-positive cancers to treatment [90].

8.4.4 Socioeconomic Status (SES)

A meta-analysis published in 2008 reviewed previous studies to establish an association between OC risk and SES. It included 41 case-control studies from around the world and identified low SES as a risk factor for OC in both high- and lower-income countries. When compared to population belonging to high SES strata, the pooled ORs for risk of developing OC were 1.85 (95% CI 1.60, 2.15; n = 37 studies) for those with low educational attainment, 1.84 (1.47, 2.31; n = 14) for those with low occupational social class, and 2.41 (1.59, 3.65; n = 5) for those with low income [91]. This data is useful for public health policy makers to focus screening and preventive measures against OC in the lower SES population.

8.4.5 Diet

Approximately 30% of cancers in Western countries have been associated with dietary factors [92]. In developing countries it is estimated to account for about 20% of malignancies [93]. A case-control study in the UK revealed that a diet deficient in fruits and vegetables is an important risk factor for OC in young individuals [94]. Another study from Kerala, India, showed that BMI was inversely related to risk of leukoplakia (p value 0.007) [95]. A meta-analysis published in 2006 estimated that each portion of fruit or vegetable consumed per day can reduce the risk of OC by 50% [96].

Some interventional studies have also provided useful insights into the role of diet and nutrition in development and progression of premalignant lesions and OC. An open-ended trial in Pakistan was conducted to see the effect of micronutrient supplementation in 117 patients with OSF. Significant improvement in symptoms, notably intolerance to spicy food, burning sensation, and mouth opening, was observed at the end (1–3 years) [97]. In a double-blind placebo trial conducted in Kerala, India, the supplementation of beta-carotene for 12 months resulted in regression of leukoplakia in one third of the study subjects [98]. This data provides substantial evidence that diet rich in fruits and vegetables can be a protective factor against development of oral cancer.

8.4.6 Oral Hygiene

Poor dentition and lack of good oral hygiene have been found to have some association with developing OC [99, 100]; however these factors are confounded by the presence of alcohol and tobacco use and not clearly indicated as an independent risk factor. Poor oral hygiene may contribute to increased exposure of carcinogen in individuals already exposed to other risk factors; hence this might just be a risk factor in high-risk individuals.

8.5 Primary Prevention

OC is largely induced by modifiable risk factors [101]. Primary prevention strategies aim at limiting the use of the major risk factors: tobacco, alcohol, and betel nut chewing. Several steps were taken to reduce the habit of tobacco smoking, and the practice has been socially discouraged. Cigarette manufacturers are required to put mandatory warnings on the products before selling, and media played a vital role to spread awareness regarding health effects of tobacco smoke. This led to a decrease in the practice of tobacco smoking. Similar steps need to be taken for betel quid. It is a challenging task due to the sociocultural importance of betel products. A joint effort by governments, public health organizations, law-enforcing agencies, physicians, and the community itself is required to have the maximum impact. In India the government has taken steps to ban the manufacturing and selling of pan masala and gutka. In 2002, the state of Maharashtra imposed a ban on these products, and a recommendation has been made to the government of India by the Central Committee on Food Safety to ban it nationwide. Special considerations need to be made to stop use of these products in the younger population. They are more vulnerable to long-term use after getting addicted to this product at a younger age. More is known about harms of alcohol and tobacco when compared to knowledge pertaining to risks of betel nut chewing in the general population. In the USA, the FDA has imposed an import alert on unsafe food additives. In 1976, the US government announced a ban on interstate traffic of betel nut. Many products of betel sold in several countries do not have any written warnings about the health hazards associated with it. Media and health campaigns can play an important role in creating more awareness about the health risks of betel [102].

8.6 Secondary Prevention: Screening Methods

When primary prevention fails, early detection of lesions can potentially provide survival benefit. The 5-year survival for early localized disease is more than 80%. It decreases to about 20% for cancers extending beyond oral cavity and involving lymph nodes [76]. Identification and treatment of cancer at early stage can also result in better outcomes after surgery and improved quality of life. There are certain issues that need to be taken into account before a screening method can be implemented: the cost-effectiveness and resource allocation, the availability of treatment options after diagnosis of a potentially malignant disorder (PMD), and the possible outcomes and unnecessary workup in case of false positives. Visual screening method has been widely tested for its sensitivity and specificity and involves examination of the oral cavity through visual inspection under adequate light and palpation to look for signs for any potentially premalignant or malignant disorder [76]. A Cochrane review published in 2013 stated, "using the conventional oral examination for screening for PMD and OC has a variable degree of sensitivity (greater than 0.70 in six studies) and a consistently high value for specificity (greater than 0.90 in eight studies)" [103]. The review suggested that compared to other methods, visual screening was the best option. There are studies to support the benefits of screening in high-risk groups. The detection of premalignant lesions can also be used to discourage further use of the causative agent. In a cluster-randomized control trial in Kerala, India, consisting of four cycles for a period of 15 years, a reduction of 24% mortality was identified among high-risk groups (alcohol and tobacco users) [104]. The American Dental Association (ADA) recommended that clinicians look for signs of premalignant lesions or early-stage cancer of the oral cavity while performing routine visual screening, particularly in those who use tobacco, alcohol, or both. The ADA also stated that the lifesaving benefits of early detection of treatable lesions outweigh the harms incurred by false positives [105].

Conclusion

OC is largely a preventable disease. The pathogenesis is strongly associated with chemicals from tobacco, alcohol, and betel quid. Practice of tobacco smoking has been discouraged, and a similar mind-set is needed to reduce the habit of quid, tobacco, and gutka chewing. Many individuals are unaware of the consequences and continue this habit for years. These products have several chemicals that are involved in causing cell damage and subsequent development of premalignant disorders which may transform into frank OSCC. Another important factor that has been emerging in younger population is HPV. The high-risk type 16 has been well documented in many cases. In cervical cancer it is a well-established risk factor and known to spread from sexual contact. HPV vaccine has shown to decrease incidence in cervical cancer and widely used for its prevention in sexually active individuals. A similar approach is being investigated to prevent HPV-positive OSCC. Oral hygiene and diet may play an important role in high-risk individuals. A diet poor in vegetables and fruits and lack of oral hygiene can potentiate the carcinogenic effects of alcohol, tobacco, and betel nut. We can therefore conclude that avoiding frequent use of these agents combined with maintaining a healthy nutritious diet can prevent majority of OCs.

References

1. Bray F, Ren JS, Masuyer E, Ferlay J. Global estimates of cancer prevalence for 27 sites in the adult population in 2008. Int J Cancer. 2013;132(5):1133–45. doi:10.1002/ijc.27711. Epub 2012 Jul 26
2. Ferlay J, Soerjomataram I, Dikshit R, Eser S, Mathers C, Rebelo M, Parkin DM, Forman D, Bray F. Cancer incidence and mortality worldwide: sources, methods and major patterns in GLOBOCAN 2012. Int J Cancer. 2015;136(5):E359–86. doi:10.1002/ijc.29210. Epub 2014 Oct 9
3. Krishna Rao SV, Mejia G, Roberts-Thomson K, Logan R. Epidemiology of oral cancer in Asia in the past decade – an update (2000–2012). Asian Pac J Cancer Prev. 2013;14(10): 5567–77.
4. IARC. IARC monographs on the evaluation of carcinogenic risks to humans, volume 85: Betel quid and areca nut derived nitrosamines. Lyon: IARC; 2004.
5. Howlader N, Ries LA, Mariotto AB, Reichman ME, Ruhl J, Cronin KA. Improved estimates of cancer-specific survival rates from population-based data. J Natl Cancer Inst. 2010;102(20):1584–98. doi:10.1093/jnci/djq366. Epub 2010 Oct 11
6. Sant M, Allemani C, Santaquilani M, Knijn A, Marchesi F, Capocaccia R, EUROCARE Working Group. EUROCARE-4. Survival of cancer patients diagnosed in 1995–1999. Results and commentary. Eur J Cancer. 2009;45(6):931–91. doi:10.1016/j.ejca.2008.11.018. Epub 2009 Jan 24
7. Sankaranarayanan R, Swaminathan R, Jayant K, Brenner H. An overview of cancer survival in Africa, Asia, the Caribbean and Central America: the case for investment in cancer health services. IARC Sci Publ. 2011;162:257–91.
8. Sankaranarayanan R, Swaminathan R, Brenner H, et al. Cancer survival in Africa, Asia, and Central America: a population-based study. Lancet Oncol. 2010;11(2):165–73. doi:10.1016/S1470-2045(09)70335-3. Epub 2009 Dec 10
9. Bhurgri Y, Bhurgri A, Usman A, Pervez S, Kayani N, Bashir I, Ahmed R, Hasan SH. Epidemiological review of head and neck cancers in Karachi. Asian Pac J Cancer Prev. 2006;7(2):195–200.
10. Radoï L, Luce D. A review of risk factors for oral cavity cancer: the importance of a standardized case definition. Community Dent Oral Epidemiol. 2013;41:97–109.
11. Johnson NW, Warnakulasuriya S, Gupta PC, Dimba E, Chindia M, et al. Global oral health inequalities in incidence and outcomes for oral cancer: causes and solutions. Adv Dent Res. 2011;23(2):237–46.

12. Marshall M. An overview of drugs in oceania. In: Lindstorm L, editor. Drugs in Western Pacific societies: relations of substance. Association for Social Anthropology in Oceania Monograph 11. Lanham: University Press of America; 1987. p. 15–21.
13. Boucher BJ, Mannan N. Metabolic effects of the consumption of Areca catechu. Addict Biol. 2002;7:103–10.
14. Zain RB, Ikeda N, Gupta PC, Warnakulasuriya S, van Wyk CW, Shrestha P, Axéll T. Oral mucosal lesions associated with betel quid, areca nut and tobacco chewing habits: consensus from a workshop held in Kuala Lumpur, Malaysia, November 25–27, 1996. J Oral Pathol Med. 1999;28(1):1–4. Review
15. Gardner S, Sidisunthorn P, Ee L. Heritage trees of Penang. Penang: Areca Books; 2011. p. 206. ISBN 978-967-57190-6-6.
16. Norton SA. Betel: consumption and consequences. J Am Acad Dermatol. 1998;1:38.
17. Gupta PC, Warnakulasuriya KAAS. Global epidemiology of areca nut use. Addict Biol. 2002;7:77–83.
18. Raghavan V, Baruah HK. Arecanut: India's popular masticatory history, chemistry and utilization. Econ Bot. 1958;12:315–45.
19. Pindborg JJ, Murthi PR, Bhonsle RB, Gupta PC. Global aspects of tobacco use and its implications for oral health. In: Gupta PC, Hamner J III, Murti P, editors. Control of tobacco-related cancers and other disease. Proceedings of an international symposium; 1990 Jan 15–19. Mumbai: Oxford University Press; 1992. p. 13–23.
20. Lee CH, Ko AM, Warnakulasuriya S, Yin BL, et al. Intercountry prevalence and practices of betel-quid use in south, southeast and eastern Asia regions and associated oral pre-neoplastic disorders: an international collaborative study by Asian betel-quid consortium of south and east Asia. Int J Cancer. 2011;129(7):1741–51. doi:10.1002/ijc.25809. Epub 2011 Mar 8
21. Talonu NT. Observations on betel nut use, habituation, addiction and carcinogenesis in Papua New Guineans. P N G Med J. 1989;32:195–7.
22. Chandra PS, Mullah U. Areca nut: the hidden Indian 'gateway' to future tobacco use and oral cancers among youth. Indian J Med Sci. 2007;61(6):319–21.
23. Amarasinghe HK, Usgodaarachchi US, Johnson NW, Lalloo R, Warnakulasuriya S. Public awareness of oral cancer, of oral potentially malignant disorders and of their risk factors in some rural populations in Sri Lanka. Community Dent Oral Epidemiol. 2010;38:540–8.
24. Nair U, Bartsch H, Nair J. Alert for an epidemic of oral cancer due to use of the betel quid substitutes, gutka and pan masala: a review of agents and causative mechanisms. Mutagenesis. 2004;19(4). UK Environmental Mutagen Society.
25. Amonkar AJ, Padma PR, Bhide SV. Protective effect of hydroxychavicol, a phenolic component of betel leaf, against the tobacco-specific carcinogens. Mutat Res. 1989;210(2): 249–53.
26. Padma PR, Lalitha VS, Amonkar AJ, Bhide SV. Anticarcinogenic effect of betel leaf extract against tobacco carcinogens. Cancer Lett. 1989;45(3):195–202.
27. Gupta PC. Gutka: a major new tobacco hazard in India. Tob Control. 1999;8(2):134.
28. Mahapatra S, Kamath R, Shetty BK, Binu VS. Risk of oral cancer associated with gutka and other tobacco products: a hospital-based case control study. J Cancer Res Ther. 2015;11(1): 199–203.
29. Gupta PC. Mouth cancer in India: a new epidemic? J Indian Med Assoc. 1999;97:370–3.
30. Dongre A, Deshmukh P, Murali N, Garg B. Tobacco consumption among adolescents in rural Wardha: where and how tobacco control should focus its attention? Indian J Cancer. 2008;45:100–6.
31. Gupta PC, Ray CS. Smokeless tobacco and health in India and South Asia. Respirology. 2003;8(4):419–31.
32. Javed F, Altamash M, Klinge B, Engstrom PE. Peridontal conditions and oral symptoms in gutka-chewers with and without type 2 diabetes. Acta Odontol Scand. 2008;66: 268–73.
33. Ali NS, Khuwaja AK, Ali T, Hameed R. Smokeless tobacco use among adult patients who visited family practice clinics in Karachi, Pakistan. J Oral Pathol Med. 2009;66:268–73.

34. Javed F, et al. Oral mucosal disorders associated with the habitual gutka usage: a review. Oral Surg Oral Med Oral Pathol Oral Radiol Endod. 2010;109:857–64.
35. Gangane N, Chawla S, Anshu, Gupta SS, Sharma S. Reassessment of risk factors for oral cancer. Asian Pac J Cancer Prev. 2007;8:243–8.
36. Guha N, Warnakulasuriya S, Vlaanderen J, Straif K. Betel quid chewing and the risk of oral and oropharyngeal cancers: a meta-analysis with implications for cancer control. Int J Cancer. 2014;135(6):1433–43. doi:10.1002/ijc.28643. Epub 2014 May 14
37. Bhide SV, Shivapurkar NM, Gothoskar SV, Ranadive KJ. Carcinogenicity of betel quid ingredients: feeding mice with aqueous extract and the polyphenolic fraction of betel nut. Br J Cancer. 1979;40:922–6.
38. Ranadive KJ, Gothoskar SV, Rao AR, Tezabwalla BU, Ambaye RY. Experimental studies on betel nut and tobacco carcinogenicity. Int J Cancer. 1989;43:728–32.
39. Surki K, Goldman HM, Wells H. Carcinogenic effect of a dimethyl sulphoxide extract of betel nut on the mucosa of the hamster buccal pouch. Nature. 1971;230:383–4.
40. Wary KK, Sharan RN. Cytotoxic and cytostatic effects of arecoline and sodium nitrite on human cells in vitro. Int J Cancer. 1991;47:396–400.
41. Wary KK, Sharan RN. Aqueous extract of betel-nut of Northeastern India induces DNA strand breaks and enhances rate of cell proliferation in vitro. J Cancer Res Clin Oncol. 1988;114:579–82.
42. Lai KC, Lee TC. Genetic damage in cultured human keratinocytes stressed by long term exposure to areca nut extracts. Mutat Res. 2006;599:66–75.
43. Chen YJ, Chang JT, Liao CT, Wang HM, Yen TC, Chiu CC, Lu YC, Li HF, Cheng AJ. Head and neck cancer in the betel quid chewing area: recent advances in molecular carcinogenesis. Cancer Sci. 2008;99(8):1507–14. doi:10.1111/j.1349-7006.2008.00863.x.
44. Jeng JH, Chang MC, Hahn LJ. Role of areca nut in betel quid associated chemical carcinogenesis: current awareness and future perspectives. Oral Oncol. 2001;37:477–92.
45. Shirname LP, Menon MM, Nair J, Bhide SV. Correlation of mutagenicity and tumorigenicity of betel quid and its ingredients. Nutr Cancer. 1983;5:87–91.
46. Mathew AG. Formation of red color on chewing areca nut with slaked lime. J Food Sci Technol. 1971;8:140–2.
47. Reichart PA, Lenz H, Becker J, Mohr U. The black layer on the teeth of betel quid chewers: a light microscopic, micro-radiographic and electron microscopic study. J Oral Pathol. 1985;14:466–75.
48. Yeh CJ. Fatigue root fracture: a spontaneous root fracture non-endodontically treated teeth. Br Dent J. 1997;182:261–6.
49. Thomas SJ, Harris R, Ness AR, Taulo J, Maclennan R, Howes N, Bain CJ. Betel quid not containing tobacco and oral leukoplakia: A report on across-sectional study in Papua New Guinea and a meta-analysis of current evidence. Int J Cancer. 2008;123:1871–6.
50. Hashibe M, Mathew B, Kuruvilla B, Thomas G, Sankaranarayanan R, Maxwell Parkin D, Zhang Z-F. Chewing tobacco, alcohol, and the risk of erythroplakia. Cancer Epidemiol Biomark Prev. 2000;9:639–45.
51. Tilakaratne WM, Klinikowski MF, Saku T, Peters TJ, Warnakulasuriya S. Oral submucous fibrosis: review on etiology and pathogenesis. Oral Oncol. 2006;42:561–8.
52. Reichart PA, Schmidtberg W, Scheifele CH. Betel chewers mucosa in elderly Cambodian women. J Oral Pathol Med. 1996;25:367–70.
53. Gupta PC, Mehta FS, Dk D, Pindborg JJ, Bhonsle RB, Jalanwalla PN, et al. Incidence of oral cancer and natural history of oral pre-cancerous lesions in a 10year follow-up study of Indian villagers. Community Dent Oral Epidemiol. 1980;8:283–333.
54. Daftary DK, Bhonsle RB, Murti RB, Pindborg JJ, Mehta FS. An oral lichen planus-like lesion in Indian betel-tobacco chewers. Scand J Dent Res. 1980;88:244–9.
55. Anand R, Dhingra C, Prasad S, Menon I. Review article: betel nut chewing and its deleterious effects on oral cavity. J Cancer Res Ther. 2014;10(3):499–505.
56. Thomas SJ, Harris R, Ness AR, Taulo J, Maclennan R, Howes N, Bain CJ. Betel quid not containing tobacco and oral leukoplakia: Areport on a cross-sectional study in Papua New Guinea and a meta-analysis of current evidence. Int J Cancer. 2008;123:1871–4.

57. Lee CH, Ko YC, Huang HL, Chao YY, Tsai CC, Shieh TY, et al. The pre-cancer risk of betel quid chewing, tobacco use, and alcohol consumption in oral leukoplakia in aborgines of Taiwan. J Oral Pathol Med. 2001;30:213–9.
58. Walker DM, Boey G, Mcdonald LA. The pathology of oral cancer. Pathology. 2003;35:376–83.
59. Bouquot JE, Ephros H. Erythroplakia: the dangerous red mucosa. Prac Peridontics Aesthet Dent. 1995;6:9–17.
60. Pindborg JJ, Sirsat SM. Oral submucous fibrosis. Oral Surg Oral Med Oral Pathol. 1966;22:764–79.
61. Chung CH, Yang YH, Wang TY, Shieh TY, Warnakulasuriya S. Oral pre-cancerous disorders associated with areca quid chewing, smoking and alcohol drinking in southern Taiwan. J Oral Pathol Med. 2005;34:460–6.
62. Yang YH, Lien YC, Ho PS, Chen CH, Chang JS, Cheng TC, et al. The effects of chewing areca/betel quid with and without cigarette smoking on oral submucous fibrosis and oral mucosal lesions. Oral Dis. 2005;11:88–94.
63. Arakeri G, Brennan PA. Oral submucous fibrosis: an overview of the etiology, pathogenesis, classification, and principles of management. Br J Oral Maxillofac Surg. 2013;51:587–93.
64. Haider SM, Merchant AT, Fikree FF, Rahbar MH. Clinical and functional staging of oral submucous fibrosis. Br J Oral Maxillofac Surg. 2000;38:12–5.
65. Gupta MK, Mhaske S, Ragavendra R, Imtiaz. Oral submucous fibrosis- current concepts in etiopathogenesis. People's J Sci Res. 2008;1:39–44.
66. Jhonson NW. A global view of the epidemiology of oral cancer. Cambridge: Cambridge University Press; 1991. p. 3–326.
67. Orr IM. Oral cancer in betel chewers in Travancore, it's etiology, pathology and treatment. Lancet. 1933;2:575–80.
68. Fells A. Cance of the mouth in Southern India. A summary of 1700 cases. Br Med J. 1908;37:414.
69. Tobacco habits other than smoking; betel quid and areca nut chewing; and some related nitrosamines. IARC working group. Lyon, 23–30 October 1984. IARC Monogr Eval Carcinog Risk Chem Hum. 1985;37:1–268.
70. Gupta B, Johnson NW. Systematic review and meta-analysis of association of smokeless tobacco and of betel quid without tobacco with incidence of oral cancer in South Asia and the Pacific. PLoS One. 2014;9(11):e113385. doi:10.1371/journal.pone.0113385.
71. Burnell AC, Yule HA. In: Crooke W, editor. Hobson-Jobson: a glossary of colloquial Anglo Indian words; 1903.
72. Winstock AR, Trivedy CR, Warnakulasuriya KAAS, Peters TJ. A dependency syndrome related to areca nut use: some medical and psychological aspects among areca nut users in the UK. Addict Biol. 2000;5:173–9.
73. Benegal V, Rajkumar RP, Muralidharan K. Does areca nut use lead to dependence? Drug Alcohol Depend. 2008;97(1–2):114–21.
74. Yamada T, Hara K, Kadowaki T. Chewing betel quid and risk of metabolic disease, cardiovascular disease, and all-cause mortality: a meta-analysis. PLOS ONE. 2013;8(8):e70679.
75. IARC. IARC monographs on the evaluation of carcinogenic risks to humans, Volume 83: Tobacco smoke and involuntary smoking. Lyon: IARC; 2004.
76. IARC. IARC monographs on the evaluation of carcinogenic risks to humans, volume 96: Alcohol consumption and ethyl carbonate. Lyon: IARC; 2010.
77. Sankaranarayanan R, Ramadas K, Amarasinghe H, Subramanian S, Jhonson N. Cancer: disease control priorities, Third Edition (Volume 3). Washington: The International Bank for Reconstruction and Development/The World Bank; 2015. Chapter 5
78. IARC. IARC monographs on the evaluation of carcinogenic risks to humans, volume 89: Smokeless tobacco and some tobacco-specific N-Nitrosamines. Lyon: IARC; 2007.
79. Ali SMA, Awan MS, Ghaffar S, Salahuddin I, Khan S, Mehraj V, Pervez S. Human Papillomavirus infection in oral squamous cell carcinoma: correlation with histologic variables and survival outcome in a high risk population. Oral Surg. 2008;1(2):96–105. ISSN 1752-2441

80. IARC. IARC monographs on the evaluation of carcinogenic risks to humans, volume 64: Papillomavirus. Lyon: IARC; 1995.
81. Werness BA, Levine AJ, Howley PM. Association of human papillomavirus type 16 and 18 E6 proteins with p53. Science. 1990;248:76–9.
82. Chaturvedi AK, Engels EA, Anderson WF, Gillison ML. Incidence trends for human papillomavirus-related and -unrelated oral squamous cell carcinomas in the United States. J Clin Oncol. 2008;26(4):612–9.
83. Ang KK, Harris J, Wheeler R, Weber R, Rosenthal DI, Nguyen-Tân PF, Westra WH, Chung CH, Jordan RC, Lu C, Kim H, Axelrod R, Silverman CC, Redmond KP, Gillison ML. Human papillomavirus and survival of patients with oropharyngeal cancer. N Engl J Med. 2010;363(1):24–35.
84. Zur Hausen H. Human papillomavirus and their possible role in squamous cell carcinomas. Curr Top Microbiol Immunol. 1977;78:1–30.
85. Franceschi S, Munoz N, Bosch XF, Snijders PJ, Walboomers JM. Human papillomavirus and cancers of the upper aerodigestive tract: a review of epidemiological and experimental evidence. Cancer Epidemiol Biomark Prev. 1996;5:567–75.
86. Kreimer AR, Clifford GM, Boyle P, Franceschi S. Human papillomavirus types in head and neck squamous cell carcinomas worldwide: a systematic review. Cancer Epidemiol Biomark Prev. 2005;14:467–75.
87. Termine N, Panzarella V, Falaschini S, Russo A, Matranga D, Lo ML, et al. HPV in oral squamous cell carcinoma vs head and neck squamous cell carcinoma biopsies: a meta-analysis (1988–2007). Ann Oncol. 2008;19:1681–90.
88. Deschler DG, Richmon JD, Khariwala SS, Ferris RL, Wang MB. The "new" head and neck cancer patient-young, nonsmoker, nondrinker, and HPV positive: evaluation. Otolaryngol Head Neck Surg. 2014;151(3):375–80.
89. Shukla S, Bharti AC, Mahata S, et al. infection of human papillomavirus in cancers of different human organ sites. Indian J Med Res. 2009;130:222–33.
90. Young D, Xiao CC, Murphy B, Moore M, Fakhry C, Day TA. Increase in head and neck cancer in younger patients due to human papillomavirus (HPV). Oral Oncol. 2015;51(8):727–30. doi:10.1016/j.oraloncology.2015.03.015. Epub 2015 Jun 9
91. Conway DI, Petticrew M, Marlborough H, Berthiller J, Hashibe M, Macpherson LMD. Socioeconomic inequalities and oral cancer risk: a systematic review and meta-analysis of case-control studies. Int J Cancer. 2008;122:2811–9.
92. Stewart BW, Kleihues P. The cause of: cancer in world cancer report. Lyon: IARC Press; 2003. p. 62–5.
93. Key TJ, Schatzkin A, Willett WC, Allen NE, Spencer EA, Travis RC. Diet, nutrition and the prevention of cancer. Public Health Nutr. 2004;7(1A):187–200.
94. Llewellyn CD, Linklater K, Bell J, Johnson NW, Warnakulasuriya S. An analysis of risk factors for oral cancer in young people: a case-control study. Oral Oncol. 2004;40:304–13.
95. Hashibe M, Sankaranarayanan R, Thomas G, et al. Alcohol drinking, body mass index and the risk of oral leukoplakia in an Indian population. Int J Cancer. 2000;88:129–34.
96. Pavia M, Pileggi C, Nobile CG, Angelillo IF. Association between fruit and vegetable consumption and oral cancer: a meta-analysis of observational studies. Am J Clin Nutr. 2006;83:1126–34.
97. Maher R, Aga P, Johnson NW, Sankaranarayanan R, Warnakulasuriya S. Evaluation of multiple micronutrient supplementation in the management of oral submucous fibrosis in Karachi, Pakistan. Nutr Cancer. 1997;27:41–7.
98. Sankaranarayanan R, Mathew B, Varghese C, et al. Chemoprevention of oral leukoplakia with vitamin A and beta carotene: an assessment. Oral Oncol. 1997;33:231–6.
99. Zheng TZ, Boyle P, Hu HF, et al. Dentition, oral hygiene and risk of oral cancer: a case control study in Beijing, Peoples Republic of China. Cancer Causes Control. 1990;1:235–41.
100. Marshall JR, Graham S, Haughey BP, et al. Smoking, alcohol, dentition and epidemiology of oral cancer. Eur J Cancer B Oral Oncol. 1992;28B:9–15.

101. World Health Organization. Control of oral cancer in developing countries. Bull World Health Org. 1984;62:817–30.
102. IARC. International Agency for Research on Cancer (IARC) – Summaries & evaluations: betel-quid and areca-nut chewing. IARC monograph evaluating carcinogenic risk from chemicals to humans, volume 85. Lyon: IARC; 2004. p. 39.
103. Walsh T, Liu JL, Brocklehurst P, Glenny AM, Lingen M, Kerr AR, Ogden G, Warnakulasuriya S, Scully C. Clinical assessment to screen for the detection of oral cavity cancer and potentially malignant disorders in apparently healthy adults. Cochrane Database Syst Rev. 2013;11:CD010173. doi:10.1002/14651858.CD010173.pub2.
104. Subramanian S, Sankaranarayanan R, Bapat B, Somanathan T, Thomas G, Matthew B, et al. Cost-effectiveness of oral cancer screening: results from a cluster randomized controlled trial in India. Bull World Health Organ. 2009;87(3):200–6.
105. Rethman MP, Carpenter W, Cohen EE, et al. Evidence-based clinical recommendations regarding screening for oral squamous cell carcinomas. J Am Dent Assoc. 2010;141(5): 509–20.

Role of Qat Chewing and Mate Consumption in Human Oral Carcinogenesis

9

Amal Kassab and Ala-Eddin Al Moustafa

9.1 Introduction

Oral and oropharyngeal (base of tongue and tonsillar) cancer are a part of the head and neck (HN) cancer group, which includes malignancies of the oral cavity, larynx, hypopharynx, oropharynx, and nasopharynx, with over 50% of these cancer cases arising in the oral cavity [1]. Oral and oropharyngeal cancer together represent the sixth most common cancer worldwide with an estimate of 300,000 new cancer cases in 2012 and approximately 145,000 deaths worldwide [2]. Survival rate of this malignancy is still around 50–60%, which is mostly due to high recurrence rate and the delay in diagnosis which is attributed to the visual similarity between benign and cancerous oral lesions at its early stages [3].

As the oral cavity represents one of the intake orifices of the human body, it is vulnerable for environmental and external pollutants. Thus, naturally the most important risk factors related to oral and oropharyngeal cancers are oral hygiene [4], tobacco use [5], betel quid chewing [6], and excessive alcohol [7], Qat [8], and mate consumption [9], in addition to bacteria/virus infections such as HPV and EBV [10] as well as *H. pylori* [11]. Vulnerability of oral cancer to environmental conditions has resulted in interesting observations over the past two decades, as reduction of smoking caused a slight decrease in oral cancer cases, followed by an increase in oropharyngeal cancer, particularly in men, which can be attributed to HPV and EBV infections; this was associated with a slow decrease in the age median for HN

A. Kassab
Concordia University, Montreal, QC, Canada

A.-E. Al Moustafa (✉)
College of Medicine & Biomedical Research Centre, Qatar University, Doha, Qatar

Oncology Department, McGill University, Montreal, QC, Canada

Syrian Research Cancer Centre of the Syrian Society Against Cancer, Aleppo, Syria
e-mail: aalmoustafa@qu.edu.qa; ala-eddin.almoustafa@mcgill.ca

A.-E. Al Moustafa (ed.), *Development of Oral Cancer*,
DOI 10.1007/978-3-319-48054-1_9

cancer diagnosis from 60 years, with more cases being detected in less than 40-year-old patients [12].

In general, management modalities of this cancer involve surgery followed by chemo-/radiotherapy, which is known to badly affect the quality of life of patients due to the resulting complications in basic daily actions such as chewing, swallowing, and speaking [12]. Therefore, given the complexities associated with this malignancy, it is obvious that preventive strategies to reduce the number of cancer cases or limit their aggressiveness represent a valid and an important avenue to fight this cancer.

Among the various risk factors of oral carcinogenesis is the excessive use of Qat and mate; both are herbal pastime products that are heavily used in certain regions of the world. These two substances have been associated with higher incidence of oral cancers, and due to immigration, their use is becoming more popular in different areas of the world. Therefore, it is important to understand how these products effect malignancies of the oral cavity and/or stimulate carcinogenesis in order to be able to draw a successful prevention campaign and reduce their adverse effects on human health.

This chapter is dedicated to these two risk factors (Qat and mate), their chemical composition, distribution, toxicity, and relation with oral cancer.

9.2 Qat and Oral Cancer

The scientific name of Qat is *Catha edulis*, but it is also known as khat, chat, jaad, qaad, miraa, and mirungi due to its spread in several African and Asian countries. This evergreen shrub or tree is a member of the Celastraceae family (Fig. 9.1a) and is found mostly in East and South Africa, the Arabian Peninsula, and particularly in Yemen; it is also found sporadically in Afghanistan, Israel, Syria, and Turkistan. Recently this shrub has been found in North America and Europe, particularly among immigrants and refugees from countries where the use of this plant is common, mainly Somalia, Ethiopia, and Yemen [13].

Historically, the use of this plant as a medicinal substance dates back to ancient Ethiopians and Egyptians, who associated it with the gods and considered it a "divine food" [14]. This is mainly due to the chemical composition of the plant that contains alkaloids of the phenylpropylamine type, in particular the two psychoactive components: cathinone and cathine. These two substances affect the two main neurochemical pathways, dopamine and noradrenalin, which give an effect similar to amphetamine [13]. Therefore, chewing Qat leaves increases alertness, suppresses the appetite, and induces a feeling of euphoria. Apart from these two main components, Qat leaves also contain about 40 alkaloids, glycosides, tannins, terpenoids, fatty acids, and five flavonoids, in addition to small amounts of ethereal oil, sterols, and triterpenes [15]. However, since the most important component of Qat leaves, cathinone, is unstable and oxidizes at room temperature within a few days of harvesting, the plant is consumed fresh, soon after it is picked up as it loses its potency

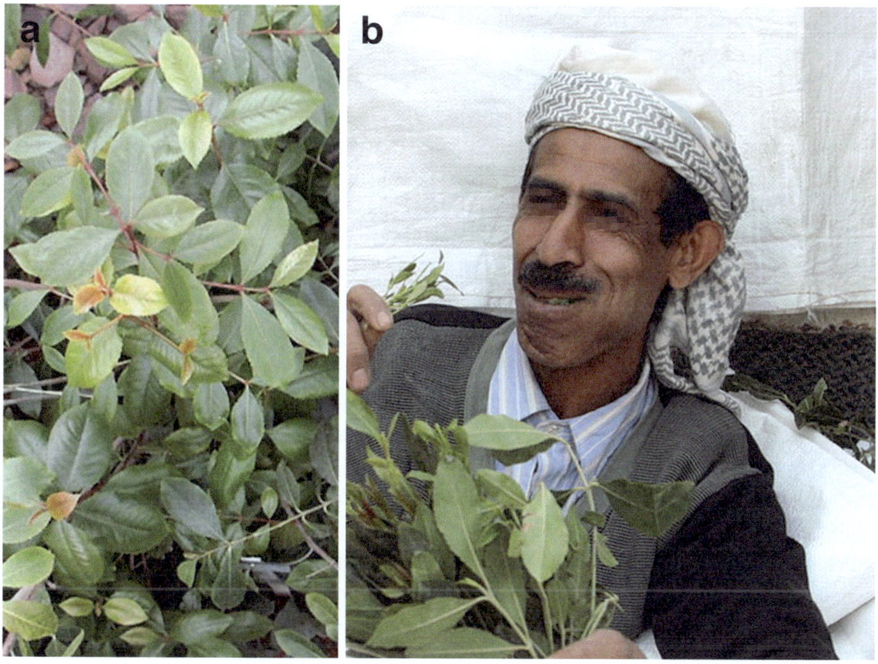

Fig. 9.1 (**a**) The Qat shrub that is common in Yemen. (**b**) The mode of raw Qat consumption by chewing and making a bolus of the plant that is preserved for hours on one side of the oral cavity

within 36 h. In 1980, the World Health Organization classified Qat as a drug of abuse that can cause mild to moderate degrees of psychological dependency but to a lesser extent than tobacco and alcohol [16]. In 2006, an estimate of 78% of males and 53% of females in Yemen chew Qat, while in Ethiopia 40% of men and 18% of women use this substance [17], and approximately one third of Somali communities in the UK also chew Qat on regular basis [18].

Qat is consumed by chewing fresh leaves and stems of the plant; the chewed fresh leaves are then stuffed into the inner cheek of one side of the mouth using the tongue (Fig. 9.2b). Chewing then continues slowly squeezing the juice of the plant while simultaneously consuming more leaves. Thus, Qat chewers form a bulge in their cheek where the Qat bolus is kept during consumption; one session usually lasts for several hours, a process that causes a drying effect on the oral mucosa and therefore is often supplemented with nonalcoholic fluid consumption and, in some cases, is accompanied with tobacco smoking.

Regular use of Qat is associated with rise of blood pressure and pulse rate, in addition to periodontal pocket formation, gingivitis, loose teeth, xerostomia, liver damage, and cardiac disease [19, 20]. Once Qat-induced stimulation is over, usually within 3 h, a depressive state follows with side effects that include insomnia, gastric disorders, depression, and anorexia [19]. Although psychotic reactions are far less in Qat users compared with amphetamine addicts, however, paranoid delusions are known to happen. Nevertheless, Qat use is generally not associated with long-term dependence like other stimulants.

Based on the mode of consumption, it is estimated that almost 90% of the alkaloid content of Qat that is extracted during the chewing session is absorbed through the oral mucosa [21], exposing the tissue to high levels of toxins. Accordingly, 20–50% [22–26] of Qat users suffer from oral mucosal keratosis, or keratotic white lesions, on the side where the Qat bolus is kept, which is identified as a precancerous lesion that can potentially develop into oral cancer. Additionally, further indication of possible Qat involvement in oral carcinogenesis is implied by the studies that associate Qat use with the genotoxic effects it has on the buccal epithelial cells among Qat chewers, which appears to be dose-related [26, 27].

In general, studies on the relation between Qat chewing and oral cancer are scarce but represent a useful base for future investigations into this risk factor. Few retrospective cohort studies were conducted in Saudi Arabia and Yemen. One large study that included 300 males (150 Qat chewers and a control group of non-chewers) in Yemen [28] found that 4% of Qat chewers had atypical cytological changes, while 16% had hyperkeratosis in the buccal mucosa, none of these hitches were observed in non-chewers; therefore the study concluded that Qat chewing is a risk factor for cytological atypia and hyperkeratosis in the buccal mucosa which are seen in premalignant or malignant oral lesions. Also, based on a study by Kassie et al. [29], Qat consumption, especially when accompanied by alcohol and tobacco use, might be a potential cause of oral malignancy. This result was based on a micronucleus test to determine the genetic damage in buccal and bladder mucosa cells of Qat consumers (20 subjects) in comparison with a control group of nonusers (10 subjects); in addition, Qat/cigarette/alcohol users (25 subjects) were compared with a group that consumed only tobacco/alcohol (25 subjects) and a control group that did not consume any of these drugs (25 subjects). They noted eightfold increase in micronucleated buccal mucosa cells among Qat consumers. However, in the second study, the compounded effect of Qat, tobacco, and alcohol was found to be additive, since the frequency of buccal mucosa cells with micronucleus was higher in the first group than those consuming only alcohol and tobacco.

Additionally, a cross-sectional study in Yemen was conducted on a group of 162 women, 67% of whom were Qat chewers [30]. It was observed that among Qat chewers, 75.2% had white lesions on the chewing side of the oral cavity, while 5.5% also presented with white lesions on the opposite side; additionally 13.2% of non-chewers had white lesions too. The study correlated the duration of Qat chewing and water-pipe and cigarette smoking with the appearance of white lesions and concluded that Qat chewing duration was highly significant as opposed to water-pipe and cigarette smoking. This result was confirmed in another cross-sectional study [23], where 490 (75.4%) Qat chewers from Yemen were examined; the author reported that white patches on the buccal or gingival mucosa were found in 94.7% of Qat chewers at the chewing site and in 8% of non-chewers. Also noted were red patches on the buccal and gingival mucosa in 3.8% of Qat chewers compared to none in the control group. Surprisingly, even though 60% of Qat chewers also used water pipe or cigarette, nevertheless when the data was stratified by tobacco use, the association between Qat chewing and white patches on oral mucosa was exclusive, particularly since these only manifested at the chewing site, instead of appearing anywhere at the oral cavity. Similarly, such results were confirmed in several other studies as well. Qat chewing was linked with leukoplakia, as it was observed on the chewing side in 83% of Qat chewers in comparison with 16% of non-chewers regardless whether the chewers also smoked [31]. Qat was also linked with hyper-orthokeratosis (12%), hyperparakeratosis (67%), and epithelial dysplasia (30%) which all appeared on the chewing side of Qat users [32].

These studies indicate clearly that Qat use is associated with several oral conditions, namely, hyperkeratosis in the buccal mucosa, leukoplakia, hyperorthokeratosis, hyperparakeratosis, and epithelial dysplasia. Several of these conditions are considered premalignant that can develop into oral malignancy with the help of another risk factor such as oncoviruses (HPV and EBV) or onco-bacteria (*H. pylori*). Nevertheless, it is worth noting that these lesions are concentrated on the side where the Qat bolus is kept for the entire duration of the chewing session, lasting typically for several hours a day (3–5 h), which suggests that the way Qat is consumed is far more concerning than the herb itself, not to mention that these studies cannot foresee additional toxic factors such as the effect of pesticides and insecticides on the oral cavity of chewers. Thus, in order to isolate the effect of Qat on normal oral cells, some studies were conducted to identify the effect of organic Qat extract on oral fibroblast and keratinocyte (epithelial) cells.

It was shown by Lukandu et al. that organic Qat extract can induce tumor suppressor proteins and G1 cell cycle arrest in normal human oral fibroblast (NOF) and normal human oral keratinocytes (NOK) cells [33]. Additionally, Qat extract inhibit the proliferation of both cell types in a dose- and time-dependent manner. It also increases the expression of p53 protein after 24 h. In NOK cells Qat extract increases p16 significantly and causes morphological changes. On the other hand, in NOF cells there was an increase in the expression of p21 accompanied by growth inhibition of these cells. Finally, the study suggested a possible effect of Qat on p38 MAP kinase pathways, due to the premature differentiation of NOK cells. The authors have continued their investigation in the kinetics of the events leading the Qat-induced cell death; their study revealed that within half an hour to an hour of exposure to Qat, NOK and NOF cells exhibited a decrease in the mitochondrial inner transmembrane potential which preceded all other biochemical and morphological changes [34]. Therefore, the authors believe that the apoptosis-inducing factor was released from mitochondria into cytosol until it reached the nucleus. Qat-associated cell death was also attributed to the activation of a family of cysteine proteases called caspases (caspase-1, caspase-3, and caspase-8) in human leukemia cells. This apoptotic cell death that took place within 8 h of exposure was partially reversed after removal of Qat as the effect was dependent on de novo protein synthesis. This was confirmed as cell death was blocked by a pan-caspase inhibitor Z-VAD-fmk (8×10^{-7} M) and submicromolar concentrations of Z-YVAD-fmk (2×10^{-7} M) and Z-IETD-fmk (8×10^{-7} M) which are inhibitors of caspase-1 and caspase-8, respectively [34, 35]. Although these results are very interesting, nevertheless the exact role of Qat extract on cell differentiation and cancer progression is yet to be defined, particularly in junction with other risk factors.

So far, studies on the effect of Qat on oral carcinogenesis have been mostly conducted in Yemen, most of which concentrate on the compounded effect of Qat chewing combined with tobacco or water-pipe smoking or shamma (tobacco leaves) chewing [22–30]. One important criticism for this method is that it fails to isolate other important risk factors such as oral hygiene routines or more significantly the possible cross contamination with pesticides; this is particularly important since several studies indicate the use of banned products such as DDT in several African and Asian countries including Yemen [36]; additionally, the recommended concentration of pesticide is often not respected, neither the harvest wait period of pesticide use [37–40]. Luckily there have been few studies that took this factor into consideration. Al-Akwa et al. examined the association between Qat chewing and the level of free radicals [41]. This comparative study between 20 chronic Qat chewers and an age-matched control group of 20 non-chewers showed clearly that Qat consumption inhibited serum free radical scavenging enzymes that lead to significant increase in free radical loads. However, acetylcholinesterase serum was significantly inhibited in the Qat chewing group which indicates the exposure of Qat chewers to carbamate and organophosphate insecticides that makes them vulnerable against oral cancer. Nevertheless, the effect of Qat itself on the inhibition of critical antioxidant enzymes and free radical scavenger proteins by reactive oxygen and nitrogen species might also be a leading cause of lower total serum antioxidant capacity [41].

In conclusion, given the various secondary factors associated with Qat chewing that might contribute to the effects observed in the oral cavity of Qat chewers in general, such as pesticide toxicity, the effect of mechanical friction during chewing that can be aggravated by the long duration and direct contact of the herb to oral cavity tissues [13], in addition to the need to corroborate the epidemiological studies conducted so far in various other countries where Qat chewing is common; it is obvious that more experimental data are necessary to elucidate the exact role of Qat extract and how this might interact with other factors to induce neoplastic transformation and consequently cancer formation, particularly in the oral cavity.

9.3 Mate Drinking and Its Role in Oral Carcinogenesis

Mate, also known as yerba maté, maté, Jesuit's tea, chimarrão, or Paraguayan tea, is a brewed hot herbal beverage that comes from the dried leaves of the *Ilex paraguariensis* perennial tree (Fig. 9.2a). Mate is a very common beverage in several countries in South America (in particular Argentina, Bolivia, Brazil, Chile, Ecuador, Paraguay, and Uruguay); however, its use has spread to several other countries in the Mediterranean such as Syria, Lebanon, and Northern Israel, in addition to Germany [9]. It is often drunk out of a straw-like metal called bombilla, as shown in Fig. 9.2b; dried leaves are packed inside the cup and hot water is poured over them; this process is repeated several times without changing the dried leaves with as much as 1 L of water. However, it is important to keep in mind that this herbal tea is not

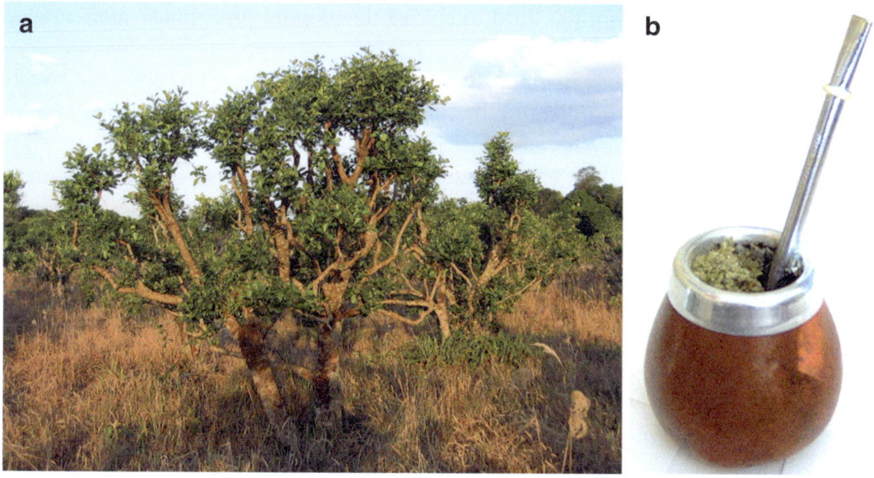

Fig. 9.2 (**a**) The yerba mate tree. (**b**) The bombilla and special cup where dried mate leaves are kept and hot water is poured in a drinking session that can take on up to 1 L of hot water

consumed as a raw product; in fact it is processed as it undergoes blanching, drying, and aging before it is packaged and ready for the consumer. The processing conditions vary wildly from one producer to another based on the desired flavor and style. But in general fresh leaves are flash heated (500° C) over wood or propane fire for a period that can last for up to 3 min in order to break the epidermis and the stomas and halt the oxidation and leaf enzymes, then the leaves are dried either using filtered or unfiltered smoke and heat (100° C) for approximately 8–24 h, after which the dry product is aged by placing it in cement or cedar aging chamber for approximately 12 months in order to develop a special flavor [42]. As such, studies on the raw mate plant extract may differ from the effects of the final product given the various stages and chemical alterations that the plant leaves undergo.

The two most prominent chemical compounds of mate are polyphenols (chlorogenic acid) and xanthines (caffeine and theobromine) followed by purine alkaloids, flavonoids, amino acids, minerals (P, Fe, Ca), and vitamins (C, B1, B2), in addition to a high concentration of bioactive compounds [42–47].

Studies on this beverage are controversial; while it has been highly publicized on some occasions for its health benefits, at other times it is associated with several cancers including oral. It has been reported that mate is a hypocholesterolemic, a hepatoprotective, a stimulant of the central nervous system [42], a benefit for the cardiovascular system [48], a protector of DNA oxidation [49], a diuretic [50], and an antioxidant [51]; in addition it is also implicated in the potential management of obesity [52]. It has been reported that mate is cytotoxic to human cancer hepatoma cells (HepG2) and can act as a catalytic inhibitor of topoisomerase II [53]. However, several investigations reported an association between the consumption of mate and an increased risk of various cancers, including oral [54], oropharyngeal [55], esophageal [56], laryngeal [57], bladder [58], and lung [59]. This is mainly due to the high prevalence of these cancers in the same region where mate drinking is common, with Brazilian males being the third in risk of developing oral cancer after France and India [60].

The involvement of mate in human carcinogenesis in general has been controversial, with most research implicating this beverage as a risk factor for cancer being epidemiological in form, whereas most research show its anticancer role in vitro [53]. However, and based on epidemiological studies, mate was found to increase the risk of laryngeal cancer by threefolds [57]. Its consumption was also associated with 2.5 relative risk of developing tongue cancer [61]. Additionally, exposure to mate caused fivefold increase in oropharyngeal cancer [62]. It has been proposed that mate consumed at high temperatures may act as a solvent for chemical carcinogens in tobacco or that mate itself can contain some phenolic compounds that can act as a carcinogenic element [63, 64]. Mate aqueous extracts (100–750 μg/ml) were linked with increased chromosome aberrations in human peripheral lymphocytes; however this was not corroborated in vivo on Wistar rats' bone marrow cells [65]. Additionally, mate infusion was found not be clastogenic or aneugenic in human lymphocyte and had no genotoxic effects on the liver, kidney, and bladder cells of male Swiss mice [66]. In fact, mate was shown to increase DNA resistance to H_2O_2-induced DNA breakage and improved DNA repair in male Swiss mice after regular ingestion of mate infusion [67].

Among the various epidemiological studies implicating the association between mate and oral cancer is a case control study in Brazil that dates back to 1989 [68]. The study encompassed three major cities from different geographical locations, São Paulo (southeast), Curitiba (south), and Goiânia (central west). Their aim was to quantify risk factors in these cities as the incidence rate of oral cancer was only second to select areas in France and India, with approximately 7.4 and 8.0 per 100,000 in São Paulo. Thus, exposure to smoking and drinking in addition to dietary factors, employment history, and general oral health characteristics were reviewed. A total of 232 oral cancer patients that have been referred to HN surgery services were studied in comparison with a 464 age- and sex-matched control group from the same hospitals except for patient with neoplastic disease or mental disorder. The study found positive cancer risk association with coffee and mate; however, when these factors were adjusted for use of alcohol and smoking, their effect visibly reduced the magnitude of the level-specific RR estimates. The temperature of the hot beverages was also examined, and there was no indication of such an effect on the general outcome. The study concludes that the most prominent risk factors are alcohol consumption and smoking, while other risk factors that were less dominant include mate, use of wood stove for cooking, and frequent consumption of charcoal-grilled meat and manioc. Similarly, another case control study of oral and pharyngeal cancer that involved 108 cancer cases versus 286 control ones in Uruguay suggests that the combined effect of black tobacco smoking with wine and mate ingestion is strongly related with risk of oral cancer [62].

Nevertheless, it is very hard to conclusively determine the exact role of mate in oral carcinogenesis. Particularly since available epidemiological data do not include the possible effect of oncoviruses such as HPV and EBV nor onco-bacteria (*H. pylori*), additionally, possible sources of contamination of mate with polycyclic aromatic hydrocarbons (PAHs) in different samples of commercial mate leaves have been previously reported [69]. On the other hand, most available experimental research on the association between mate and HN carcinogenesis has concentrated so far on its role in esophageal cancer with only few dedicated to oral and oropharyngeal cancers [9].

So far, experimental data regarding the role of mate brew on carcinogenesis have not been in support of the claims of its complicity in cancer progression. Da Silva et al. (2009) evaluated the modifying effects of mate on primary DNA damages in rat peripheral blood leukocytes and the development of esophageal preneoplastic and neoplastic lesions in male Wistar rats treated with carcinogen diethylnitrosamine (DEN) and submitted to thermal injury by instillation of hot water at 65° C, positive control groups treated with green tea were included. The results show that mate reduced DNA damage levels in peripheral blood leukocytes and esophageal carcinogenesis induced by DEN/thermal injury protocol; it also inhibited liver carcinogenesis induced by DEN, which was similar in its effect to that of green tea [70].

In another investigation, Gonzalez de Mejia et al. studied the phenolic content of mate tea products (MT) and evaluated its capacity to inhibit topoisomerase I (topo I) and II (topo II) activities in oral cancer cells. Topoisomerase inhibition was determined by a clone-forming assay, which uses yeast strains as model, while cytotoxicity was studied using a non-tumorigenic human keratinocyte cell line and two human squamous cancer cell lines. The results of this study indicated that MT was a rich source of phenolic compounds; however its concentration levels were significantly different from one product to another based on its origin. In addition, MT showed dose-dependent cytotoxicity against all squamous cell lines tested, resulting in up to 50% inhibition of net cell growth in human oral cancer cell line, which indicates that far from being an oral cancer risk factor, mate can actually inhibit oral cancer proliferation [71].

Based on these limited amounts of published studies, it is very hard to discern the exact role of mate involvement in oral carcinogenesis, particularly in conjunction with other known risk factors, which obviously begs for more investigations dedicated to this important and common beverage.

Conclusion

This chapter reviewed available information to date on two lesser known risk factors of oral cancer: Qat, which is a plant that is chewed raw in various parts of East Africa and the Middle East, particularly Yemen, and mate, a hot beverage that is processed and brewed in various parts of South America and the Middle East. The complicity of both plants in oral carcinogenesis lacks sufficient evidence, with most indication in support of this claim derived from local epidemiological studies. However, there appears to be a clear association between Qat and precancerous white lesions in the oral cavity; the concentration of these lesions in the area of the chewing side and the lack of these lesions at the rest of the oral cavity suggest that ingestion of the plant itself may not be a risk factor, rather the method it is consumed in. This is particularly important if we consider other possible risk factors that can be associated with Qat chewing such as the effect of pesticides and the combination of alcohol and tobacco smoking, in addition to other contaminants that might be present following the level of hygiene during the various sessions, such as possible contamination of oncoviruses or oncobacteria. Nevertheless, presently published data on the effect of Qat extract on oral and oropharyngeal carcinogens are not conclusive. The same can be said about mate, where even more controversy is evidenced, with most experimental data supporting claims of a positive role of the mate brew in cancer prevention, which is in contrast to most epidemiological findings. Once again, lack of association of oral cancer prevalence with risk factors that encompass alcohol and cigarette consumption, such as viral or bacterial infection, not to mention the effect of certain contamination in some processing methods of mate, may reduce confidence in the epidemiological data in this regard.

Based on these facts, these two plants cannot be fully considered as risk factors for oral and oropharyngeal carcinogenesis without proper understanding of their real role in human oral normal and cancer cells. Nevertheless, since use of Qat is presented with several toxic effects on the human body, we believe it is important to avoid the use of this plant as a prevention strategy for oral cancer development.

References

1. Forastiere A, Koch W, Trotti A, Sidransky D. Head and neck cancer. N Engl J Med. 2001;345(26):1890–900.
2. Torre LA, Bray F, Siegel RL, Ferlay J, Lortet-Tieulent J, Jemal A. Global cancer statistics, 2012. CA Cancer J Clin. 2015;65(2):87–108.
3. Jo JA, Applegate BE, Park J, Shrestha S, Pande P, Gimenez-Conti IB, Brandon JL. In vivo simultaneous morphological and biochemical optical imaging of oral epithelial cancer. IEEE Trans Biomed Eng. 2010;57(10):2596–9.
4. Zheng T, Boyle P, Hu H, Duan J, Jiang P, Ma D, Shui L, Niu S, Scully C, MacMahon B. Dentition, oral hygiene, and risk of oral cancer: a case-control study in Beijing, People's Republic of China. Cancer Causes Control. 1990;1(3):235–41.
5. Warnakulasuriya S, Sutherland G, Scully C. Tobacco, oral cancer, and treatment of dependence. Oral Oncol. 2005;41(3):244–60.
6. Lee HC, Yin PH, Yu TN, Chang YD, Hsu WC, Kao SY, Chi CW, Liu TY, Wei YH. Accumulation of mitochondrial DNA deletions in human oral tissues—effects of betel quid chewing and oral cancer. Mutat Res Genet Toxicol Environ Mutagen. 2001;493(1):67–74.
7. Moreno-Lopez LA, Esparza-Gomez GC, Gonzalez-Navarro A, Cerero-Lapiedra R, Gonzalez-Hernandez MJ, Domınguez-Rojas V. Risk of oral cancer associated with tobacco smoking, alcohol consumption and oral hygiene: a case-control study in Madrid, Spain. Oral Oncol. 2000;36(2):170–4.
8. Soufi HE, Kameswaran M, Malatani T. Khat and oral cancer. J Laryngol Otol. 1991;105(08): 643–5.
9. Dasanayake AP, Silverman AJ, Warnakulasuriya S. Maté drinking and oral and oro-pharyngeal cancer: a systematic review and meta-analysis. Oral Oncol. 2010;46(2):82–6.
10. Herrero R, Castellsagué X, Pawlita M, Lissowska J, Kee F, Balaram P, Rajkumar T, Sridhar H, Rose B, Pintos J, Fernández L. Human papillomavirus and oral cancer: the International Agency for Research on Cancer multicenter study. J Natl Cancer Inst. 2003;95(23):1772–83.

11. Dayama A, Srivastava V, Shukla M, Singh R, Pandey M. Helicobacter pylori and oral cancer: possible association in a preliminary case control study. Asian Pac J Cancer Prev. 2011;12(5):1333–6.
12. Ribeiro IP, Barroso L, Marques F, Melo JB, Carreira IM. Early detection and personalized treatment in oral cancer: the impact of omics approaches. Mol Cytogenet. 2016;9(1):85.
13. El-Zaemey S, Schüz J, Leon ME. Qat chewing and risk of potentially malignant and malignant oral disorders: a systematic review. Int J Occup Environ Med. 2015;6(3 July):537–129.
14. Balint EE, Falkay G, Balint GA. Khat–a controversial plant. Wien Klin Wochenschr. 2009;121(19–20):604–14.
15. Al-Meshal IA, Tariq M., Hifnawy MS, Mekkawi AG, Muhtadi FJ. Characterization and evaluation of Saudi Arabian khat. In: International Council on Alcohol and Addictions, editors. First international conference on Khat, Lausanne, Switzerland; 1983. p. 110–134.
16. World Health Organization Expert Committee on Drug Dependence. Assessment of khat (Catha edulis forsk). In: Proceedings of the 34th meeting, Expert Committee on drug dependence; 2006. p. 9.
17. World Bank. Yemen towards qat demand reduction. Country Development III. Sustainable Development Department, Middle East and North Africa Region; 2007.
18. Patel SL, Murray R, Britain G. Khat use among Somalis in four English cities. London: Home Office; 2005.
19. Nencini P, Ahmed AM. Khat consumption: a pharmacological review. Drug Alcohol Depend. 1989;23(1):19–29.
20. Cox G, Rampes H. Adverse effects of khat: a review. Adv Psychiatr Treat. 2003;9(6):456–63.
21. Toennes SW, Harder S, Schramm M, Niess C, Kauert GF. Pharmacokinetics of cathinone, cathine and norephedrine after the chewing of khat leaves. Br J Clin Pharmacol. 2003;56(1):125–30.
22. Macigo FG, Mwaniki DL, Guthua SW. The association between oral leukoplakia and use of tobacco, alcohol and that based on relative risks assessment in Kenya. Eur J Oral Sci. 1995;103(5):268–73.
23. Al-sharabi AK. Condition of oral mucosa due to takhzeen al qat. Yemeni J Med Sci. 2011;5:1–6.
24. Ibrahim EM, Satti MB, Al Idrissi HY, Higazi MM, Magbool GM, Al Quorain A. Oral cancer in Saudi Arabia: the role of alqat and alshammah. Cancer Detect Prev. 1985;9(3–4):215–8.
25. Ali AA, Al-Sharabi AK, Aguirre JM, Nahas R. A study of 342 oral keratotic white lesions induced by qat chewing among 2500 yemeni. J Oral Pathol Med. 2004;33(6):368–72.
26. Halboub E, Dhaifullah E, Abdulhuq M. Khat chewing and smoking effect on oral mucosa: a clinical study. Acta Med (Hradec Kralove). 2009;52(4):155–8.
27. Lukandu OM, Neppelberg E, Vintermyr OK, Johannessen AC, Costea DE. Khat alters the phenotype of in vitro-reconstructed human oral mucosa. J Dent Res. 2010;89(3):270–5.
28. Ahmed HGE, Omer ASA. Cytological study of exfoliative buccal mucosal cells of qat chewers in Yemen. Diagn Cytopathol. 2011;39(11):796–800.
29. Kassie F, Darroudi F, Kundi M, Schulte-Hermann R, Knasmüller S. Khat (Catha edulis) consumption causes genotoxic effects in humans. Int J Cancer. 2001;92(3):329–32.
30. Schmidt-Westhausen AM, Al Sanabani J, Al-Sharabi AK. Prevalence of oral white lesions due to qat chewing among women in Yemen. Oral Dis. 2014;20(7):675–81.
31. Yarom N, Epstein J, Levi H, Porat D, Kaufman E, Gorsky M. Oral manifestations of habitual khat chewing: a case-control study. Oral Surg Oral Med Oral Pathol Oral Radiol Endod. 2010;109(6):e60–6.
32. Ali AA. Histopathologic changes in oral mucosa of yemenis addicted to water-pipe and cigarette smoking in addition to takhzeen al-qat. Oral Surg Oral Med Oral Pathol Oral Radiol Endod. 2007;103(3):e55–9.
33. Lukandu OM, Costea DE, Dimba EA, Neppelberg E, Bredholt T, Gjertsen BT, Vintermyr OK, Johannessen AC. Khat induces G1-phase arrest and increased expression of stress-sensitive p53 and p16 proteins in normal human oral keratinocytes and fibroblasts. Eur J Oral Sci. 2008;116(1):23–30.

34. Lukandu OM, Bredholt T, Neppelberg E, Gjertsen BT, Johannessen AC, Vintermyr OK, Costea DE. Early loss of mitochondrial inner transmembrane potential in khat-induced cell death of primary normal human oral cells. Toxicology. 2009;263(2):108–16.
35. Lukandu OM, Costea DE, Neppelberg E, Johannessen AC, Vintermyr OK. Khat (Catha edulis) induces reactive oxygen species and apoptosis in normal human oral keratinocytes and fibroblasts. Toxicol Sci. 2008;103(2):311–24.
36. Food and Agriculture Organization (FAO), Ministry of Agriculture & Irrigation (MAI). Production of qat in Yemen, water use and the competitive alternatives available to policy change. In: FAO, editor. Arabica, Cairo, Egypt; 2008.
37. Al-Hadrani AM, Thabet AMM. Acute adverse health effects of pesticides sprayed on khat trees. J Pestic Control Environ Sci. 2000;8(1):97–106.
38. Abdulaziz M. An assessment of possible health risks of using DDT and Farmers' Perception towards toxicity of pesticides used on Khat (Catha edulis): In Haromaya Woreda, Ethiopia [dissertation]. AAU; 2010.
39. Al-Haj M, Nasser A, Anis A. Survey of pesticides used in qat cultivation in dhale and yafe and their adverse effects. J Nat Appl Sci. 2005;9:103–10.
40. Daba D, Hymete A, Bekhit AA, Mohamed AMI, Bekhit AEDA. Multi residue analysis of pesticides in wheat and khat collected from different regions of Ethiopia. Bull Environ Contam Toxicol. 2011;86(3):336–41.
41. Al-Akwa AA, Shaher M, Al-Akwa S, Aleryani SL. Free radicals are present in human serum of Catha edulis forsk (khat) abusers. J Ethnopharmacol. 2009;125(3):471–3.
42. Heck CI, De Mejia EG. Yerba mate tea (Ilex paraguariensis): a comprehensive review on chemistry, health implications, and technological considerations. J Food Sci. 2007;72(9): R138–51.
43. Chandra S, Gonzalez de Mejia E. Polyphenolic compounds, antioxidant capacity, and quinone reductase activity of an aqueous extract of Ardisia compressa in comparison to mate (Ilex paraguariensis) and green (Camellia sinensis) teas. J Agric Food Chem. 2004;52(11):3583–9.
44. Dall'Orto § VC, Vago JM, Carballo RR, Rezzano IN. Comparison of tyrosinase biosensor and colorimetric method for polyphenol analysis in different kinds of teas. Anal Lett. 2005;38(1):19–33.
45. Carini M, Facino RM, Aldini G, Calloni M, Colombo L. Characterization of phenolic antioxidants from Maté (Ilex paraguayensis) by liquid chromatography/mass spectrometry and liquid chromatography/tandem mass spectrometry. Rapid Commun Mass Spectrom. 1998;12(22): 1813–9.
46. Bastos DH, Saldanha LA, Catharino RR, Sawaya A, Cunha IB, Carvalho PO, Eberlin MN. Phenolic antioxidants identified by ESI-MS from yerba mate (Ilex paraguariensis) and green tea (Camellia sinensis) extracts. Molecules. 2007;12(3):423–32.
47. Turkmen N, Sari F, Velioglu YS. Effects of extraction solvents on concentration and antioxidant activity of black and black mate tea polyphenols determined by ferrous tartrate and folin–ciocalteu methods. Food Chem. 2006;99(4):835–41.
48. Schinella G, Fantinelli JC, Mosca SM. Cardioprotective effects of Ilex paraguariensis extract: evidence for a nitric oxide-dependent mechanism. Clin Nutr. 2005;24(3):360–6.
49. Bracesco N, Dell M, Rocha A, Behtash S, Menini T, Gugliucci A, Nunes E. Antioxidant activity of a botanical extract preparation of Ilex paraguariensis: prevention of DNA double-strand breaks in Saccharomyces cerevisiae and human low-density lipoprotein oxidation. J Altern Complement Med. 2003;9(3):379–87.
50. Gonzalez A, Ferreira F, Vazquez A, Moyna P, Paz EA. Biological screening of uruguayan medicinal plants. J Ethnopharmacol. 1993;39(3):217–20.
51. Filip R, Ferraro GE. Researching on new species of "mate": Ilex Brevicuspis. Eur J Nutr. 2003;42(1):50–4.
52. Andersen T, Fogh J. Weight loss and delayed gastric emptying following a South American herbal preparation in overweight patients. J Hum Nutr Diet. 2001;14(3):243–50.
53. Ramirez-Mares MV, Chandra S, de Mejia EG. In vitro chemopreventive activity of Camellia sinensis, Ilex paraguariensis and Ardisia Compressa tea extracts and selected polyphenols. Mutat Res Fundam Mol Mech Mutagen. 2004;554(1):53–65.

54. Deneo-Pellegrini H, De Stefani E, Boffetta P, Ronco AL, Acosta G, Correa P, Mendilaharsu M. Maté consumption and risk of oral cancer: case-control study in Uruguay. Head Neck. 2013;35(8):1091–5.
55. Goldenberg D. Maté: a risk factor for oral and oropharyngeal cancer. Oral Oncol. 2002;38(7):646–9.
56. Rolon PA, Castellsague X, Benz M, Munoz N. Hot and cold mate drinking and esophageal cancer in Paraguay. Cancer Epidemiol Biomark Prev. 1995;4(6):595–605.
57. De Stefani E, Correa P, Oreggia F, Leiva J, Rivero S, Fernandez G, Deneo-Pellegrini H, Zavala D, Fontham E. Risk factors for laryngeal cancer. Cancer. 1987;60(12):3087–91.
58. De Stefani E, Boffetta P, Deneo-Pellegrini H, Correa P, Ronco AL, Brennan P, Ferro G, Acosta G, Mendilaharsu M. Non-alcoholic beverages and risk of bladder cancer in Uruguay. BMC Cancer. 2007;7(1):1.
59. De Stefani E, Fierro L, Correa P, Fontham E, Ronco A, Larrinaga M, Balbi J, Mendilaharsu M. Mate drinking and risk of lung cancer in males: a case-control study from Uruguay. Cancer Epidemiol Biomark Prev. 1996;5(7):515–9.
60. Wünsch-Filho V, de Camargo EA. The burden of mouth cancer in Latin America and the Caribbean: epidemiologic issues. Semin Oncol. 2001;28(2):158–68.
61. Oreggia F, de Stefani E, Correa P, Fierro L. Risk factors for cancer of the tongue in Uruguay. Cancer. 1991;67(1):180–3.
62. De Stefani E, Correa P, Oreggia F, Deneo-Pellegrini H, Fernandez G, Zavala D, Carzoglio J, Leiva J, Fontham E, Rivero S. Black tobacco, wine and mate in oropharyngeal cancer. A case-control study from Uruguay. Revue d'epidemiologie et de sante publique. 1987;36(6): 389–94.
63. Muñoz SE, Chatenoud L, La Vecchia C, Negri E, Levi F. Trends in cancer mortality in Argentina, 1966–91. Eur J Cancer Prev. 1998;7(1):37–44.
64. De Barros SG, Ghisolfi ES, Luz LP, Barlem GG, Vidal RM, Wolff FH, Magno VA, Breyer HP, Dietz J, Grüber AC, Kruel CD. High temperature "mate" infusion drinking in a population at risk for squamous cell carcinoma of the esophagus. Arq Gastroenterol. 1999;37(1):25–30.
65. Fonseca CA, Otto SS, Paumgartten FJ, Leitão AC. Nontoxic, mutagenic, and clastogenic activities of mate-chimarrao (Ilex paraguariensis). J Environ Pathol Toxicol Oncol. 1999;19(4): 333–46.
66. Alves RJV, Jotz GP, do Amaral VS, Montes TMH, Menezes HS, de Andrade HHR. The evaluation of maté (Ilex paraguariensis) genetic toxicity in human lymphocytes by the cytokinesis-block in the micronucleus assay. Toxicol In Vitro. 2008;22(3):695–8.
67. Miranda DD, Arçari DP, Pedrazzoli J, Carvalho PDO, Cerutti SM, Bastos DH, Ribeiro ML. Protective effects of mate tea (Ilex paraguariensis) on H2O2-induced DNA damage and DNA repair in mice. Mutagenesis. 2008;23(4):261–5.
68. Franco EL, Kowalski LP, Oliveira BV, Curado MP, Pereira RN, Silva ME, Fava AS, Torloni H. Risk factors for oral cancer in Brazil: a case-control study. Int J Cancer. 1989;43(6): 992–1000.
69. Zuin VG, Montero L, Bauer C, Popp P. Stir bar sorptive extraction and high-performance liquid chromatography–fluorescence detection for the determination of polycyclic aromatic hydrocarbons in mate teas. J Chromatogr A. 2005;1091(1):2–10.
70. da Silva JF, Bidinotto LT, Furtado KS, Salvadori DMF, Rivelli DP, de Moraes Barros SB, Rodrigues MAM, Barbisan LF. Maté attenuates DNA damage and carcinogenesis induced by diethylnitrosamine and thermal injury in rat esophagus. Food Chem Toxicol. 2009;47(7): 1321–9.
71. Gonzalez de Mejia E, Song YS, Ramirez-Mares MV, Kobayashi H. Effect of yerba mate (Ilex paraguariensis) tea on topoisomerase inhibition and oral carcinoma cell proliferation. J Agric Food Chem. 2005;53(6):1966–73.

Photodynamic Diagnosis and Therapy for Oral Potentially Malignant Disorders and Cancers

10

Sara A. Abdel Gaber

10.1 Introduction

Oral lesions can be either benign—off scope—pre-malignant, or malignant ones. Precancerous lesions include oral leukoplakia (OL)—either homogenous or nonhomogenous—and erythroplakia. For both of them, epithelial dysplasia occurrence exacerbates the situation and indicates a high probability for transformation into tumor lesions [1]. On the other hand, 90% of the malignant lesions are squamous cell carcinoma (SCC), and the rest are lymphomas and verrucous and minor salivary gland carcinomas [2]. Tumor-node-metastasis (TNM) system is exploited in lesion staging where T indicates the tumor size, N describes the involvement of lymph nodes, and M indicates the metastatic status; each is numerically subdivided in accordance with severity [3]. Detecting the tumor lesions at early stages may save patient's life and ultimately improve the oral cancer 5-year survival that is sadly only 50% [4].

Photodynamic diagnosis (PDD) and photodynamic therapy (PDT) are diagnostic and therapeutic modalities with excellent outcome in the dentistry field for both non-oncologic conditions such as the control of oral plaques caused by biofilm-forming bacteria [5] and inflammatory diseases such as lichen planus [6] in addition to oncologic ones which are the scope of this chapter. The exploitation of PDD and PDT is dependent on pre-administration of a photosensitizer (PS) which is either a naturally occurring or a chemically synthesized inert compound. PS light activation promotes fluorescence emission or generation of reactive oxygen species (ROS) with destructive repercussion on tumor cells [7].

S.A. Abdel Gaber
Pharmaceutical Biology Department, Photochemistry and Photodynamic Therapy Research Group, German University in Cairo (GUC), Cairo, Egypt
e-mail: Sara.abdel-gaber@guc.edu.eg

A.-E. Al Moustafa (ed.), *Development of Oral Cancer*,
DOI 10.1007/978-3-319-48054-1_10

10.2 Brief History

The utilization of light in the treatment of several diseases mainly the dermatological ones is old dated (3000–1000 BC) as confirmed by the supporting evidences proving that the ancient Egyptian, Chinese, and Indian civilizations were familiar with it [8, 9]. It was only in the last century when this science was brought back into focus, thanks to great efforts exerted by several scientists [10]. For example, the term (photodynamic action) was first introduced in 1904 by the German pharmacologist Prof. Dr. Hermann von Tappeiner and his coworkers [11]. He conducted the first clinical application of PDT on six patients using the PS eosin to treat facial basal cell carcinoma such as those located in the lower lip and showed complete response in four of them [12]. In 1910 for the first time, the phototoxicity of the PS hematoporphyrin was tested on paramecia and mice by the biologist Prof. Dr. W. Hausmann [13]. Later in 1924, the French physician Albert Policard was the first to detect an intense red fluorescence in experimentally introduced rat sarcoma cells in comparison to the surrounding normal tissues after hematoporphyrin administration [14]. The diagnostic properties of hematoporphyrin was confirmed only in 1960 when the same observation was reported after applying fluorescence endoscopy to diagnose different cancer types in 15 patients [15]. In 1967, the diagnostic and cytotoxic effects of hematoporphyrin were combined in a clinical study performed on a female patient suffering from recurrent ulcerative cancer of the mammary glands [16]. A purified form of hematoporphyrin was introduced in 1987 [17], and it successfully treated—either completely or partially—111 patients out of 113 suffering from either cutaneous or subcutaneous cancer located in different sites such as the breast, colon, prostate, and many other body regions [18]. Finally, the clinical use of the purified hematoporphyrin form commercially known as Photofrin® was approved in Canada in 1993, and 2 years later, PDT using Photofrin gained the US Food and Drug Administration (FDA) approval for the clinical use as a palliative treatment of esophageal cancer [19].

10.3 Concept Behind PDD and PDT

In contrast to normal cells, "enhanced permeability and retention (EPR)" is a key feature of cancer cells [20] which grants—to a great extent—a preferential accumulation of PS after administration. Both PDD and PDT protocols involve illuminating a previously administered PS with a light of an appropriate wavelength. According to the first law of thermodynamics, the gained energy coming from the used light will never be lost, but rather converted into another form. Depending on the wavelength used for exciting PS electrons, one of the many processes might take place while returning to the ground state. For PDD, the excited electrons undergo "internal conversion" in which they replace their electronic energy with a vibrational one so that they release the gained energy in a form of fluorescence. For PDT, PSs have a high "intersystem crossing" yield meaning that they undergo a spin flip and move from singlet energy levels to the triplet ones. There, one of two chemical reactions, is taking place for these excited electrons to move down from the triplet to the ground state. The first is known as "Type I "reaction in which the excited PS reacts with nearby molecules such as cell membrane components and converts them into radicals. The latter react with molecular oxygen and produces reactive oxygen species (ROS). On the other hand, in "Type II" reaction, the excited PS reacts directly with molecular oxygen converting it to ROS where the latter react with surrounding molecules [7, 21, 22]. Examples of the mechanisms through which the produced ROS impose their deleterious cellular effects are lipid peroxidation [23] and protein carbonylation [24]. A schematic illustration for both PDD and PDT is shown in Fig. 10.1.

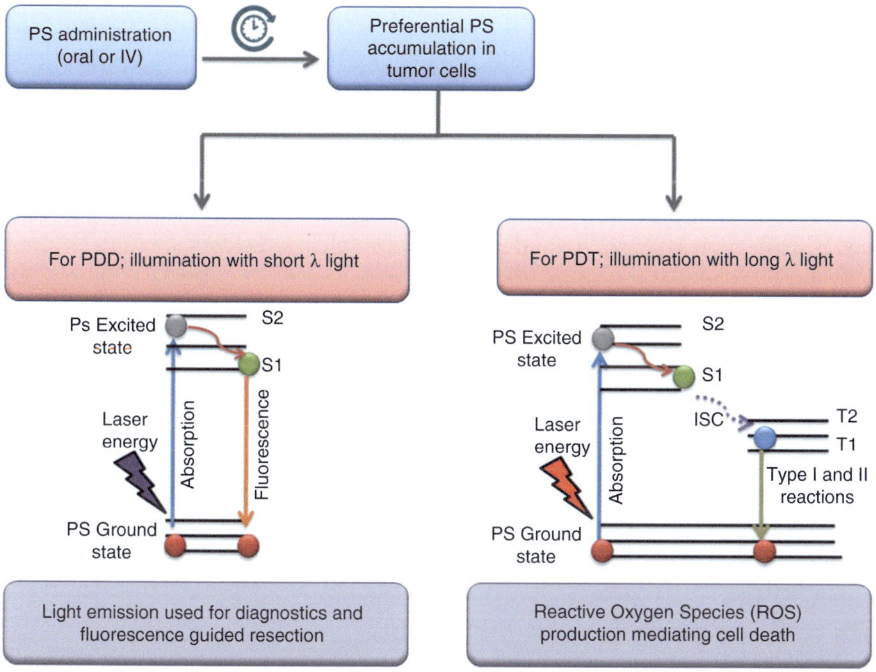

Fig. 10.1 Schematic illustration of PDD and PDT accompanied with modified Jablonski diagrams. PS is administered either orally or intravascular followed by waiting time that differs from one PS to the other to allow preferential PS tumor accumulation. For diagnostic purposes, PS is activated using light of short wavelength. Excited PS undergoes internal conversion to return from singlet energy levels (S1 and S2) back to the ground state accompanied by light emission used for tumor visualization. For therapeutic applications, PS is activated using long wavelength light. Excited PS undergoes intersystem crossing from singlet energy levels to triplet ones (T1 and T2). Either type I or II reactions take place for PS to return to the ground state with concurrent production of toxic reactive oxygen species (Phosphorescence might take place instead of type I and II reaction, but it is not depicted in the figure.)

10.4 Elements of PDD and PDT

As illustrated above, the pillars for PDD are PS and light, while PDT is a three-component system as it involves the simultaneous existence of Ps, light, and tissue oxygen. What follows is a brief discussion for each element.

10.4.1 Photosensitizer (PS)

PS is an inert chromophore with a highly conjugated chemical structure which enables it to absorb the energy from the exciting light. An ideal PS should fulfill some criteria from the biological, photochemical, and photophysical perspectives. From the biological point of view, being free of dark toxicity, highly selective, free of side effects, and rapidly cleared from the body are among the essential requirements. Meanwhile, chemical purity, stability on storage along with good aqueous, and lipid solubility are on the top of the needed features from the photochemical angle. Compounds with a high quantum yield and a long lifetime of the triplet state are photophysically considered ideal PSs mainly for PDT [25–27].

Due to the huge diversity of available PSs, they are classified according to various classification systems. According to their chemical structures, they are grouped into three broad classes: porphyrin (tetrapyrrole nucleus), chlorins (chlorophyll-like), and dyes. With respect to their developmental stage, they are grouped into first, second, and third generations where the preceding ones overcome previously observed limitations [26]. For instance, third-generation PSs—unlike first and second ones—seek active targeted delivery; thus they are conjugated to targeting moieties such as monoclonal antibodies [28] and albumin [29].

This chapter emphasizes on three frequently used PSs for oral cavity cancer PDD and PDT. Namely, they are 5,10,15,20 meta-tetra(hydroxyphenyl)chlorin (m-THPC) which is commercially sold under the name of Foscan® and commonly referred to as temoporfin, porfimer sodium, and 5-aminolevulinic acid (5-ALA)-induced protoporphyrin IX (PPIX) whose trade names are Photofrin® and Levulan©, respectively. Their chemical structures are shown in Fig. 10.2.

M-THPC is a second-generation PS that showed the highest potency among a various series of chlorin derivatives [30]. It has an absorption peak near the far end of the red region (at 650 nm) which is used for PDT application 3–4 days after either topical or intravenous (0.1–0.15 mg/kg) administration [31–33]. In 2001, it gained the European approval to be used as a palliative treatment for head and neck cancers. Compared to standard therapeutic options for advanced head and neck cancers such as palliative surgery and chemotherapy, m-THPC-PDT significantly elongated patients' life expectancy and was found to be cost-effective [34]. Foslip® is an available m-THPC liposomal formulation with elevated water solubility, but similar PDT potency [35].

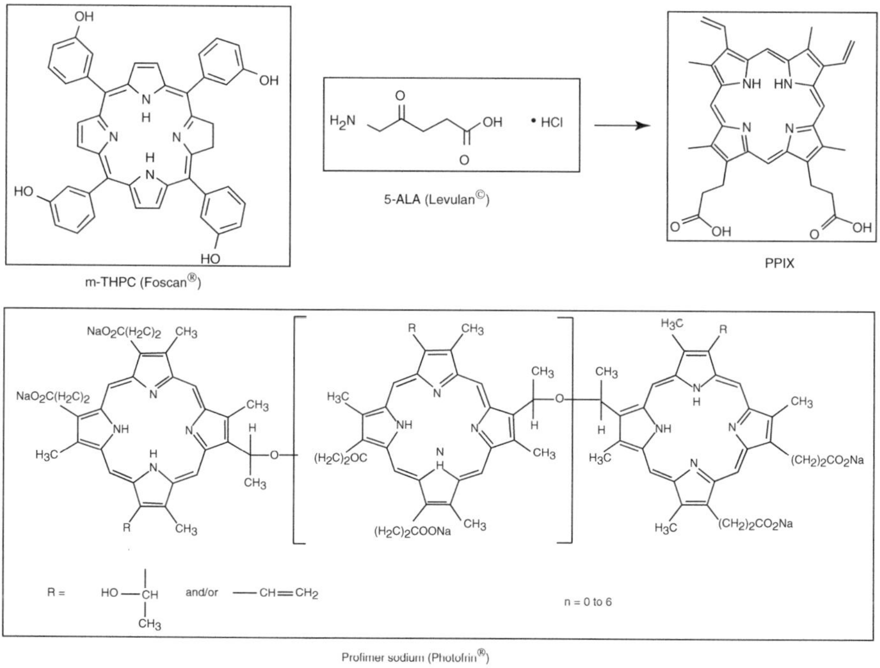

Fig. 10.2 Chemical structure of some photosensitizers commonly used in oral cancer. *M-THPC* 5,10,15,20 meta-tetra (hydroxyphenyl)chlorin, *5-ALA* 5-aminolevulinic acid, *PPIX* protoporphyrin IX

Although porfimer sodium is the first approved PS, it is not a single chemical compound. It is rather an oligomer of up to eight porphyrin units connected together by ether and ester linkages making up almost 85% of the total composition, and the rest are either monomers or dimmers of hematoporphyrin in addition to other 60 compounds [36, 37]. This first-generation PS has several absorption peaks, but the one used for PDT is at 630 nm. It is administered intravenously (2 mg/kg) and illumination takes place 50 up to 70 h later [38]. In addition to its previously mentioned FDA approval for esophageal cancer, it is approved for non-small lung cancer and recently for Barrett's esophagus.

Unlike m-THPC and porfimer sodium, 5-ALA is naturally synthesized in the body and resembles the first step in heme biosynthesis. Its exogenous administration fosters its enzymatic conversion and leads to cellular accumulation of PPIX within 2–6 h after administration which is the active PS [39]. This prodrug behavior accounts greatly to its associated high selectivity [40]. Oral and systemic routes of administrations are feasible in addition to preparations designed for topical application. Similar to porfimer sodium, PPIX has several absorption peaks; among them, 635 nm is the one used for PDT. In 1999, it was approved by FDA to be used for actinic keratosis treatment, but expansion of its use is intensively studied [41].

10.4.2 Light

Optical properties of PSs, the characteristics of desired illumination site (such as location and anatomical nature), and the application purpose determine to a great extent the light delivery system selected for irradiation. For instance, the previously listed PSs have a strong and broad absorption band known as Soret band between 400 and 430 nm and another absorption band (usually smaller than Soret band) at above 550 nm known as Q band [26]. This limits the "therapeutic window" between 400 and 800 nm [21]. For PDD purposes, 370–450 nm light—matching absorption of Soret band—is applied, while for PDT applications, longer wavelengths, matching Q bands, are preferred to guarantee deep tissue penetration [42]. The depth of tissue penetration does not depend solely on the wavelength of the applied light but also on the anatomical composition of the desired tissue [43].

Used light sources in clinical PDD and PDT are broadly classified according to coherency into laser and non-laser ones. Argon laser and argon-pumped dye lasers are on the top of commonly used continuous laser light sources. They fit more for endoscopic applications and are famous for their high irradiance, but suffer from their continuous need for technical support. Another laser light source is the metal vapor laser which provides a pulsed irradiation and can cover large illumination surface areas without using beam expanders. On the other hand, diode lasers are portable and easy to operate and provide both continuous and pulsed irradiation. The major limitation for laser light sources is their expensive cost. Consequently, non-laser light sources such as lamps (i.e., xenon arc, tungsten filament quartz halogen, and metal halide) are utilized. To narrow their spectrum, filters such as narrowband ones which select the desired wavelength, longpass filters that eliminate high-power UV wavelengths, and shortpass filter that cut IR radiation to avoid hyperthermic effects are usually combined with the lamps. Some delivery systems are FDA approved. Examples include the laser along with its optic fiber manufactured by QuadraLogic Technologies which is designed for esophageal cancer Photofrin-PDT [44–46]. Interestingly, there was no significant difference in the clinical outcome of oral verrucous hyperplasia patients treated with 5-ALA-PDT using either coherent or noncoherent light sources [47].

To maximize the illuminated surface area, access deep-lying tissues, and maintain to a great extent the homogeneity of the delivered light over a large surface area, interstitial PDT (iPDT) is applied. IPDT involves inserting several optical fibers into the tumor mass. Such a setup of irradiation following Photofrin® administration has completely cured two of three patients diagnosed with SCC of the tongue without any complications [48]. Using m-THPC-iPDT eliminated the functional disabilities in breathing or swallowing for patients diagnosed with advanced or recurrent stage IV tongue base carcinoma [49, 50]. The location of the optical fibers can be assigned by means of magnetic resonance (MR) [51, 52] or ultrasound [53] guidance. Currently, there is a running phase II clinical trial by Roswell Park Cancer Institute in collaboration with the National Cancer Institute (NCI) for iPDT during chemotherapy as a palliative treatment of advanced head and neck cancers.

10.4.3 Tissue Oxygen

Adequate tissue oxygenation during PDT is crucial for an efficient therapeutic outcome [54]. Currently, tissue oxygen level can be monitored by various techniques such as near-infrared spectroscopy [55] and polarographic sensitive electrodes [56]. During PDT, oxygen can be promptly consumed. Slow illumination fluence rate [57] and fractionated light [58] are among the strategies followed to oppose rapid oxygen depletion and thus are correlated with better treatment efficiency. However, hypoxic tumors would not benefit from either of them. In such cases, coadministration of anticoagulants such as heparin improves blood perfusion and thus tumor response [59]. Alternatively, the percentage of oxygen in the surrounding atmosphere can be increased. Among various oxygen supplements, it was concluded that breathing hyperbaric oxygen for 1 h before irradiation provided the best Photofrin®-PDT efficiency in treating mammary cancer mice model [60] and significantly decreased the recurrence rate to only 20% in 2 months [61].

10.5 Cell Death Mechanisms After PDT

Following PDT, several signal transduction pathways are activated, and a cluster of cellular responses ranging from cell survival to cell death usually takes place [62]. They are broadly grouped into three major processes (direct cell killing by apoptosis, necrosis, or autophagy, vascular shutdown, and indirect prolonged death mechanism due to immunostimulation) as illustrated in Fig. 10.3. They occur simultaneously rather than separately ending up in most cases with cell death. Clinically, slough, ulceration, vascular congestion, and necrotic tissues are frequently observed following PDT as reported from 19 patients suffering from oral cavity malignant lesions and treated using m-THPC-PDT [63]. With emphasis on oral cancer PDT, each cell death mechanism is deliberated.

10.5.1 Apoptosis, Necrosis, and Autophagy

Apoptosis is a programmed energy-dependent cell death mode that is characterized by cell bubbling, chromatin condensation, and DNA fragmentation. It serves as a homeostatic mechanism in physiological processes such as growth. On the other hand, necrosis is an energy-independent process characterized by cell swelling and disrupted cell membranes that is stimulated by cell injuries. [64]. In contrast to apoptosis and necrosis that deal with whole cells, autophagy involves engulfment of

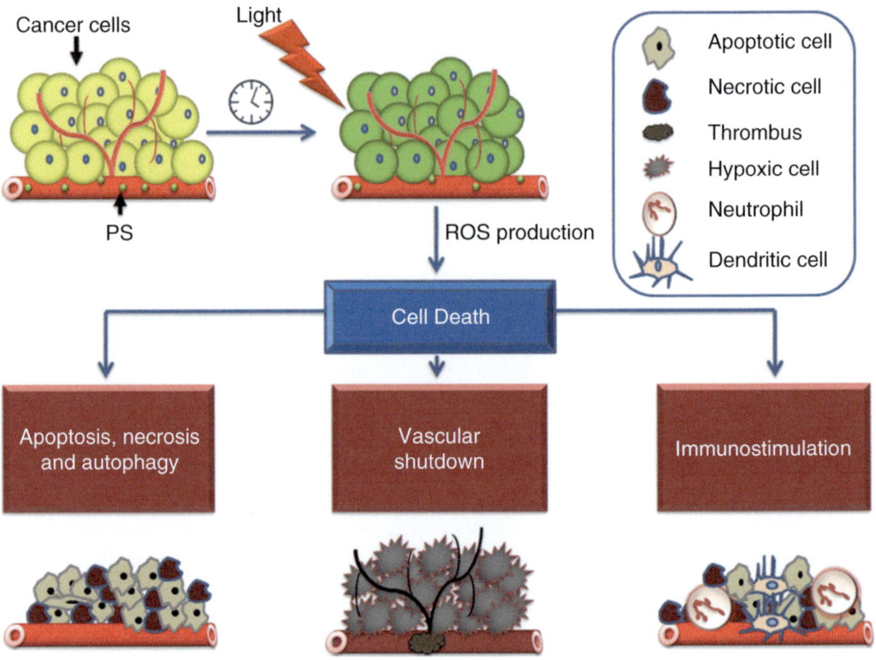

Fig. 10.3 Summary of cell death mechanisms following PDT. Protocols involve drug-light intervals after PS administration to allow preferential PS accumulation in tumor cells. Subsequent illumination leads to ROS production that mediates cell death. A direct cell death through apoptosis, necrosis, or sometimes autophagy can take place. Vascular congestion, stasis, and subsequent hypoxia-mediated cell death may occur. Moreover, a delayed indirect antitumor effect can be exerted after immunostimulation

damaged cellular components and their subsequent lysosomal degradation. Paradoxically, it can serve as either a survival or cell death mode [65].

A certain statement about the mode of cell death cannot be declared with respect to a certain PS or cell line. Several factors decide whether cells die or survive and if to die, then through which mode. Death mode can shift from apoptosis to necrosis in response to PS concentration used in PDT as demonstrated by the study of Garg et al. When they treated premalignant and malignant oral epithelial cells, DOK and H357, respectively, with low concentration erythrosine-PDT, apoptosis was the dominant cell death mode. On the other hand, when erythrosine concentration was 16 times more, morphological studies confirmed a necrotic death mode [66]. The studied model characteristics play as well a role in determining the cell death mode. Human oral squamous carcinoma cells (YD10B) treated with hexenyl 5-ALA-PDT showed elevated levels of apoptosis executors; Caspase3/Caspase7 and their activity was confirmed by the presence of cleaved ADP-ribose polymerase (PARP). Moreover, a high level of cytochrome c was detected along with low levels of the antiapoptotic Bcl-2 protein. These findings together supported that hexenyl 5-ALA-PDT induced a mitochondrial-dependent apoptotic cell death mode [67]. The mode of cell death was shifted to necrosis when oral SCC was replaced with human salivary gland adenocarcinomas cells (SGT) as indicated by elevated lactate dehydrogenase level and staining with the necrotic propidium iodide dye. The necrotic mode was also observed when SGT cells inoculated in chorioallantoic membrane were treated as necrotic bodies were visible [68].

The involvement of key mediators of these cell death modes following PDT is intensively studied. 5-ALA-PDT was reported to exert its cytotoxic effect on human oral cancer cells (Ca9-22) through activating NF-κB-JNK pathway as shown by the escalation of Caspase 8 and 9 levels following PDT [69]. Studying the molecular basis of 5-ALA-PDT on SCC cell line (A431 and COLO-16) elucidated that the exerted cytotoxic effect was mediated through the intrinsic pathway of apoptosis, namely, activating signal transducer and activator of transcription 3 (STAT3). The consequences were lowering the protein level of the antiapoptotic regulator Bcl-2 and increasing the protein level of the proapoptotic regulator Bax [70, 71]. Likewise, apoptosis was observed when human oral squamous KB cells were treated using the PS indocyanine green (ICG)-mediated PDT [72].

Hematoporphyrin-PDT antitumor activity against human mouth epidermal carcinoma KB cells was found to be mediated through both apoptotic and necrotic death modes. Precisely, a mitochondrial-dependent apoptotic pathway was proven by Western blot analysis [73]. Recently, it was reported that hematoporphyrin monomethyl ether exerted a potent cytotoxic effect on human tongue carcinoma cell line (Tca8113) after illumination using 530 nm and subsequent ROS production. The mode of cell death was mainly apoptotic as proved by means of imaging and an elevation in Caspase 3 activity [74]. On the other hand, a second-generation PS called talaporfin-induced necrosis in experimentally induced SCC in the tongue of six nude mice (10 mg/kg) 2 h after illumination using 664 nm diode laser [75]. Talaporfin got the approval from the Japanese health authorities in 2004 for centrally located early-stage lung cancer PDT. Commercially, it is sold under the name Laserphyrin, and structurally, it is a mono-L-aspartyl chlorin e6 [76]. Another chlorin-based PS called pheophorbide a suppressed the proliferation of human oral SCC YD-10B cells, and this growth inhibitory effect was associated with mitochondrial membrane depolarization. Subsequently, Bax/Bcl-2 ratio increased leading to cytochrome c release which activated Caspase 3/Caspase 7 as being apoptosis executors that ultimately cleaved PARP. These findings collectively proved a mitochondrial-dependent apoptotic cell death mode. In addition to this, it was reported that at the molecular level, the induced apoptosis was supported by a decline in the phosphorylated extracellular signal-regulated kinases (ERK) [77].

At the in vivo level, when fractionated 5-ALA-PDT was applied on chemically induced leukoplakia in female Wistar rats, elevation in Caspase 3 activity, DNA fragmentation, and epithelial atrophy were reported 6, 24, and 48 h post PDT, respectively. Such findings indicated apoptotic death mode following the first PDT cycle. It is worth mentioning that cell proliferation was concurrently observed as indicated by elevated level of proliferating cell nuclear antigen (PCNA) [78]. On the other hand, non-fractionated 5-ALA-PDT applied on the same animal model showed necrotic tissues 24 h after treatment [79]. Deep ulceration, mucosal degeneration, eosinophilic tissue lacking both nucleus, and membrane integrity were histopathologically confirmed 24 h after treating Swiss mice inoculated with Ehrlich cells in the mouth with liposomal aluminum-chloro-phthalocyanine-mediated PDT. Necrotic tissues represented 90% of the analyzed histological section of the treated group [80]. Analogously, treating premalignant and malignant hamster cheek pouch model with porfimer sodium-PDT resulted in ulceration and necrotic tissues [81].

In general, autophagy is more allied to resistance than to cytotoxicity. Treating human oral SCC YD-10B with pheophorbide a-PDT exerted its tumoricidal impact by virtue of mitochondrial-dependent apoptosis. Concurrently, autophagy evident by formation of autophagosome, elevation of microtubule-associated protein 1A/1B-light chain 3 (LC3) in its phosphatidylethanolamine form referred to as LC3II, and presence of acidic vesicular organelles was observed. Inhibiting autophagy increased the sensitivity of the cells to PDT which indicates the death inhibitory role played by autophagy [77].

10.5.2 Vascular Cessation

The most famous PS that causes vascular destruction is the second-generation benzoporphyrin derivative commonly known as verteporfin. It is FDA approved for the treatment of age-related macular degeneration. Its mechanism of action involves ROS-mediated damage to the endothelial lining of blood vessels, recruitment of platelets, and leukocytes followed by release of vasoconstrictors and thrombus formation stimulators. The consequence is a vascular blood clot accompanied with blood stasis [82]. From one side, this vascular shutdown causes hypoxia which is positively contributing to cell death [83]. From the other side, this endothelial dysfunction creates gaps in the endothelial barrier increasing macromolecule extravasation to the tumor microenvironment which ultimately enhances drug delivery [84]. Verteporfin antivascular effects were confirmed in treating dogs that naturally developed oral and nasal cancers. Dogs were illuminated using 690 nm shortly after verteporfin intravenous administration, and post-PDT vascular damage was confirmed by means of angiogenic computed tomography [85].

5-ALA is one of the PSs that is reported to cause vascular cessation, but when ultrasound stimulation rather than light illumination is applied in a system known as sonodynamic therapy (SDT). The antiangiogenic effect of 5-ALA-SDT was evaluated in vitro using primary human umbilical vein endothelial cells (HUVECs) and in vivo using BALB/c mice model for human tongue carcinoma cells (SAS). A significant reduction in HUVEC cell proliferation, migration, and tube formation ability was reported. Moreover, a remarked tumor regression, damped microvessel density, and diminished vascular endothelial growth factor (VEGF) expression were confirmed in the treated mice [86].

PS pharmacokinetics and extent of vascular accumulation at the illumination time define its ability to induce a detrimental effect on the blood vessels as proved by a study conducted on a xenograft model for human squamous cells. It was observed that m-THPC localized in the blood vessels 3 h after administration. Thus, when irradiation took place at this time point, tumor hypoxia was observed. It was also concluded that this treatment protocol was correlated with a better therapeutic outcome in terms of lowered recurrence and improved cure rate than the standard one in which illumination was performed 48 h after administration [87]. The vascular shutdown effect of m-THPC-PDT was confirmed clinically. The tumor microvasculature of ten patients diagnosed with oral squamous carcinoma of the tongue, soft palate, buccal mucosa, labial mucosa, and floor of the mouse was examined after m-THPC-PDT. 90% of the patient experiences micro-hemorrhage during or 15 min post illumination which was indicative for tumor microvasculature rupture. Blood stasis was imaged in the tumor mega-vasculature 15 min post illumination [88].

10.5.3 Immunostimulation

PDT is a revolutionary tumor treatment modality, thanks to its associated immunostimulatory effect [89, 90] that is proven by an exponentially increasing number of reports. Damaged cells release pro-inflammatory mediators and cell death-associated molecular pattern (cDAMP) that alert innate immune system and trigger the recruitment of dendritic cells, neutrophils, and macrophages. Being antigen-presenting cell, dendritic cells mature and trigger an adaptive immune response through stimulating $CD4^+$ T helper cells and $CD8^+$ cytotoxic T lymphocyte. Eventually, $CD8^+$ effector and memory T cell are generated and sustain the antitumor effect of PDT for a prolonged duration [91, 92].

Paradoxically, the infiltration of immune cells is not always observed as illustrated by the study of Dube et al. They treated hamster cheek pouch with chlorin p6-PDT after systemic administration of either 2 or 4 mg/kg in accordance with tumor volume. Low-dose PDT imposed its cytotoxic effect through a necrotic pathway, while on the other hand, high-dose PDT showed an apoptotic one. Importantly, infiltration of immune cells along with an inflammatory response was evident only in low-dose PDT protocol [93]. As previously mentioned, PDT-induced endothelial damage of microvasculature initiates recruitment of various blood cells. It was reported that exposing human neutrophils to mono-L-aspartyl chlorin e6-mediated PDT resulted in three times overexpression of CD11b receptor which promotes leukocyte adhesion followed by migration to the injury site and thus plays an integral role in provoking an immune response. C11b overexpression was accompanied by two times increase in the level of the chemotactic agent leukotriene B4 [94].

Interestingly, Sharma et al. demonstrated a significantly higher sensitivity of macrophages to 5-ALA-PDT while either cocultured with or separated from human OSCC, NT8e and 4451. This reflects the major role played by immune cells in PDT-mediated cell death [95].

At the in vivo level, the elevation of cytokines such as interleukin-1β and tumor necrosis factor-α in tumor regions following PDT using liposomal aluminum chloride phthalocyanine was recently proved [96]. Clinically, patients diagnosed with basal cell carcinoma were treated with either 5-ALA or porfimer sodium PDT. Blood samples were collected before and 7–10 days post PDT to be screened for the presence of an immunologic response. Post-PDT blood samples showed an elevation in the level of the cytokine interferon gamma which is crucial for innate and adaptive immunity. Furthermore, the tumor-associated antigen (Hip1) was better recognized indicating the generation of a systemic immune response and clinically confirming the PDT-mediated immunostimulatory effect [97].

The immunostimulatory effect of PDT is exploited in PDT-generated vaccines. Verteporfin-PDT was applied—in vitro—on mouse squamous cell carcinoma (SCCVII) cells followed by x-ray. These cells were then directly peritumorally injected in mice bearing the same tumor, and mice were monitored for 4–5 days afterward. In addition to a significantly higher tumor cure rate, a marked increase in lymph node immune cells was observed, namely, 5–6 times increase in T lymphocyte along with CD44+ memory phenotype, more than 10 times increase in dendritic cells, and more than 17 times increase in B lymphocytes. At the injection, cells expressed heat shock protein 70 and complement C3 protein. The involvement of host immune cells was confirmed by the lack of curative effects when immunodeficient mice were tested [98]. PDT-generated vaccine could protect mice through T lymphocytes against cancer rechallenge when chlorin e6-PDT-treated cells were cultured for further 16 h postirradiation before being injected into SCCVII tumor-bearing mice [99].

10.6 Major Advantages of PDD and PDT in Oral Cancer Diagnosis and Therapy

10.6.1 Easily Combined with Standard Diagnostics and Therapies

Combining 5-ALA-PDD with rigid confocal endoscopy resulted in a better living tissue diagnosis where structural elements such as keratinized epithelium, filiform papillae, and fungiform papillae were visible along with cancer transformation-related structural changes [100]. Moreover, 5-ALA-PDT and cryotherapy synergistic effect in treating man with late-stage large verrucous hyperplasia located in the buccal mucosa was recently reported [101]. Likewise, pretreating oral cancer mice models with chemotherapeutics such as methotrexate or cisplatin before 5-ALA-PDT or porfimer sodium PDT, respectively, augmented the antitumor activity and significantly lowered the number of treatment session to reach complete cure [102, 103]. PDT can serve as an adjuvant therapy to surgery also. Quon et al. combined Photofrin®-PDT with transoral robotic surgery (TORS) to treat a 46-year-old patient suffering from a 2.5 cm diffuse carcinoma of the right tonsil [104].

10.6.2 Better Selectivity and Less Side Effects

PDT implies the concept of prodrug as it involves the use of chemically inert compounds in darkness. In other words, selectivity is imposed by selective illumination for the desired body region which results in selective destruction and spares the rest of the body. Experimentally, the safety of PDT using various PSs on the normal mucosa of healthy 133 rats was investigated. Histopathological examinations revealed intact healthy tissues up to 15 days after illumination which was the longest tested period in the study [105]. Clinically, for a total of 128 patients diagnosed with recurrent squamous cell carcinoma in the head and neck and treated with m-THPC-PDT, none showed signs of major toxicities [106]. The frequently observed side effects are acute ones such as pain, erythema, and edema. Usually, they resolve in few weeks, and the use of nonsteroidal pain relievers shortens the pain sensation period [107]. Photosensitivity in forms of sunburns and blisters is commonly observed. It is a consequence of PS accumulation in the skin and subsequent activation upon sun exposure. They can be avoided by staying in the darkness. Patients treated using PSs characterized with slow clearance rate, and thus prolonged photosensitivity periods such as Photofrin® are required to stay longer in dark rooms [108]. Alternatively, it was reported that a special type of fabric protected 100% of 5-ALA-PDT-treated mice from associated photosensitivity [109].

10.6.3 Repetitive Treatment Does Not Evoke Cancer Resistance

Multiple treatment sessions are commonly scheduled, and generally such a treatment protocol yields a better clinical outcome. Chen et al. concluded that two treatment sessions per week of topical 5-ALA-PDT show a significantly better clinical outcome for the treatment of 24 patients diagnosed with oral leukoplakia than once per week. In both groups, a total of eight treatment sessions was scheduled [110]. The same group reported that fractionated 3 min irradiation following 1.5 h of topical 20% 5-ALA-PDT required six sessions to completely cure oral verrucous hyperplasia of buccal mucosa in a 56-year-old male patient [111]. In accordance with this, the hematoporphyrin derivative (photosan)-PDT completely cured chemically induced oral moderate to severe dysplasia in male Syrian golden hamsters after 3–5 treatment sessions, and importantly, these repetitive sessions were not associated with resistance as indicated by remaining disease-free for 50 weeks post-PDT [112].

10.6.4 Noninvasive Method for Both Diagnosis and Treatment

PDD and PDT of oral cavity cancers are an outpatient practice that does not need general anesthesia. Optimum drug-light interval to have maximum signal contrast between neoplastic and health tissues after 1.5 h in case of topical administration [113] which concurs with good patient compliance as the whole treatment is done in one visit. Being noninvasive is associated with a better cosmetic outcome and lack of functional disabilities as reported when 25 patients suffering from SCC in the lip were treated using m-THPC-PDT [114]. 5-ALA-PDT for 48 patients suffering from leukoplakia was compared to cryotherapy applied to 37 patients diagnosed with the same disease. Clinically, they were eqi-effective, but PDT privileged in being "less painful and more esthetic" [115].

10.6.5 Early Stage of Cancer Development Can Be Diagnosed Accurately and Treated

Unlike conventional diagnostic methods, PDD allows the detection of early stages of cancer development. Leunig et al. diagnosed dysplasia, carcinoma in situ, and cancer branches in 13.8% of 58 oral cavity cancer patients enrolled in a clinical PDD study in which 0.4% topical 5-ALA was applied [113]. Applying porfimer sodium-PDD for a total of 20 patients diagnosed with premalignant and malignant oral lesions was correlated with sensitivity up to almost 94% and specificity up to 97.5% [116]. Surprisingly, PDT can attenuate cancer stem cells and weaken invasion, migration, and angiogenesis capabilities of the treated cancerous cells which remarkably restrain cancer progression. 5-ALA-PDT could diminish the self-renewal ability and CD44 expression of sphere-enriched cancer stem cells of tongue squamous cell carcinoma (SAS) and oral carcinoma cells (Ca9-22) along with primary head and neck cells derived from patients. Moreover, it rendered the cells more sensitive to cisplatin chemotherapy [117]. Furthermore, it was reported that treating human OSCC cells (H376 and VB6) with m-THPC-PDT resulted in a significant suppression of invasion and metastasis-promoting enzymes such as both latent and active metalloproteinases MMP9 and MMP2, respectively, in addition to vascular endothelial growth factor (VEGF) level [118]. Similarly, 5-ALA or chlorin e6-PDT-treated human tongue squamous cell carcinoma, SCC-4, demonstrated relative migration ability of only 4.4%. Studying their genotype revealed a significant suppression of proliferative and angiogenic genes such as CLIC4, MMP2, and MMP9 [119].

10.7 Clinical Studies of PDT and PDD in Oral Cancer Management

One of the largest conducted clinical trials included 121 patients diagnosed with primary oral cancer located in several sites of the oral cavity such as lips, interior tongue, hard palate, soft palate, and floor of the tongue. They were treated with intravenous m-THPC-PDT and results were impressive. Complete response was reported for 85% of them with no recurrence over 1 year for 85% and over 2 years for 77% [120]. In 2007, Biel M.A. reported about his massive experience in PDT that extended over 16 years from 1990 till 2006. A total of 276 patients diagnosed with early carcinoma in the head and neck underwent porfimer sodium-PDT. Out of them, 161 had oral cavity lesions ranging from carcinoma in situ to T1-T3/N0. They all showed complete cure after one PDT session. For a minority of them, salvage treatment was required due to recurrence, and it is worth mentioning that they all showed a normal healing post-PDT process [121].

Not only cancerous lesions but also the precancerous ones should be treated. In a follow-up study lasting for 11 years and including 54 patients, it was found that 70% of patients diagnosed with proliferative verrucous leukoplakia developed squamous cell carcinoma in less than 8 years which indicates the importance of treating such precancerous cases [122]. In a clinical trial including five patients diagnosed with oral leukoplakia representing homogenous, verrucous, and erythro-leukoplakia types, PDT was applied after the failure of oral prophylaxis. Patients received 10% 5-ALA emulsion for 3 h before illumination. Complete response was observed in 40% of the patients, and those showing partial response had at least 20% reduction in the lesion size after 1 month of treatment. For both groups, no recurrence was observed for a total of 1 year after treatment [123].

Concerning PDD, 5-ALA-induced PPIX was topically applied (40 mg/ml) for the detection of oral cancers in a total of 85 patients. PPIX fluorescence intensity in tumor cells was greater than the one emitted from normal mucosa, and the superficial margin of the tumor was easily identified [124]. Such a diagnostic method required only 1.5 h of incubation and resulted in 99% sensitivity in addition to a contrast ratio of 10:1 between neoplastic and healthy surrounding tissues [113, 125]. In one of the many porfimer sodium-PDD clinical trials, 20 patients diagnosed with oral neoplasm were enrolled. PS was topically administered and, 3 h later, biopsies were collected, and fluoresce contrast between healthy and tumor cells was calculated where the illumination modes were red, green, blue, or gray scale. Sensitivity was 92.45% and specificity was 95.65% for all lights combined [116]. Below is a table of selected clinical studies conducted from 2010 till 2016 (Table 10.1).

Table 10.1 Summary of some clinical PDT and PDD studies conducted from 2010 till 2016

PS	*n*	Patient characteristics	Main finding	Year	Ref.
5-ALA	80	40 (OVH) and 40 (OEL)	All OVH had CR after 3.6 session, but only 38 of OEL had CR and the rest was PR	2010	[126]
m-THPC	39	-Recurrent SCC -For 21 patients, the primary cancer was located in the oral cavity	60% CR and 28.5% PR	2010	[127]
Porfimer sodium	30	SCC (Tis-T2N0M0) in the oral cavity or oropharynx	80% CR and the rest PR 46% were disease-free for 2 years	2010	[128]
5-ALA	147	Premalignant homogenous/ nonhomogenous leukoplakia and erythroplakia in different oral cavity sites	81% CR, 8% RP, and 3.4% SD	2011	[129]
m-THPC	170	56% 1^{ry} cancers and 44% 2^{ry}/recurrent ones in oral cavity and oropharynx	-Treatment efficiency declined with progression of case severity and 1^{ry} cancers responded better than non-primary ones -Overall response rate was 90.7% and CR rate was 70.8% -Lesion in the tongue and floor of the mouth showed better therapeutic outcomes	2011	[130]
m-THPC	38	Oral SCC (T1/T2 N0). 31.6%, 42%, and 26.3% were well, moderately, and poorly differentiated, respectively	68% CR and 5-year survival was 84.2%	2011	[131]
m-THPC	20	Recurrent SCC in the base of the tongue underwent MR-guided iPDT	-At 6 months, 45% CR -Mean overall survival was 25.5 months	2012	[52]

Table 10.1 (continued)

PS	*n*	Patient characteristics	Main finding	Year	Ref.
5-ALA	11	Histologically confirmed OL enrolled for phase 1 trial for PDT safety using 585 nm laser	Up to 4 J/cm^2, no significant toxicity is observed	2013	[132]
m-THPC	15	Recurrent SCC and 12 patients had lesion in oral cavity	-93% CR and rest PR -Overall survival after 12 months was 72%	2013	[133]
Porfimer sodium	25	Early SCC or dysplasia in oral cavity	-96% CR and the rest PR -Disease-specific survival rate was 95.8%	2013	[134]
5-ALA	50	60% malignant and 40% premalignant late-stage lesions (T3-T4/N0-N2a) in oral cavity enrolled for PDD	-Tongue tumor extensions up to 5 mm was detected -Sensitivity was 95.7%, specificity was 100%, positive predictive value was 100%, and negative predictive value was 60%	2015	[135]
5-ALA	5	OL (pilot study)	40% CR, 40% RP, and 10% no response after 1 month	2015	[123]
m-THPC	2	Recurrent SCC in the base of the tongue after transoral robotic surgery (TORS)	-100% CR and restoration of functional activities -Disease-free for up to 42 months	2015	[136]
Porfimer sodium	34	Oral cavity Cis or SCC	After 6 months, 88.2% CR and 8.6% PR	2016	[107]

OVH oral verrucous hyperplasia, *OEL* oral erythroleukoplakia, *CR* complete response, *PR* partial response, *SCC* squamous cell carcinoma, *SD* stable disease, *MR* magnetic resonance, *iPDT* interstitial PDT, *OL* oral leukoplakia, *Cis* carcinoma in situ (The duration for defining the clinical response varies from one study to the other.)

10.8 Where Does PDD/PDT Currently Stand?

PDD and PDT are steadily making their way to the clinics for oral premalignant and malignant lesions. Saini et al. have discussed the current progress for PDT as a topical therapy, a primary treatment, an adjuvant/combined modality, a palliative, and a maintenance of cancer-free status approaches [137]. The accumulated results from the previously conducted clinical trials along with the expected data from the currently ongoing ones pave this road more. Among the nowadays active clinical trials are an open-label phase 1 clinical trial using 2-(1-hexyloxyethyl)-2-devinyl pyropheophorbide a (HPPH)-PDT for the treatment of dysplasia and oral cancer SCC (NCT01140178)[31], a randomized phase 1 clinical trial for 5-ALA-PDT treating premalignant head and neck lesions (NCT00978081)[3], and a phase 3 clinical trial for 5-ALA/methyl 5-ALA-PDT treating premalignant oral lesions (NCT01497951)[3].

More attention is drawn toward combination therapy. An ongoing phase 1 clinical trial for HPPH-PDT treating recurrent stage I and II head and neck cancers (NCT00470496)[3] investigates the combination of PDT and tumor resection surgery. Sixteen patients have been recruited where six of them have oral cavity cancer. The safety of administering HPPH at a concentration of 4 mg/m^2 followed by 655 nm irradiation up to 75 J/cm^2 has been confirmed [138].

10.9 Limitations and Possible Side Effects

Patrice T. has listed three main obstacles rendering the wide spread of PDT. The first lies in the nature of PDT itself, whereas the therapeutic response relies on the PS kinetic at the time of the irradiation. The latter is widely variable from one model to the other or even between adjacent cells and up till now is poorly studied. Furthermore, the involvement of several death mediators and lack of sufficient explanation for the observed high degree of selectivity oppress advocating PDD/PDT. On the other hand, the second and third main obstacle are the clinicians' rejection to new modalities and the economic burden PDT resembles to the pharmaceutical companies producing standard therapeutic agents [139]. With special regard to oral cavity cancer, PDD and PDT are limited to premalignant and early malignant superficial lesions where the success rates in deep or late-stage lesions are not that high [137].

It was concluded from nearly all conducted clinical trials that patients do not experience serious or chronic side effects. For example, in the clinical study for using mTHPC-PDT for head and neck cancer, 114 patients were recruited, and 82% of them suffered from mild to moderate pain at the site of treatment. The use of opiate along with NSAD was sufficient to relieve this pain. Swelling was observed in 10% of the patients along with a temporary rise in the white blood cell count, and 13% of them witnessed skin phototoxicity as they exposed themselves to direct light after treatment. Only one patient required skin grafting to resolve the burn [120].

[1] Retrieved from www.clinicaltrials.gov visited on 12.1.2017.

10.10 Future Aspects

10.10.1 Photochemical Internalization (PCI)

The benefits of ROS generated during PS illumination are not limited to direct therapeutic applications only. If precisely controlled, it can aid in elevating the therapeutic outcome of other drugs especially those characterized by their cellular uptake via endocytosis. Examples include—and are not limited to—macromolecules i.e., nucleic acids [140] and nanoparticles [141]. Photochemical internalization (PCI) involves using PSs accumulating favorably in the membranes of endosomes. Illuminating them leads to endocytic vesicle rupture as in this way PCI acts a platform for macromolecules release in the cytosol and the consequent escape from the otherwise associated lysosomal degradation [142]. The effectiveness of PCI in treating human oral squamous cells was proved at the in vitro level using a conjugate made of the chlorin derivative: disulfonated tetraphenylchlorin ($TPCS_{2a}$) and the ribosome-inactivating protein (saporin) [143].

10.10.2 New Drug Delivery Systems: The Road for Third-Generation PS

To prolong the buccal mucosa retention time and enhance 5-ALA mucosal penetration, a mucoadhesive chitosan film loaded with various 5-ALA concentrations was prepared. In vivo studies for the formulation containing 10% 5-ALA using pig buccal mucosa showed 4 times increase in 5-ALA permeation and 17 times increase in mucosal retention relative to the control [144]. Such improvements are expected to concur with enhanced PDD and PDT responses. Recently, metalloproteinase-activated beacons were utilized as a very smart and highly selective delivery system for oral cancer pyropheophorbide-PDD-guided resection. As malignant cells are characterized with overexpression of metalloproteinases for angiogenic purposes, no beacon cleavage and thus no fluorescence signal were evident in normal cells as confirmed by fluorescence and confocal images of the athymic nude mice xenograft model for human oral carcinoma cell line UM-SCC-1. This delivery system provided a precise fluorescence-guided resection of tumor lesion located in the cheek of a hamster model for oral cancer [145].

Another drug delivery system was designed for m-THPC-targeted delivery. It consisted of micelles conjugated with folic acid. Two times increase in the concentration of internalized m-THPC and an elevated fluorescence signal in comparison to the control were reported in the in vitro studies on the folate receptor overexpressing human mouth epidermal KB. The selective targeting was confirmed by in vivo studies of KB cell mice model where a tumor-to-muscle ratio was twice that observed for the control. This uptake enhancement was reflected on the tumoricidal effect where a significantly more reduction in the tumor volume was reported for the conjugate without affecting imposing any toxicity on the mice as proven by normal body weight [146]. Another novel PS delivery system adopted the biocompatible and biodegradable hyper branched poly-ether ester macromolecule to deliver a covalently bound PS—namely, chlorin e6—to human tongue carcinoma CAL-27 cells. The conjugate shifted the absorption band 12 nm in the red region and localized in the cytoplasm, and its associated tumoricidal effect was 3–4 times more potent [147].

As an example of multimodal systems, gold nanoparticles were coated with Raman dye and a stabilized form of the PS hypericin. The conjugate served both diagnostic and treatment purposes successfully when tested using human oral cell line SCC4. Treatment was mediated by either photodynamic therapy after hypericin activation or photothermal therapy after nanoparticle activation [148]. Magnetic resonance imaging, phthalocyanine-mediated PDT, and fibronectin-mimetic peptide-mediated active targeting were all three accomplished using a synthesized conjugate. Results of head and neck cancer cells (M4E, 686LN, and TU212) along with their xenograft nude mice model confirmed the superiority of the conjugate in terms of potency—ten times less concentration was needed—and selectivity [149].

10.10.3 Administration of PDD and PDT Response: Enhancers

Potentiating PDD and PDT is feasible through opposing factors positively associated with PDD interference or PDT resistance. Human oral carcinoma cell lines (SSC4 and SAS) were incubated with calcium-phosphate nanoparticles loaded with small interfering RNA (siRNA) for hypoxia-inducible factor 1 alpha (HIF-1α) followed by photosan-PDT. Normally, HIF-1α expression promotes cell proliferation and resistance to apoptosis. Opposing HIF-1α by its siRNA along with photosan-PDT corresponded to three times increase in the cytotoxic activity in comparison to either PDT or HIF-1α-siRNA alone. This augmented cellular progression-inhibitory effect was also evident at the in vivo level through an apoptotic cell death mode [150]. The same group delivered vascular endothelial growth factor (VEGF) siRNA using the same delivery system and reported a selective and enhanced PS delivery accompanied with a better therapeutic effect at both in vitro and in vivo levels [151]. Likewise, coadministration of the selective cyclooxygenase (COX)-2 inhibitor; nimesulide along with 5-ALA-PDT synergized the antitumor activity against COX-2 overexpressing human oral carcinoma cells HSC-2 [152].

The use of antibodies is also reported as a way for PDD and PDT enhancement. Conjugating monoclonal antibodies with fluorescent dyes for diagnostic purposes is known as immunophotodiagnosis and to a PS for therapeutic purposes is known as photoimmunotherapy. As oral cancer cells overexpress epidermal growth factor receptor (EGFR), it was the marker of choice. Human epidermoid SCC A431 and HCPC-1 were diagnosed using EGFR monoclonal antibody (C225) covalently bound to the fluorescent dye Cy5.5. This conjugate granted a selective tumor to normal tissue fluorescence intensity that was correlated with severity and allowed the detection of the otherwise not visible dysplastic area. In the same study, C225 was conjugated with chlorin e6, and PDT successfully cured oral cancerous lesions of hamster cheek pouch model [153]. Antibody administration can precede PDT by few hours. Chlorin e6-PDT was applied on epithelial EGFR overexpressing human oral squamous cell lines HSC-3 and SCC-25 after administration of EGFR human monoclonal antibodies, nimotuzumab and cetuximab. Both cells and xenograft model studies demonstrated a remarkable decrease in tumor proliferation and angiogenic behavior in comparison to PDT alone [154].

Especially 5-ALA-PDD and PDT can be modulated through interfering PPIX synthetic pathway. For instance, coadministration of the iron chelator deferoxamine mesylate (DFO) lowered the production rate of hematoporphyrin and favored the accumulation of PPIX. This was reflected as a higher fluorescence signal (2–4 times increase according to cell line) and an expected better antitumor action against human oral SCC (HSC-2, HSC-3, HSC-4, Ca9-22, and SAS) along with their respective scid mice model [155]. In another trial to improve 5-ALA-PDT, it was combined with either ferrochelatase or ATP-binding cassette G2 (ABCG2) inhibitors. The first inhibited iron utilization and thus elevated PPIX accumulation by fivefolds, and the latter blocked an efflux pump that otherwise lowers intracellular levels of PPIX and inhibiting it was correlated with 5.2 times increase in accumulated PPIX in the absence of serum. The antiproliferative effect against human tongue carcinoma cells (HSC-4) and human OSCC (HSC-2) has significantly improved after co-administration of either inhibitor and was the highest when both inhibitors were combined [156]. Interestingly, it was reported that vitamin D derivative, calcipotriol, upregulates PPIX synthesis rate-limiting enzyme, coproporphyrinogen oxidase. This explained the rationale behind pretreating human tongue carcinoma SCC4, oral carcinoma SAS cells, and hamster check pouch model with calcipotriol before 5-ALA-PDD and PDT. Results were in favor for a potentiating effect. Calcipotriol pretreatment increased significantly the fluorescence ratio between tumor and healthy oral lesions. Furthermore, a significantly lower number of treatment sessions were needed in case of calcipotriol pretreated group to reach complete cure in comparison to 5-ALA-PDT alone [157].

Conclusion

Oral cancer lesion's late diagnosis exacerbates case prognosis and raises associated mortality. Both photodynamic diagnosis (PDD) and photodynamic therapy (PDT) are effective, noninvasive, patient friendly, and highly precise modalities. The outcome of conducted clinical studies is very promising and promotes their utilization as standard and adjuvant interventions.

References

1. Reibel J. Prognosis of oral pre-malignant lesions: significance of clinical, histopathological, and molecular biological characteristics. Crit Rev Oral Biol Med. 2003;14(1):47–62.
2. Daley T, Darling M. Nonsquamous cell malignant tumours of the oral cavity: an overview. J Can Dent Assoc. 2003;69(9):577–82.
3. Patel SG, Shah JP. TNM staging of cancers of the head and neck: striving for uniformity among diversity. CA Cancer J Clin. 2005;55(4):242–58. quiz 61-2, 64

4. Silverman S Jr. Demographics and occurrence of oral and pharyngeal cancers. The outcomes, the trends, the challenge. J Am Dent Assoc. 2001;132(Suppl):7S–11S.
5. Tahmassebi JF, Drogkari E, Wood SR. A study of the control of oral plaque biofilms via antibacterial photodynamic therapy. Eur Arch Paediatr Dent. 2015;16(6):433–40.
6. Sobaniec S, Bernaczyk P, Pietruski J, Cholewa M, Skurska A, Dolinska E, Duraj E, Tokajuk G, Paniczko A, Olszewska E, Pietruska M. Clinical assessment of the efficacy of photodynamic therapy in the treatment of oral lichen planus. Lasers Med Sci. 2013;28(1):311–6.
7. Dolmans DE, Fukumura D, Jain RK. Photodynamic therapy for cancer. Nat Rev Cancer. 2003;3(5):380–7.
8. Daniell MD, Hill JS. A history of photodynamic therapy. Aust N Z J Surg. 1991;61(5):340–8.
9. McDonagh AF. Phototherapy: from ancient Egypt to the new millennium. J Perinatol. 2001;21(Suppl 1):S7–S12.
10. Moan J, Peng Q. An outline of the hundred-year history of PDT. Anticancer Res. 2003;23(5A):3591–600.
11. Tappeiner H, Jodlbauer A. Über Wirkung der photodynamischen (fluoreszierenden) Stoffe auf Protozoan und Enzyme. [On the effect of photodynamic (fluorescent) substances on protozoa and enzymes]. Dtsch Arch Klin Med. 1904;80(427–487).
12. Jesionek A, Tappeiner H. Zur Behandlung der Hautkarzinome mit fluoreszierenden Stoffen. Dtsch Arch Klin Med. 1905;82:223–9.
13. Hausman W. Die sensibilisierende wirkung des hematoporphyrins. Biochem Z. 1911;30:276.
14. Policard A. Etudes sur les aspects offerts par des tumeurs experimentales examinees a la lumiere de Wood. Cr Soc Biol. 1924;91:1423–8.
15. Lipson RL, Baldes EJ. The photodynamic properties of a particular hematoporphyrin derivative. Arch Dermatol. 1960;82:508–16.
16. Lipson RL, Baldes EJ, Gray MJ. Hematoporphyrin derivative for detection and management of cancer. Cancer. 1967;20(12):2255–7.
17. Kessel D, Thompson P. Purification and analysis of hematoporphyrin and hematoporphyrin derivative by gel exclusion and reverse-phase chromatography. Photochem Photobiol. 1987;46(6):1023–5.
18. Dougherty TJ, Kaufman JE, Goldfarb A, Weishaupt KR, Boyle D, Mittleman A. Photoradiation therapy for the treatment of malignant tumors. Cancer Res. 1978;38(8):2628–35.
19. Dougherty TJ, Gomer CJ, Henderson BW, Jori G, Kessel D, Korbelik M, Moan J, Peng Q. Photodynamic therapy. J Natl Cancer Inst. 1998;90(12):889–905.
20. Azzi S, Hebda JK, Gavard J. Vascular permeability and drug delivery in cancers. Front Oncol. 2013;3:211.
21. Zhu TC, Finlay JC. The role of photodynamic therapy (PDT) physics. Med Phys. 2008;35(7):3127–36.
22. Castano AP, Demidova TN, Hamblin MR. Mechanisms in photodynamic therapy: part one-photosensitizers, photochemistry and cellular localization. Photodiagn Photodyn Ther. 2004;1(4):279–93.
23. Halliwell B, Chirico S. Lipid peroxidation: its mechanism, measurement, and significance. Am J Clin Nutr. 1993;57(5 Suppl):715S–24S; discussion 24S-25S
24. Dalle-Donne I, Giustarini D, Colombo R, Rossi R, Milzani A. Protein carbonylation in human diseases. Trends Mol Med. 2003;9(4):169–76.
25. Abrahamse H, Hamblin MR. New photosensitizers for photodynamic therapy. Biochem J. 2016;473(4):347–64.
26. Allison RR, Downie GH, Cuenca R, XH H, Childs CJ, Sibata CH. Photosensitizers in clinical PDT. Photodiagn Photodyn Ther. 2004;1(1):27–42.
27. Allison RR, Sibata CH. Oncologic photodynamic therapy photosensitizers: a clinical review. Photodiagn Photodyn Ther. 2010;7(2):61–75.
28. van Dongen GA, Visser GW, Vrouenraets MB. Photosensitizer-antibody conjugates for detection and therapy of cancer. Adv Drug Deliv Rev. 2004;56(1):31–52.

29. Jeong H, Huh M, Lee SJ, Koo H, Kwon IC, Jeong SY, Kim K. Photosensitizer-conjugated human serum albumin nanoparticles for effective photodynamic therapy. Theranostics. 2011;1:230–9.
30. Bonnett R, White RD, Winfield UJ, Berenbaum MC. Hydroporphyrins of the meso-tetra(hydroxyphenyl)porphyrin series as tumour photosensitizers. Biochem J. 1989; 261(1):277–80.
31. de Visscher SA, Dijkstra PU, Tan IB, Roodenburg JL, Witjes MJ. mTHPC mediated photodynamic therapy (PDT) of squamous cell carcinoma in the head and neck: a systematic review. Oral Oncol. 2013;49(3):192–210.
32. Huang Z. A review of progress in clinical photodynamic therapy. Technol Cancer Res Treat. 2005;4(3):283–93.
33. Senge MO, Brandt JC. Temoporfin (Foscan(R), 5,10,15,20-tetra(m-hydroxyphenyl)chlorin)- a second-generation photosensitizer. Photochem Photobiol. 2011;87(6):1240–96.
34. Hopper C, Niziol C, Sidhu M. The cost-effectiveness of Foscan mediated photodynamic therapy (Foscan-PDT) compared with extensive palliative surgery and palliative chemotherapy for patients with advanced head and neck cancer in the UK. Oral Oncol. 2004;40(4):372–82.
35. Kiesslich T, Berlanda J, Plaetzer K, Krammer B, Berr F. Comparative characterization of the efficiency and cellular pharmacokinetics of Foscan-and Foslip-based photodynamic treatment in human biliary tract cancer cell lines. Photochem Photobiol Sci. 2007;6(6):619–27.
36. Dougherty TJ. Studies on the structure of porphyrins contained in Photofrin II. Photochem Photobiol. 1987;46(5):569–73.
37. Byrne CJ, Marshallsay LV, Ward AD. The composition of Photofrin II. J Photochem Photobiol B. 1990;6(1–2):13–27.
38. Moan J, Sommer S. Action spectra for hematoporphyrin derivative and Photofrin II with respect to sensitization of human cells in vitro to photoinactivation. Photochem Photobiol. 1984;40(5):631–4.
39. Yang X, Palasuberniam P, Kraus D, Chen B. Aminolevulinic acid-based tumor detection and therapy: molecular mechanisms and strategies for enhancement. Int J Mol Sci. 2015;16(10):25865–80.
40. Musiol R, Serda M, Polanski J. Prodrugs in photodynamic anticancer therapy. Curr Pharm Des. 2011;17(32):3548–59.
41. Wachowska M, Muchowicz A, Firczuk M, Gabrysiak M, Winiarska M, Wańczyk M, Bojarczuk K, Golab J. Aminolevulinic Acid (ALA) as a prodrug in photodynamic therapy of cancer. Molecules. 2011;16:4140–64.
42. Pansare V, Hejazi S, Faenza W, Prud'homme RK. Review of long-wavelength optical and NIR imaging materials: contrast agents, fluorophores and multifunctional nano carriers. Chem Mater. 2012;24(5):812–27.
43. Shackley DC, Whitehurst C, Moore JV, George NJ, Betts CD, Clarke NW. Light penetration in bladder tissue: implications for the intravesical photodynamic therapy of bladder tumours. BJU Int. 2000;86(6):638–43.
44. Brancaleon L, Moseley H. Laser and non-laser light sources for photodynamic therapy. Lasers Med Sci. 2002;17(3):173–86.
45. Mang TS. Lasers and light sources for PDT: past, present and future. Photodiagn Photodyn Ther. 2004;1(1):43–8.
46. Yoon I, Li JZ, Shim YK. Advance in photosensitizers and light delivery for photodynamic therapy. Clin Endosc. 2013;46(1):7–23.
47. CH Y, Lin HP, Chen HM, Yang H, Wang YP, Chiang CP. Comparison of clinical outcomes of oral erythroleukoplakia treated with photodynamic therapy using either light-emitting diode or laser light. Lasers Surg Med. 2009;41(9):628–33.
48. Tanaka H, Hashimoto K, Yamada I, Masumoto K, Ohsawa T, Murai M, Hirano T. Interstitial photodynamic therapy with rotating and reciprocating optical fibers. Cancer. 2001;91(9):1791–6.

49. Jerjes W, Upile T, Hamdoon Z, Abbas S, Akram S, Mosse CA, Morley S, Hopper C. Photodynamic therapy: the minimally invasive surgical intervention for advanced and/or recurrent tongue base carcinoma. Lasers Surg Med. 2011;43(4):283–92.
50. Jerjes W, Upile T, Radhi H, Hopper C. Photodynamic therapy and end-stage tongue base cancer: short communication. Head Neck Oncol. 2011;3:49.
51. Jager HR, Taylor MN, Theodossy T, Hopper C. MR imaging-guided interstitial photodynamic laser therapy for advanced head and neck tumors. AJNR Am J Neuroradiol. 2005;26(5):1193–200.
52. Karakullukcu B, Nyst HJ, van Veen RL, Hoebers FJ, Hamming-Vrieze O, Witjes MJ, de Visscher SA, Burlage FR, Levendag PC, Sterenborg HJ, Tan IB. mTHPC mediated interstitial photodynamic therapy of recurrent nonmetastatic base of tongue cancers: development of a new method. Head Neck. 2012;34(11):1597–606.
53. Osher J, Jerjes W, Upile T, Hamdoon Z, Morley S, Hopper C. Adenoid cystic carcinoma of the tongue base treated with ultrasound-guided interstitial photodynamic therapy: a case study. Photodiagn Photodyn Ther. 2011;8(1):68–71.
54. Chen Q, Chen H, Hetzel FW. Tumor oxygenation changes post-photodynamic therapy. Photochem Photobiol. 1996;63(1):128–31.
55. Scheeren TW, Schober P, Schwarte LA. Monitoring tissue oxygenation by near infrared spectroscopy (NIRS): background and current applications. J Clin Monit Comput. 2012;26(4):279–87.
56. Nordsmark M, Loncaster J, Aquino-Parsons C, Chou SC, Ladekarl M, Havsteen H, Lindegaard JC, Davidson SE, Varia M, West C, Hunter R, Overgaard J, Raleigh JA. Measurements of hypoxia using pimonidazole and polarographic oxygen-sensitive electrodes in human cervix carcinomas. Radiother Oncol. 2003;67(1):35–44.
57. Coutier S, Bezdetnaya LN, Foster TH, Parache RM, Guillemin F. Effect of irradiation fluence rate on the efficacy of photodynamic therapy and tumor oxygenation in meta-tetra (hydroxyphenyl) chlorin (mTHPC)-sensitized HT29 xenografts in nude mice. Radiat Res. 2002;158(3):339–45.
58. Xiao Z, Halls S, Dickey D, Tulip J, Moore RB. Fractionated versus standard continuous light delivery in interstitial photodynamic therapy of dunning prostate carcinomas. Clin Cancer Res. 2007;13(24):7496–505.
59. Yang L, Wei Y, Xing D, Chen Q. Increasing the efficiency of photodynamic therapy by improved light delivery and oxygen supply using an anticoagulant in a solid tumor model. Lasers Surg Med. 2010;42(7):671–9.
60. Huang Z, Chen Q, Shakil A, Chen H, Beckers J, Shapiro H, Hetzel FW. Hyperoxygenation enhances the tumor cell killing of photofrin-mediated photodynamic therapy. Photochem Photobiol. 2003;78(5):496–502.
61. Chen Q, Huang Z, Chen H, Shapiro H, Beckers J, Hetzel FW. Improvement of tumor response by manipulation of tumor oxygenation during photodynamic therapy. Photochem Photobiol. 2002;76(2):197–203.
62. Broekgaarden M, Weijer R, van Gulik TM, Hamblin MR, Heger M. Tumor cell survival pathways activated by photodynamic therapy: a molecular basis for pharmacological inhibition strategies. Cancer Metastasis Rev. 2015;34(4):643–90.
63. Fan KF, Hopper C, Speight PM, Buonaccorsi GA, Bown SG. Photodynamic therapy using mTHPC for malignant disease in the oral cavity. Int J Cancer. 1997;73(1):25–32.
64. Elmore S. Apoptosis: a review of programmed cell death. Toxicol Pathol. 2007;35(4):495–516.
65. Glick D, Barth S, Macleod KF. Autophagy: cellular and molecular mechanisms. J Pathol. 2010;221(1):3–12.
66. Garg AD, Bose M, Ahmed MI, Bonass WA, Wood SR. In vitro studies on erythrosine-based photodynamic therapy of malignant and pre-malignant oral epithelial cells. PLoS One. 2012;7(4):e34475.

67. Moon YH, Park JH, Kim SA, Lee JB, Ahn SG, Yoon JH. Anticancer effect of photodynamic therapy with hexenyl ester of 5-aminolevulinic acid in oral squamous cell carcinoma. Head Neck. 2010;32(9):1136–42.
68. Park JH, Moon YH, Kim DJ, Kim SA, Lee JB, Ahn SG, Yoon JH. Photodynamic therapy with hexenyl ester of 5-aminolevulinic acid induces necrotic cell death in salivary gland adenocarcinoma cells. Oncol Rep. 2010;24(1):177–81.
69. Chen HM, Liu CM, Yang H, Chou HY, Chiang CP, Kuo MY. 5-Aminolevulinic acid induce apoptosis via NF-kappaB/JNK pathway in human oral cancer Ca9-22 cells. J Oral Pathol Med. 2011;40(6):483–9.
70. Qiao L, Mei Z, Yang Z, Li X, Cai H, Liu W. ALA-PDT inhibits proliferation and promotes apoptosis of SCC cells through STAT3 signal pathway. Photodiagn Photodyn Ther. 2016;14:66–73.
71. Qiao L, Xu C, Li Q, Mei Z, Li X, Cai H, Liu W. Photodynamic therapy activated STAT3 associated pathways: targeting intrinsic apoptotic pathways to increase PDT efficacy in human squamous carcinoma cells. Photodiagn Photodyn Ther. 2016;14:119–27.
72. Lim HJ, Oh CH. Indocyanine green-based photodynamic therapy with 785 nm light emitting diode for oral squamous cancer cells. Photodiagn Photodyn Ther. 2011;8(4):337–42.
73. Choi H, Lim W, Kim JE, Kim I, Jeong J, Ko Y, Song J, You S, Kim D, Kim M, Kim BK, Kim O. Cell death and intracellular distribution of hematoporphyrin in a KB cell line. Photomed Laser Surg. 2009;27(3):453–60.
74. Lai X, Ning F, Xia X, Wang D, Tang L, Hu J, Wu J, Liu J, Li X. HMME combined with green light-emitting diode irradiation results in efficient apoptosis on human tongue squamous cell carcinoma. Lasers Med Sci. 2015;30(7):1941–8.
75. Kobayashi W, Liu Q, Nakagawa H, Sakaki H, Teh B, Matsumiya T, Yoshida H, Imaizumi T, Satoh K, Kimura H. Photodynamic therapy with mono-L-aspartyl chlorin e6 can cause necrosis of squamous cell carcinoma of tongue: experimental study on an animal model of nude mouse. Oral Oncol. 2006;42(1):46–50.
76. Usuda J, Kato H, Okunaka T, Furukawa K, Tsutsui H, Yamada K, Suga Y, Honda H, Nagatsuka Y, Ohira T, Tsuboi M, Hirano T. Photodynamic therapy (PDT) for lung cancers. J Thorac Oncol. 2006;1(5):489–93.
77. Ahn MY, Yoon HE, Kwon SM, Lee J, Min SK, Kim YC, Ahn SG, Yoon JH. Synthesized Pheophorbide a-mediated photodynamic therapy induced apoptosis and autophagy in human oral squamous carcinoma cells. J Oral Pathol Med. 2013;42(1):17–25.
78. Barcessat AR, Huang I, Rosin FP, dos Santos Pinto D Jr, Maria Zezell D, Correa L. Effect of topical 5-ALA mediated photodynamic therapy on proliferation index of keratinocytes in 4-NQO-induced potentially malignant oral lesions. J Photochem Photobiol B. 2013;126:33–41.
79. Rosin FC, Barcessat AR, Borges GG, Correa L. Effect of 5-ALA-mediated photodynamic therapy on mast cell and microvessels densities present in oral premalignant lesions induced in rats. J Photochem Photobiol B. 2015;153:429–34.
80. Longo JP, Lozzi SP, Simioni AR, Morais PC, Tedesco AC, Azevedo RB. Photodynamic therapy with aluminum-chloro-phthalocyanine induces necrosis and vascular damage in mice tongue tumors. J Photochem Photobiol B. 2009;94(2):143–6.
81. Kingsbury JS, Cecere W, Mang TS, Liebow C. Photodynamic therapy for premalignant lesions in DMBA-treated hamsters: a preliminary study. J Oral Maxillofac Surg. 1997;55(4):376–81, discussion 81-2
82. Schmidt-Erfurth U, Hasan T. Mechanisms of action of photodynamic therapy with verteporfin for the treatment of age-related macular degeneration. Surv Ophthalmol. 2000;45(3):195–214.
83. Lenihan CR, Taylor CT. The impact of hypoxia on cell death pathways. Biochem Soc Trans. 2013;41(2):657–63.

84. Chen B, Pogue BW, Luna JM, Hardman RL, Hoopes PJ, Hasan T. Tumor vascular permeabilization by vascular-targeting photosensitization: effects, mechanism, and therapeutic implications. Clin Cancer Res. 2006;12(3 Pt 1):917–23.
85. Osaki T, Takagi S, Hoshino Y, Okumura M, Kadosawa T, Fujinaga T. Efficacy of antivascular photodynamic therapy using benzoporphyrin derivative monoacid ring A (BPD-MA) in 14 dogs with oral and nasal tumors. J Vet Med Sci. 2009;71(2):125–32.
86. Gao Z, Zheng J, Yang B, Wang Z, Fan H, Lv Y, Li H, Jia L, Cao W. Sonodynamic therapy inhibits angiogenesis and tumor growth in a xenograft mouse model. Cancer Lett. 2013;335(1):93–9.
87. Triesscheijn M, Ruevekamp M, Aalders M, Baas P, Stewart FA. Outcome of mTHPC mediated photodynamic therapy is primarily determined by the vascular response. Photochem Photobiol. 2005;81(5):1161–7.
88. Milstein DM, van Kuijen AM, Copper MP, Karakullukcu B, Tan IB, Lindeboom JA, Fokkens WJ, Ince C. Monitoring microcirculatory alterations in oral squamous cell carcinoma following photodynamic therapy. Photodiagn Photodyn Ther. 2012;9(1):69–75.
89. Garg AD, Nowis D, Golab J, Agostinis P. Photodynamic therapy: illuminating the road from cell death towards anti-tumour immunity. Apoptosis. 2010;15(9):1050–71.
90. Castano AP, Mroz P, Hamblin MR. Photodynamic therapy and anti-tumour immunity. Nat Rev Cancer. 2006;6(7):535–45.
91. Reginato E, Wolf P, Hamblin MR. Immune response after photodynamic therapy increases anti-cancer and anti-bacterial effects. World J Immunol. 2014;4(1):1–11.
92. Wachowska M, Muchowicz A, Demkow U. Immunological aspects of antitumor photodynamic therapy outcome. Cent Eur J Immunol. 2015;40(4):481–5.
93. Dube A, Sharma S, Gupta PK. Tumor regression induced by photodynamic treatment with chlorin p(6) in hamster cheek pouch model of oral carcinogenesis: dependence of mode of tumor cell death on the applied drug dose. Oral Oncol. 2011;47(6):467–71.
94. Kobayashi W, Liu Q, Matsumiya T, Nakagawa H, Yoshida H, Imaizumi T, Satoh K, Kimura H. Photodynamic therapy upregulates expression of Mac-1 and generation of leukotriene B(4) by human polymorphonuclear leukocytes. Oral Oncol. 2004;40(5):506–10.
95. Sharma S, Jajoo A, Dube A. 5-Aminolevulinic acid-induced protoporphyrin-IX accumulation and associated phototoxicity in macrophages and oral cancer cell lines. J Photochem Photobiol B. 2007;88(2–3):156–62.
96. Mijan MC, Longo JPF, Melo LNDd, Simioni AR, Tedesco AC, Azevedo RB. Vascular shutdown and pro-inflammatory cytokine expression in breast cancer tumors after photodynamic therapy mediated by nano-sized liposomes containing aluminium-chloride-phthalocyanine. J Nanomed Nanotechnol. 2014;5(218).
97. Kabingu E, Oseroff AR, Wilding GE, Gollnick SO. Enhanced systemic immune reactivity to a basal cell carcinoma associated antigen following photodynamic therapy. Clin Cancer Res. 2009;15(13):4460–6.
98. Korbelik M, Sun J. Photodynamic therapy-generated vaccine for cancer therapy. Cancer Immunol Immunother. 2006;55(8):900–9.
99. Korbelik M, Stott B, Sun J. Photodynamic therapy-generated vaccines: relevance of tumour cell death expression. Br J Cancer. 2007;97(10):1381–7.
100. Zheng W, Harris M, Kho KW, Thong PS, Hibbs A, Olivo M, Soo KC. Confocal endomicroscopic imaging of normal and neoplastic human tongue tissue using ALA-induced-PPIX fluorescence: a preliminary study. Oncol Rep. 2004;12(2):397–401.
101. Chang YC, Yu CH. Successful treatment of oral verrucous hyperplasia with photodynamic therapy combined with cryotherapy-report of 3 cases. Photodiagn Photodyn Ther. 2014;11(2):127–9.
102. Yang DF, Lee JW, Chen HM, Hsu YC. Topical methotrexate pretreatment enhances the therapeutic effect of topical 5-aminolevulinic acid-mediated photodynamic therapy on hamster buccal pouch precancers. J Formos Med Assoc. 2014;113(9):591–9.

103. Uehara M, Inokuchi T, Ikeda H. Enhanced susceptibility of mouse squamous cell carcinoma to photodynamic therapy combined with low-dose administration of cisplatin. J Oral Maxillofac Surg. 2006;64(3):390–6.
104. Quon H, Finlay J, Cengel K, Zhu T, O'Malley B Jr, Weinstein G. Transoral robotic photodynamic therapy for the oropharynx. Photodiagn Photodyn Ther. 2011;8(1):64–7.
105. Fontana CR, Lerman MA, Patel N, Grecco C, Costa CA, Amiji MM, Bagnato VS, Soukos NS. Safety assessment of oral photodynamic therapy in rats. Lasers Med Sci. 2013;28(2):479–86.
106. D'Cruz AK, Robinson MH, Biel MA. mTHPC-mediated photodynamic therapy in patients with advanced, incurable head and neck cancer: a multicenter study of 128 patients. Head Neck. 2004;26(3):232–40.
107. Toratani S, Tani R, Kanda T, Koizumi K, Yoshioka Y, Okamoto T. Photodynamic therapy using Photofrin and excimer dye laser treatment for superficial oral squamous cell carcinomas with long-term follow up. Photodiagn Photodyn Ther. 2016;1572(30):104–10. 30060-0
108. Dougherty TJ, Cooper MT, Mang TS. Cutaneous phototoxic occurrences in patients receiving Photofrin. Lasers Surg Med. 1990;10(5):485–8.
109. Menter JM, Hollins TD, Sayre RM, Etemadi AA, Willis I, Hughes SN. Protection against photodynamic therapy (PDT)-induced photosensitivity by fabric materials. Photodermatol Photoimmunol Photomed. 1998;14(5–6):154–9.
110. Chen HM, CH Y, PC T, Yeh CY, Tsai T, Chiang CP. Successful treatment of oral verrucous hyperplasia and oral leukoplakia with topical 5-aminolevulinic acid-mediated photodynamic therapy. Lasers Surg Med. 2005;37(2):114–22.
111. Chen HM, Chen CT, Yang H, Lee MI, Kuo MY, Kuo YS, Wang YP, Tsai T, Chiang CP. Successful treatment of an extensive verrucous carcinoma with topical 5-aminolevulinic acid-mediated photodynamic therapy. J Oral Pathol Med. 2005;34(4):253–6.
112. Chiang CP, Huang WT, Lee JW, Hsu YC. Effective treatment of 7,12-dimethylbenz(a) anthracene-induced hamster buccal pouch precancerous lesions by topical photosan-mediated photodynamic therapy. Head Neck. 2012;34(4):505–12.
113. Leunig A, Betz CS, Mehlmann M, Stepp H, Arbogast S, Grevers G, Baumgartner R. Detection of squamous cell carcinoma of the oral cavity by imaging 5-aminolevulinic acid-induced protoporphyrin IX fluorescence. Laryngoscope. 2000;110(1):78–83.
114. Kubler AC, de Carpentier J, Hopper C, Leonard AG, Putnam G. Treatment of squamous cell carcinoma of the lip using Foscan-mediated photodynamic therapy. Int J Oral Maxillofac Surg. 2001;30(6):504–9.
115. Kawczyk-Krupka A, Waskowska J, Raczkowska-Siostrzonek A, Kosciarz-Grzesiok A, Kwiatek S, Straszak D, Latos W, Koszowski R, Sieron A. Comparison of cryotherapy and photodynamic therapy in treatment of oral leukoplakia. Photodiagn Photodyn Ther. 2012;9(2):148–55.
116. Chang CJ, Wilder-Smith P. Topical application of photofrin for photodynamic diagnosis of oral neoplasms. Plast Reconstr Surg. 2005;115(7):1877–86.
117. Yu CH, Yu CC. Photodynamic therapy with 5-aminolevulinic acid (ALA) impairs tumor initiating and chemo-resistance property in head and neck cancer-derived cancer stem cells. PLoS One. 2014;9(1):e87129.
118. Sharwani A, Jerjes W, Hopper C, Lewis MP, El-Maaytah M, Khalil HS, Macrobert AJ, Upile T, Salih V. Photodynamic therapy down-regulates the invasion promoting factors in human oral cancer. Arch Oral Biol. 2006;51(12):1104–11.
119. Li P-T, Ke E-S, Chiang P-C, Tsai T. ALA-or Ce6-PDT induced phenotypic change and suppressed migration in surviving cancer cells. J Dent Sci. 2015;10(1):74–80.
120. Hopper C, Kubler A, Lewis H, Tan IB, Putnam G. mTHPC-mediated photodynamic therapy for early oral squamous cell carcinoma. Int J Cancer. 2004;111(1):138–46.
121. Biel MA. Photodynamic therapy treatment of early oral and laryngeal cancers. Photochem Photobiol. 2007;83(5):1063–8.

122. Silverman S Jr, Gorsky M. Proliferative verrucous leukoplakia: a follow-up study of 54 cases. Oral Surg Oral Med Oral Pathol Oral Radiol Endod. 1997;84(2):154–7.
123. Selvam NP, Sadaksharam J, Singaravelu G, Ramu R. Treatment of oral leukoplakia with photodynamic therapy: a pilot study. J Cancer Res Ther. 2015;11(2):464–7.
124. Betz CS, Stepp H, Janda P, Arbogast S, Grevers G, Baumgartner R, Leunig A. A comparative study of normal inspection, autofluorescence and 5-ALA-induced PPIX fluorescence for oral cancer diagnosis. Int J Cancer. 2002;97(2):245–52.
125. Leunig A, Rick K, Stepp H, Gutmann R, Alwin G, Baumgartner R, Feyh J. Fluorescence imaging and spectroscopy of 5-aminolevulinic acid induced protoporphyrin IX for the detection of neoplastic lesions in the oral cavity. Am J Surg. 1996;172(6):674–7.
126. Lin HP, Chen HM, Yu CH, Yang H, Wang YP, Chiang CP. Topical photodynamic therapy is very effective for oral verrucous hyperplasia and oral erythroleukoplakia. J Oral Pathol Med. 2010;39(8):624–30.
127. Tan IB, Dolivet G, Ceruse P, Vander Poorten V, Roest G, Rauschning W. Temoporfin-mediated photodynamic therapy in patients with advanced, incurable head and neck cancer: a multicenter study. Head Neck. 2010;32(12):1597–604.
128. Schweitzer VG, Somers ML. PHOTOFRIN-mediated photodynamic therapy for treatment of early stage (Tis-T2N0M0) SqCCa of oral cavity and oropharynx. Lasers Surg Med. 2010;42(1):1–8.
129. Jerjes W, Upile T, Hamdoon Z, Mosse CA, Akram S, Hopper C. Photodynamic therapy outcome for oral dysplasia. Lasers Surg Med. 2011;43(3):192–9.
130. Karakullukcu B, van Oudenaarde K, Copper MP, Klop WM, van Veen R, Wildeman M, Bing Tan I. Photodynamic therapy of early stage oral cavity and oropharynx neoplasms: an outcome analysis of 170 patients. Eur Arch Otorhinolaryngol. 2011;268(2):281–8.
131. Jerjes W, Upile T, Hamdoon Z, Alexander Mosse C, Morcos M, Hopper C. Photodynamic therapy outcome for T1/T2 N0 oral squamous cell carcinoma. Lasers Surg Med. 2011;43(6):463–9.
132. Wong SJ, Campbell B, Massey B, Lynch DP, Cohen EE, Blair E, Selle R, Shklovskaya J, Jovanovic BD, Skripkauskas S, Dew A, Kulesza P, Parimi V, Bergan RC, Szabo E. A phase I trial of aminolevulinic acid-photodynamic therapy for treatment of oral leukoplakia. Oral Oncol. 2013;49(9):970–6.
133. Durbec M, Cosmidis A, Fuchsmann C, Ramade A, Ceruse P. Efficacy and safety of photodynamic therapy with temoporfin in curative treatment of recurrent carcinoma of the oral cavity and oropharynx. Eur Arch Otorhinolaryngol. 2013;270(4):1433–9.
134. Ikeda H, Tobita T, Ohba S, Uehara M, Asahina I. Treatment outcome of Photofrin-based photodynamic therapy for T1 and T2 oral squamous cell carcinoma and dysplasia. Photodiagn Photodyn Ther. 2013;10(3):229–35.
135. Ramachandra M, Mohlyuddin SA, Suresh T, Sagayaraj A, Merchant S. Evaluating usefulness of 5-aminolevulinic acid induced fluorescence to guide biopsy of oral cancers and premalignant legions. Int J Head Neck Surg. 2015;6(2):64–8.
136. Vander Poorten V, Meulemans J, Nuyts S, Clement P, Hermans R, Hauben E, Delaere P. Postoperative photodynamic therapy as a new adjuvant treatment after robot-assisted salvage surgery of recurrent squamous cell carcinoma of the base of tongue. World J Surg Oncol. 2015;13:214.
137. Saini R, Lee NV, Liu KY, Poh CF. Prospects in the application of photodynamic therapy in oral cancer and premalignant lesions. Cancers (Basel). 2016;8(9). pii: E83.
138. Rigual NR, Shafirstein G, Frustino J, Seshadri M, Cooper M, Wilding G, Sullivan MA, Henderson B. Adjuvant intraoperative photodynamic therapy in head and neck cancer. JAMA Otolaryngol Head Neck Surg. 2013;139(7):706–11.
139. Patrice T. Factors in establishment and spread of photodynamic therapy. In: Patrice T, editor. Photodynamic therapy. Great Britain: Royal Society of Chemistry; 2003.
140. Malefyt AP, Walton SP, Chan C. Endocytosis pathways for nucleic acid therapeutics. Nano Life. 2012;2(3):1241005.

141. Iversena T-G, Skotlanda T, Sandviga K. Endocytosis and intracellular transport of nanoparticles: present knowledge and need for future studies. NanoToday. 2011;6(2):176–85.
142. Berg K, Weyergang A, Prasmickaite L, Bonsted A, Hogset A, Strand MT, Wagner E, Selbo PK. Photochemical internalization (PCI): a technology for drug delivery. Methods Mol Biol. 2010;635:133–45.
143. Wang JT, Berg K, Hogset A, Bown SG, MacRobert AJ. Photophysical and photobiological properties of a sulfonated chlorin photosensitiser TPCS(2a) for photochemical internalisation (PCI). Photochem Photobiol Sci. 2013;12(3):519–26.
144. Costa Idos S, Abranches RP, Garcia MT, Pierre MB. Chitosan-based mucoadhesive films containing 5-aminolevulinic acid for buccal cancer's treatment. J Photochem Photobiol B. 2014;140:266–75.
145. Burgess L, Chen J, Wolter NE, Wilson B, Zheng G. Topical MMP beacon enabled fluorescence-guided resection of oral carcinoma. Biomed Opt Express. 2016;7(3):1089–99.
146. Syu W-J, Yu H-P, Hsu C-Y, Rajan YC, Hsu Y-H, Chang Y-C, Hsieh W-Y, Wang C-H, Lai P-S. Improved photodynamic cancer treatment by folate-conjugated polymeric micelles in a KB xenografted animal model. Small. 2012;8(13):2060–9.
147. Li P, Zhou G, Zhu X, Li G, Yan P, Shen L, Xu Q, Hamblin MR. Photodynamic therapy with hyperbranched poly(ether-ester) chlorin(e6) nanoparticles on human tongue carcinoma CAL-27 cells. Photodiagn Photodyn Ther. 2012;9(1):76–82.
148. Raghavan V, Connolly JM, Fan HM, Dockery P, Wheatley A, Keogh I, Olivo M. Gold nanosensitisers for multimodal optical diagnostic imaging and therapy of cancer. J Nanomed Nanotechnol. 2014;5(6).
149. Wang D, Fei B, Halig LV, Qin X, Hu Z, Xu H, Wang YA, Chen Z, Kim S, Shin DM, Chen ZG. Targeted iron-oxide nanoparticle for photodynamic therapy and imaging of head and neck cancer. ACS Nano. 2014;8(7):6620–32.
150. Chen WH, Lecaros RL, Tseng YC, Huang L, Hsu YC. Nanoparticle delivery of HIF1alpha siRNA combined with photodynamic therapy as a potential treatment strategy for head-and-neck cancer. Cancer Lett. 2015;359(1):65–74.
151. Lecaros RL, Huang L, Lee TC, Hsu YC. Nanoparticle delivered VEGF-A siRNA enhances photodynamic therapy for head and neck cancer treatment. Mol Ther. 2016;24(1):106–16.
152. Akita Y, Kozaki K, Nakagawa A, Saito T, Ito S, Tamada Y, Fujiwara S, Nishikawa N, Uchida K, Yoshikawa K, Noguchi T, Miyaishi O, Shimozato K, Saga S, Matsumoto Y. Cyclooxygenase-2 is a possible target of treatment approach in conjunction with photodynamic therapy for various disorders in skin and oral cavity. Br J Dermatol. 2004;151(2):472–80.
153. Soukos NS, Hamblin MR, Keel S, Fabian RL, Deutsch TF, Hasan T. Epidermal growth factor receptor-targeted immunophotodiagnosis and photoimmunotherapy of oral precancer in vivo. Cancer Res. 2001;61(11):4490–6.
154. Bhuvaneswari R, Ng QF, Thong PS, Soo KC. Nimotuzumab increases the anti-tumor effect of photodynamic therapy in an oral tumor model. Oncotarget. 2015;6(15):13487–505.
155. Uekusa M, Omura K, Nakajima Y, Hasegawa S, Harada H, Morita KI, Tsuda H. Uptake and kinetics of 5-aminolevulinic acid in oral squamous cell carcinoma. Int J Oral Maxillofac Surg. 2010;39(8):802–5.
156. Yamamoto M, Fujita H, Katase N, Inoue K, Nagatsuka H, Utsumi K, Sasaki J, Ohuchi H. Improvement of the efficacy of 5-aminolevulinic acid-mediated photodynamic treatment in human oral squamous cell carcinoma HSC-4. Acta Med Okayama. 2013;67(3):153–64.
157. Yang DF, Chen JH, Chiang CP, Huang Z, Lee JW, Liu CJ, Chang JL, Hsu YC. Improve efficacy of topical ALA-PDT by calcipotriol through up-regulation of coproporphyrinogen oxidase. Photodiagn Photodyn Ther. 2014;11(3):331–41.

Role of Nutrition in Oral and Pharyngeal Cancers: From Etiology to Prevention

11

Hiba Bawadi and "Mo'ez Al-Islam" Faris

11.1 Introduction

Oral and pharyngeal cancers (OPC) are considered the sixth most common cancers with incidence of around 405,300 cases/year [1]. Epidemiological studies showed that diet may account for 20–25% of OPC in Western countries [2]. Like other types of cancers, risk of OPC is attributed to interaction between environmental exposures and genetic predisposition factors. Among the environmental determinants of OPC, diet may include a wide array of both protective and risk factors. The role of nutrition and dietary factors in the process of carcinogenesis process ranges from the preventive role of food-containing bioactive compounds to the causal role of some dietary carcinogens. According to WHO's latest statistics [3], nutritional factors related to cancer etiology include obesity and low intake of fruits and vegetables. In fact, nutritional factors are recognized among the five leading causes of cancer-related deaths [3]. Multiple risk factors are associated with the etiology of OPC, of which the most commonly documented ones include tobacco smoking and alcohol drinking [4]. On the other hand, the most documented preventive factors include the consuming diets rich in fruits and vegetables [5]. An evidence exists about the protective effect of each serving of fruits and vegetables consumed with a decreased risk of OPC by 25% [6]. The power of fruits and vegetables in reducing risk of OPC stems from their naturally occurring antioxidants content [7]. In addition to fruits and vegetables, the plant kingdom also includes legumes which have been investigated for their antiproliferative and chemopreventive effects against oral carcinogenesis [8].

H. Bawadi (✉)
Department of Human Nutrition, College of Health Sciences, Qatar University, Doha, Qatar
e-mail: hbawadi@qu.edu.qa

M.A.-I. Faris
Department of Clinical Nutrition and Dietetics, College of Health Sciences and Sharjah Institute for Medical Reseacrh (SIMR), University of Sharjah, Sharjah, United Arab Emirates

A.-E. Al Moustafa (ed.), *Development of Oral Cancer*,
DOI 10.1007/978-3-319-48054-1_11

In addition to fruits and vegetables, other plant-based foods such as legumes and olive oil were investigated as favorable ways to reduce the burden of OPC risks [9]. Western diet that is characterized by its high content of animal proteins and low plant-based proteins and fibers, with high ratios of saturated and polyunsaturated fats (PUFA) in comparison to monounsaturated fats (MUFA), had been looked at as one of the risk factors of OPC [10]. On the other hand, a Mediterranean diet that is characterized by its plant-based proteins and higher MUFA from olive oil had been found to play a protective role against OPC [11–13]. This chapter will try to highlight the role of dietary factors in the initiation and prevention of OPC and to elaborate the underlying molecular mechanisms associated with the role of dietary factors in the etiology and prevention of OPC, as revealed by the most recent published works.

11.2 Food Groups and Risk of OPC

The role of food groups in cancer prevention revolves around the concept of variety and the importance of consuming combinations of food items from all food groups and probably subgroups. The synergistic effect of different nutrients and non-nutrient phytochemicals in chemoprevention is imperative. Foods belonging to the same group share health-related attributes. Such attributes may increase or decrease the risk of OPC. Hence, the importance of consuming diets with high variety (e.g., including foods from all food groups and subgroups) seems to be imperative [9]. A case-control study was conducted in multiple centers in Italy aimed at investigating the association between risk of OPC and diet variety defined as the total number of food items at least once per week [9]. The study included 805 of histologically diagnosed OPC cases and 2081 controls. After adjusting for confounding variables, authors reported a protective effect among individuals with the highest tertile of diet variety score against risk of OPC (OR: 0.78; 95% CI: 0.61–0.98). Diet variety within the food group was also reported to be statistically significant. For instance, variety within vegetables was inversely related to risk of OPC (OR: 0.62; 95% CI: 0.49–0.78). Similar results were reported with regard to variety in fruits (OR: 0.67; 95% CI: 0.53–0.86) [9]. The association between diet variety score and protection against OPC can be explained by the higher likelihood of consuming more types of anticancer compounds in different foods that work synergistically in cancer prevention.

The following section of this chapter will discuss the OPC anti- or procarcinogenic properties of different food groups, namely, fruits and vegetables, grains, legumes, meats, and fats, on the risk of OPC. Food groups documented to exhibit OPC anticarcinogenic properties are fruits and vegetables [5], legumes [14], and unsaturated oils [15]. On the other hand, meats and animal-based foods [16] and saturated fats [17] are reported to exhibit OPC procarcinogenic properties.

11.2.1 Fruits and Vegetables

Fruits and vegetables are characterized by their high content of vitamins, minerals, and dietary fibers, along with a plethora of bioactive phytochemicals, with low caloric content and minimum fats. Consumption of vegetables and fruits has been consistently linked to reduced risk of several types of cancer including OPC [5, 18]. The anticarcinogenic feature of fruits and vegetables is the inclusion of a wide array of bioactive phytochemicals and antioxidants such as flavonoids and carotenoids. Recently, the World Cancer Research Fund reported a likely protective effect of fruits and non-starchy vegetables against OPC [19].

The role of fruits and vegetables in OPC risk reduction was reported in a meta-analysis carried out by Pavia et al. [18]. The meta-analysis included 16 epidemiological studies from which a combined adjusted OR was estimated. The daily consumption of one serving of fruits was associated with 49% risk reduction of oral cancer (OR: 0.51; 95% CI: 0.40, 0.65), and daily consumption of one serving of vegetable was associated with 50% risk reduction (OR: 0.50; 95% CI: 0.38, 0.65) [18]. Furthermore, the meta-analysis revealed that the type of fruits consumed seemed to have a greater protective effect against OPC risk. For instance, the daily consumption of one serving of citrus fruits was associated with 62% risk reduction of OPC (OR: 0.38; 95% CI: 0.26, 0.56) [18].

A recent cohort study on 120,852 participants was conducted by Maasland et al. [5] aimed to investigate the relationship between consumption of fruits and vegetables and risk of head and neck cancers, including OPC. After 20 years for the cohort, results showed an inverse relation between total consumption of fruits and vegetables with risk of overall head and neck cancers (*P*-trend = 0.002) [5]. In the UK, low consumption rates of fruits and vegetables was considered as one of the attributable factors for the development of more than one type of cancers, including oral cavity [20]. In his study, Parkin [20] found that 56% of oral cavity and pharynx cancer cases may be related to the low intake of fruits and vegetables expressed as of consuming less than five portions/servings (at least 400 g) of a variety of non-starchy vegetables and of fruits every day, with less contribution to esophageal cancer (46%) and laryngeal cancer (45%).

Different types of fruit and vegetables were found to exhibit variable abilities of protection against OPC. *Allium* species including garlic (*Allium sativum*) and onion (*Allium cepa*) are among the most common types of *Allium* vegetables and characterized by their distinguished content of organosulfur compounds that possess anti-inflammatory, antioxidant, and anticancer properties [21]. Galeone and colleagues [22] found that consumption of *Allium* vegetables has a favorable correlate with cancer risk in Europe, with ORs for the highest category of onion and garlic intake using data from an integrated network of Italian and Swiss case-control studies being, respectively, 0.16 and 0.61 for cancers of the oral cavity and pharynx and 0.12 and 0.43 for esophageal cancer [22]. Cruciferous vegetables such as cauliflower, cabbage, broccoli, and Brussels sprouts are among the vegetable types with noticeable chemopreventive effect against more than one type of cancers, including oral cancer [23]. When analyzing the studies included a total of 1468 cancers of the oral cavity/pharynx, Bosetti and co-authors [24] found that consumption of cruciferous vegetables at least once a week, when compared with no/occasional consumption, resulted in a significant reduction in the incidence of cancer of the oral cavity/pharynx, with OR of 0.83 [24].

The mechanisms of action by which fruits and vegetables may exhibit OPC preventive roles may include the presence of anticarcinogenic bioactive compounds and phytochemicals such as carotenoids and flavonoids [18]. Phytochemicals in fruits and vegetables scavenge free radicals, decrease oxidative stress, and hence protect the DNA from damage [5]. The effect of bioactive compounds in fruits and vegetables in the protection of oral and pharyngeal tissues was proposed to be both a systematic effect and local effect due to the direct contact between the tissues and the ingested compounds [5]. The mechanisms by which *Allium* vegetables exert their chemopreventive potential against oral tumorigenesis include the induction of apoptosis, suppression of angiogenesis and metastasis, and cancer cell growth inhibition [25].

The protective effect of cruciferous vegetables are characterized with their high content of bioactive flavonoids that are known to exhibit anti-inflammatory, antioxidant, and tumor-growth inhibitory effects, with particular attention toward glucosinolates which are supposed to have anticarcinogenic potential [26], in addition to the trace mineral selenium. The molecular mechanisms through which cruciferous vegetables exert their chemopreventive potential against OPC include altered estrogen metabolism, protection against reactive oxygen species (ROS), altered detoxification by induction of phase II enzymes, decreased carcinogen activation by inhibition of phase I enzymes, and slowed tumor growth and induction of apoptosis [23].

11.2.2 Legumes and Plant-Based Proteins

Plant-based proteins, including legumes, are low caloric, nutrient-dense foods with several health-enhancing attributes [27]. Studies conducted on vegetarians and risk of cancers showed a protective effect of vegetarian diets against carcinogenesis. A 12-year follow-up study was conducted by Key et al. [28] and included 61,566 participants. Investigators showed that vegetarian diets exhibited chemopreventive properties and were associated with lower risk of cancers as compared to meat-containing diets [28]. Epidemiological studies conducted on vegetarian populations such as Indians reported that vegetarian diet is among the predominant antiproliferative practices and is protective against head and neck cancers including the OPC [29]. A case-control study conducted by Bravi et al. [16] found statistically inverse trends in risk of OPC among study participants with a highest quintile of plant-based protein intake as compared to those in the lowest quantile of intake [16]. A recent large case-control study conducted in Italy by Giraldi and colleagues [14] found that legumes consumption was associated with lower risk of OPC (OR = 0.05, 95% CI: 0.01–0.25) [14].

The chemopreventive properties of legumes were assessed by Xu and Chang [8]. Different kinds of legumes such as Adzuki bean and black soybean exhibited cellular antioxidant and antiproliferative activities on different cancer cell lines [8], while lentils exhibited a potent chemopreventive effect against early colon carcinogenesis in chemically induced colon cancer [30]. The impact of legumes and plant-based proteins consumption on the prevention of the lower gastrointestinal tract tumors was documented earlier [31]. However limited research discussed the impact of legumes on the prevention of OPC. Research on soy-derived isoflavones such as glycitein, daidzein, and genistein revealed a synergistic chemopreventive effect against OPC [32]. Soy protein extract was tested for its in vitro antiproliferative effect on CAL 27 and SCC25 cell lines. Results showed that soy protein extract inhibited the growth of oral cancer cell lines [32].

11.2.3 Meats and Animal Foods

The impact of meats and animal foods on risk of OPC seems to be dependent on the type of meat. In general, studies investigated the relationship between animal-based protein and risk of OPC revealed a positive association. Bravi et al. [16] reported that OR of OPC risk was 1.57 in individuals with the highest quantile of animal protein intake as compared to individuals with the lowest quantile of intake. Similar findings were also reported in a case-control study conducted in Argentina and found a positive association between red meats consumption and risk of oral squamous cell carcinoma [33]. The association between meat consumption and risk of OPC was examined in a meta-analysis of 12 case-control studies, and one cohort study included a total of 4104 cases of OPC. Results indicated that consumption of processed meats was associate with 1.9 times increased risk of OPC (95% CI: 1.19–3.06) [34].

The mechanism of action by which red meats increase the risk of OPC is related to the content of saturated fats and nitrites and formation of toxins during meat grilling or roasting such as the heterocyclic amines and polycyclic aromatic hydrocarbons [16]. An interesting mechanism of action was proposed by Samraj et al. [35]to explain the relation of red meat with cancer initiation. Authors suggested that the presence of bound N-glycolylneuraminic acid in red processed meats is bioavailable for humans and interacts with humans' antibody which results in systemic inflammation which may in turn initiate tumors [35].

On the other hand, fish intake seems to have a prevention effect against OPC. The association between fish intake and the risk of OPC was discussed previously in several epidemiological reports [14]. Most of the findings that supported the potential chemopreventive role of fish originated from research on Mediterranean diets with fish being a chief component [14]. A meta-analysis review study included 24 studies and aimed to examine the relation between fish consumption and esophageal cancer. The summary relative risk (RR) obtained in the study was 0.81 (95% CI: 0.66–0.99) for categories with highest intakes of fish consumption versus those with lowest intakes [36]. However, the impact of fish consumption was valid only in hospital-based, not population-based, studies [36].

The antitumor effect fish is mediated by the impact of fish oil rich in DHA on inflammation and related uncontrolled cell proliferation. Alaarg et al. [37] designed an in vitro experiment aimed at examining the impact of fish oil on inflammatory cells. A nanomedicine approach was used where nanoparticles of DHA was delivered to target inflammatory immune cells. Researchers demonstrated that the release of ROS and the production of the inflammatory cytokines were strongly inhibited.

Moreover, the proliferation of head and neck tumor cells was also inhibited. Based on the finding of their experiment, authors proposed the potential benefit of fish oil on head and neck cancer prevention and treatment [37]. Other researchers reported that the impact of fish oil on cancer prevention may be explained by the process of intrinsic apoptosis [38].

11.2.4 Dietary Fats

Dietary fats are a major source of energy and essential fatty acids. Amount and type of dietary fats consumed are both crucial factors when studying the role of fats in human health and disease. Results of the investigations concerning dietary fats and risk of OPC are conflicting and are specific to the amount and type of dietary fats being investigated. In general, essential PUFA, especially omega-3 fatty acids (OFA), were linked to protection against OPC [15]. An experiment conducted using animal model demonstrated that OFA regulated cell proliferation and the expression of HNF-4α and β-catenin, indicating antiproliferative therapeutic potential of OFA [39]. A recent case-control study in Iran was conducted on 96 controls and 47 cases with esophageal cancer. Dietary data were food frequency questionnaire. After controlling for age, gender, physical activity, body mass index, gastrointestinal reflux, education, and smoking history, it was found that participants who reported the highest intakes of OFA had 68% lower risk of esophageal cancer [17].

Saturated fats are now being linked to the etiology of tumorigenesis. In a case-control study, it was reported that individuals reported with highest intake of saturated fats had 188% increased risk of esophageal cancer as compared to those with the lowest intakes of saturated fats [95%CI:1.15–3.08] [17]. In a case-control study, a group of patients with oral cancer were matched with controls for gender, age, and smoking status. The study pointed that habitual intake of foods rich in saturated fats represented a risk factor for oral cancer [40]. A recent case-control study of 768 OPC cases and 2078 controls found 118% increased risk of OPC among individuals with highest consumption of saturated fats as compared to those with the lowest intakes [16]. Plausible pathways by which saturated fats consumption is associated with increased risk of tumorigenesis include increasing the activity of lipid peroxidase and changing the composition of fatty acids in cell membranes, hence compromising the integrity of cell membranes [15].

MUFA present in olive oil seem to have a protective effect against OPC. In order to compare the effect of intake of different types of dietary fats on risk of oral cancer, OR for OPC according to the intake quintile of olive oil and other added fats was calculated. Results revealed that OR was 0.4 for olive oil, while it increased to 2.3 for butter and 1.1 for mixed seed oils [2, 41]. Thus, a compelling and accumulating body of epidemiological evidence supports that olive oil has a potent chemopreventive potential against OPC.

Olive oil is a healthy functional food with a plethora of essential nutrients and bioactive microconstituents that synergize to provide a protective effect against several types of cancers [42]. Olive oil, largely consumed in the Mediterranean countries, has also been reported to have a favorable influence on various neoplasms [11]. In a meta-analysis study on the relationship between cancer incidence rates and olive oil consumption, results from 19 case-control studies which included 13,800 cancer patients and 23,340 controls showed that the highest category of olive oil consumption was significantly associated with lower odds of having any type of cancer (OR = 0.41). Further, consumption of olive oil was found to be significantly associated with lower odds of developing cancers of the digestive system including oral cancer (OR = 0.36) [43]. In vivo studies on animal models confirmed the epidemiological evidence and revealed that olive oil is powerful in suppressing the chemically induced oral carcinogenesis in rodents. By virtue of its phenolic compounds, olive oil not only increased defense in scavenging ROS but also suppressed xanthine oxidase activity, a factor which is known to influence carcinogenesis [44]. Tanaka and colleagues have shown that the xanthine oxidase inhibitor 1-acetoxychavicol has a significant chemopreventive effect on 4-nitroquinoline-1-oxide-induced oral cancer in rats [45].

The protective effect of olive oil on cancer risk has been explained by virtue of its antioxidant properties attributable both to oleic acid itself and to the presence of other nutrients such as vitamin E and bioactive polyphenols [44]. The main phenolic compounds are hydroxytyrosol and oleuropein, phytochemicals that give extra-virgin olive oil its unique distinctive bitterness and pungent taste [46]. The anticancer effect of polyphenols had been extensively studied and reviewed elsewhere [47].

11.3 Micronutrients and Risk of Oral and Pharyngeal Cancers

11.3.1 Vitamin A

Vitamin A can be obtained directly from food as retinoids or can be synthesized in the body from its carotenoids precursors. A major function of the retinoids in the body is normal cells proliferation and differentiation and apoptosis [48]. The role of vitamin A in OPC prevention was not clearly addressed in human studies. Conflicting results were obtained in a study amid at investigating the preventive role of vitamin A against OPC [49]. Cohort studies reported a trend in lowering the risk of OPC with vitamin A intake, whereas other studies failed to find any trend [49].

In vitro, the chemopreventive effect of retinoids was clear and showed promising differentiative, antiproliferative, and proapoptotic attributes [48]. The anticancer effect of retinoids was also thought to be beyond cancer prevention. Retinoids may be considered antineoplastic agents with therapeutic potential mediated by retinoic acid and regulated by retinoic acid receptors-β (RAR-β) which is shown to arrest cancer cells growth and differentiation and induce apoptosis [48]. The significance of RARs in inhibiting the growth of cancer cells was studied in vitro by Soprano and partners [50] It was shown that the treatment of oral squamous carcinoma cell lines with retinoic acid modulated the function of RAR and, hence, inhibited the growth oral carcinoma cells.

11.3.2 Vitamin E

The role of vitamin E as antioxidant in disease prevention is well documented. A recent review was conducted to examine the association between dietary intakes of tocopherols and risk of OPC [51]. Data pooled from ten case-control studies showed inverse relationship between vitamin E intake and risk of OPC, with significant OR of 0.59 (95% CI: 0.49–0.71) between individuals with highest intake of vitamin E and those with the lowest intake [51]. A hospital-based case-control study in Iran aimed at investigating the dietary factors in relation to risk of esophageal carcinoma revealed that the most chemopreventive dietary factor was combination of high vitamin E and folate intakes with OR of 0.02 (95%CI: 0.00–0.87; $P < 0.001$) [17]. Similar results were confirmed by Hu et al. [52] where low intake of dietary vitamin E was associated with the risk of esophageal cancer.

The molecular pathway by which the protective effect of vitamin E against OPC is attributed to the antioxidation power of vitamin E in preventing oxidation of PUFA of the cell membranes [49]. In the absence of tocopherols, the oxidation of cell membrane lipids generates ROS which can reach the nucleus, damage the DNA, and increase the risk of mutagenesis [51]. Other mechanisms of action were proposed such as the synergistic effect of vitamin E with vitamin C in blocking formation of nitrosamines and preventing DNA damage in cells exposed to carcinogens [49, 51].

11.3.3 Vitamin C

Vitamin C has been linked to health and protection against oxidative stress-related diseases including cancer. The impact of adequate intake of vitamin C on risk of OPC has been examined in epidemiological studies [53, 54]. A pooled analysis of 12 case-control studies was conducted to examine the relationship between vitamin and mineral supplements with risk of head and neck cancers including OPC [53]. A significant linear inverse relation was observed between vitamin C supplement and risk of head and neck carcinoma (OR = 0.76, 95% CI = 0.59–0.96). In addition, the association between energy-adjusted vitamin C intake and risk of OPC was examined in pooled data of 5959 cases vs 12,248 controls. Individuals in the fifth highest quintile of vitamin C intake had significantly lower OR for OPC risk as compared to those in the first low quintile with OR of 0.54 (95% CI: 0.45–0.65) [54].

The proposed molecular mechanisms of the protective effect of vitamin C against malignancies were focused on, but were not limited to, the ability of vitamin C in maintaining the integrity of cell membrane and protecting the DNA from oxidative damage [54]. Vitamin C is a strong dietary antioxidant that stabilizes ROS before attacking lipids of the cell membrane. As discussed earlier, vitamin C works synergistically with vitamin E to block the formation of nitrosamines, a potent chemical carcinogen [49]. Vitamin C is also believed to possess a role in inhibiting the binding of the carcinogens to the DNA [49]. The role of vitamin C in the prevention of metastasis was attributed to its role in the formation of the extracellular collagen matrix formation around the tumor [54].

11.3.4 Selenium

Selenium is an essential nutrient to human health and a constituent of antioxidation protein system associated with the formation with several proteins such as glutathione peroxidases and thioredoxin reductases. The association between selenium and risk of OPC was reported earlier [17, 55]. The effect of selenium on the growth of head and neck squamous cell carcinoma was examined in vitro by Hassan and Webster [56]. Human dermal fibroblast cells were used for comparison. Cells were incubated with selenium nanoparticles for 3 days. Cells viability assays indicated that selenium nanoparticle induced apoptosis of head and neck cancer cells, with inducing harmful effect on normal cells [56].

Epidemiological studies confirmed the antineoplastic effect of selenium intakes. Cases of esophageal squamous cell carcinoma were compared to healthy controls in Iran. Cases reported consumption of selenium 623.5 times less than that reported by the controls [17]. Selenium status and risk of OPC among other subtypes of head and neck cancers was investigated in a cohort study in Netherlands [55]. The study cohort included about 121,000 participants who were followed up for 20 years. Selenium status was assessed by measuring toenail selenium, and risk of developing head and neck cancers was found to be 1.8 higher for individuals in the first quartile of selenium levels as compared to those in the fourth quartile (*P*-trend = 0.001) [55]. It was documented that patients diagnosed with head and neck cancers including OPC have reduced levels of selenium-binding protein 1. Reduced levels of selenium-binding protein 1 among head and neck cancer patients were associated with poor prognosis and survival rates [57].

Several mechanisms of action were hypothesized with regard to antineoplastic effect of selenium apart from being a constituent of the antioxidation selenoprotein system such as glutathione peroxidases and thioredoxin reductases [55]. The impact of selenium was on inducing apoptosis of malignant cells, which was proposed due to the association of selenium with the regulation of protein folding through the function of endoplasmic reticulum of these cells [58]. Role of selenium in maintaining the stability of DNA was also proposed as a plausible explanation of selenium in protection against cancer [58].

11.3.5 Iron

Unparalleled with the protective effect of essential micronutrients against OPC, increased iron stores have been linked recently to health-devastating conditions and increased mortality rates [59]. The association between blood iron levels and risk of oral cancer was investigated in a case-control study. Findings of the study showed a decreased risk of oral cancer among participants in the lowest tertiles of free iron and transferrin saturation versus those in the highest tertile, with OR = 0.3 and 0.4, respectively [60]. Levels of serum ferritin seem to be positively associated with risk of oral cancer, as shown in a case-control study conducted by Baharvand et al. [61]. Levels of serum ferritin among patients diagnosed with oral cancer were

267.4 ± 249.5 ng/mL compared to 106.13 ± 72.96 ng/mL in controls ($P < 0.001$). Another case-control study aimed at investigating the impact of iron intake and status was conducted on 224 cases of esophageal adenocarcinoma matched for 256 controls. The study found a significant inverse association between iron intake (OR = 0.5), nonheme iron intake (OR = 0.29), and iron status (OR = 0.4) with risk of esophageal adenocarcinoma. The study, however, found positive association between esophageal adenocarcinoma and heme iron intake with OR = 3.1 [62].

Analysis of cohort data from the National Health and Nutrition Examination Survey I showed increased risk of cancers among individuals with high levels of iron stores and iron intakes versus those with low levels (hazard ratio (HR), 2.00; 95% CI, 1.04–3.82) [59]. The link between iron status and morbidity has been attributed in most cases to the increased oxidative stress with high levels of free non-bound serum iron. Free iron is a potent pro-oxidant that leads to the increased generation of ROS which, in turn, induce lipid peroxidation, compromised cell membrane, and DNA damage [63].

11.3.6 Folate

Folate is an essential B vitamin present mainly in some legumes, citrus fruits, and dark green leafy vegetables. The role of folate in DNA synthesis, repair, and methylation explains the link between folate intake and risk of cancer. Pooled analysis of ten case-control studies with a total of 5127 cases of OPC and 13,249 controls revealed that the OR of developing OPC was significantly less among individuals in the highest quintile of folate intake as compared to individuals in the lowest quantile (0.65, 95% CI: 0.43–0.99). However, the strongest association was found between folate intake and oral cancer (OR = 0.57, 95% CI: 0.43–0.75) [64]. Similar findings were also observed in Japanese individual-based case-control study with OR for OPC of 0.53 among individuals reported with high folate intake as compared to those reported with low folate intake (P-trend = 0.003) [65]. The relation between intake of folate and esophageal cancer was studied previously in a case-control study by Torukiri and colleagues [66]. Results showed higher levels of consumed dietary folate reported by controls as compared to the levels of folate intakes reported by the cases indicating a protective effect of folate against esophageal cancer (P-trend = 0.01) [66]. Another population-based case-control study was conducted on 223 histologically confirmed esophageal adenocarcinoma cases versus 256 controls. Study results showed a decreased OR of esophageal adenocarcinoma among individuals reported with highest folate intake as compared to those reported with low folate intake with OR of 0.56 (P-trend < 0.01) [67].

Findings about folate and risk of OPC were confirmed by published cohort studies. A prospective study conducted on 492,293 individuals from both genders aimed at examining the relationship between folate intake and esophageal cancer found that individuals reported with low intake of folate had around two times higher risk of developing esophageal squamous cell carcinoma, with RR of 1.91 (95% CI: 1.17, 3.10) [68].

The plausible molecular mechanism of folate role in the prevention of OPC is related to the folate's ability to donate a methyl group required for DNA synthesis and methylation. Folate deficiency may be associated with disrupted DNA methylation, proto-oncogene activation, and altered expression of tumor suppressor genes [64]. Molecular studies conducted in individuals showed decreased activity of 5,10-methylenetetrahydrofolate reductase, the enzyme responsible for producing folate form works as a methylation co-substrate [64].

11.4 Bioactive Phytochemicals and Risk of Oral and Pharyngeal Cancers

11.4.1 Carotenoids

Carotenoids are a class of naturally occurring bioactive compounds linked to reduced risk of several types of cancers [69]. The most studied carotenoids with chemoprevention attributes are beta-carotene, lycopene, lutein, and zeaxanthin [69]. In vivo studies on rats revealed the possession of beta-carotene for a chemopreventive potential against oral cancer [69], while in vitro studies showed antiproliferative effect of lycopene and beta-carotene on oral cancer cells [70]. Moreover, it was shown that carotenoids upregulated the transcription and expression of the gap-junctional communication proteins, a key process in tissues and cells homeostasis [70].

Findings of epidemiological studies with regard to the chemoprevention potentials of carotenoids against OPC were controversial [71, 72]. Pooled data from ten case-control studies were analyzed to examine the relation between carotenoids with head and neck cancers [71]. Among all the cases, 4414 cases with OPC were included. Individuals reported with carotenoids intakes in the highest quintile had 39% OPC risk reduction as compared to those reported with intakes in the lowest quintile (95% CI 29–47%) [71]. On the other hand, no significant impact of carotenoids on risk of head and neck cancers including OPC was reported by de Munter et al. [72]. De Munter and colleagues [72] studied data of a cohort group of 120,852 healthy participants in the Netherlands who were followed up for 20 years. No statistically significant OPC risk reduction was observed with higher intakes of carotenoids [72].

Several mechanisms of actions were identified with regard to antineoplastic activities of carotenoids. Carotenoids are antioxidants and thus scavenge ROS and protect the cell membrane and DNA from damage. Carotenoids were also linked to modulating the immune system, modulating normal cell gap junction and cells communication, and increasing the activities of carcinogen detoxification enzymes [49, 69].

11.4.2 Flavonoids

Flavonoids are classes of bioactive compounds derived from plants with diseases prevention characteristics. The most studied classes of flavonoids include isoflavones, flavonols, flavanones, and anthocyanidins [73]. In a multicenter case-control study in Italy, 10,000 cases of cancers were compared with 16,000 controls with regard to their flavonoid intakes. Individuals reported with flavonoids intake in the highest quintile had reduced risk of cancers as compared to individuals with lowest intakes [74]. For instance, the OR for oral cancer and total flavonoids intake was 0.56, for total flavanones was 0.51, and for total flavonols was 0.62 ($P < 0.05$) [74].

Catechins are flavanols mainly found in green tea. A large cohort study in Japan was conducted on 20,550 men and women free of oral cancer. The cohort group was followed for about 10 years. Thirsty-seven participants were diagnosed with oral cancer during the follow-up period. Intake of green tea was reported, and HR for oral cancer for women reported drinking five cups of green per day was 0.31 compared to those reported with consumption of one cup per day [75].

Quercetin was intensively studied as the most abundant flavonoids in food. In vitro, quercetin inhibited the proliferation of oral cancer cell lines showing enzymatic inhibition of the thymidylate synthase, a key enzyme expressed by oral cancer cells [76]. Apoptotic properties of quercetin were also explained by the modulation of the Bax/Bcl-2 ratio in oral cancer cells. Quercetin was also associated with the prevention of oral cancer cell migration in several ways including the inhibiting of the expression of metalloprotease 2 and metalloprotease 9 [76]. The effect of quercetin extends beyond prevention; quercetin showed some cancer therapeutic potential. The combination of quercetin with cisplatin (a chemotherapeutic drug) induced apoptosis and decreased the cells' resistance to the chemotherapeutic medication [77].

11.5 Chemopreventive and Etiological Mechanisms of Action of Dietary Factors

Mechanisms of action by which diet can protect against imposed risk of OPC are not yet fully understood. Investigating the mechanism of action of a single nutrient is a very complicated task given the complexity of human diet with hundreds of thousands of compounds working synergistically on a cellular and molecular level. Epidemiological studies revealed some associations between food groups [16], macronutrients [49], micronutrients, and food bioactive compounds [16]; however, the mechanisms of action were mostly based on in vitro studies.

11.5.1 Etiological Mechanisms

Dietary factors accused for increasing risk of OPC include excessive iron intake, high intake of saturated fats, and high intake of red meats [15, 16, 63]. Indeed, the aforementioned dietary factors usually coexist in diet; i.e., diets high in red, especially processed, meats are usually high in iron and saturated fats. High iron intake is linked to increased free circulation and increased oxidative stress, increased lipid peroxidation, and DNA damage [63]. Intake of saturated fats is linked to increase activity of lipid peroxidase, hence the oxidation of cell membrane lipids [15]. Besides iron and saturated fat contents of red meats, red processed meats also contain carcinogen precursors which can be converted into carcinogens when exposed to dry heat such as grilling, roasting, or barbequing [16]. Figure 11.1 illustrates the OPC etiological mechanism of foods.

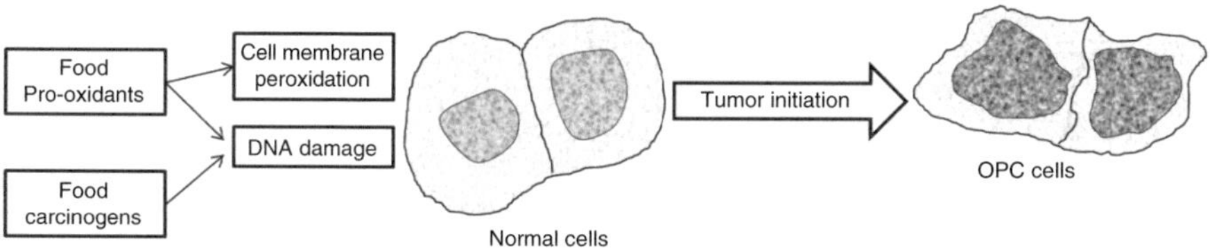

Fig. 11.1 Etiological mechanisms of foods in oral and pharyngeal cancers (OPC)

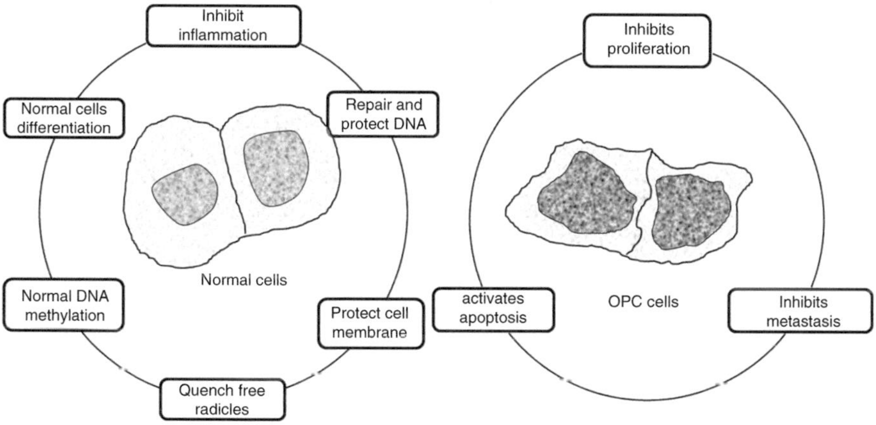

Fig. 11.2 Chemopreventive mechanisms of foods against oral and pharyngeal cancer (OPC)

11.5.2 Chemopreventive Mechanisms

Several OPC chemopreventive dietary factors were linked to diet, including consumption of foods rich in bioactive phytochemicals, antioxidants, and unsaturated fats. The chemopreventive mechanisms of action include (1) scavenging free radicals and decreasing oxidative stress [49], (2) protecting DNA from damage [5], (3) OPC cytotoxic effect and induction of apoptosis [38], (4) suppressing angiogenesis and metastasis [25], suppressing low-grade inflammation [37], (5) inhibiting OPC cells proliferation [8], and modulating normal DNA methylation and normal cells differentiation [50]. Figure 11.2 summarizes the chemopreventive mechanisms of foods against OPC.

References

1. Warnakulasuriya S. Global epidemiology of oral and oropharyngeal cancer. Oral Oncol. 2009;45(4):309–16.
2. Lucenteforte E, et al. Dietary factors and oral and pharyngeal cancer risk. Oral Oncol. 2009;45(6):461–7.
3. WHO, World Cancer Report. 2014.

4. Petti S, Masood M, Scully C. The magnitude of tobacco smoking-betel quid chewing-alcohol drinking interaction effect on oral cancer in South-East Asia. A meta-analysis of observational studies. PLoS One. 2013;8(11):e78999.
5. Maasland DH, et al. Consumption of vegetables and fruits and risk of subtypes of head–neck cancer in the Netherlands cohort study. Int J Cancer. 2015;136(5):E396–409.
6. Warnakulasuriya S, Wilson M. Food, nutrition and oral cancer. In: Food constituents and oral health: current status and future prospects CRC and Woodhead publishing limited. 2009. pp. 273–95.
7. Nagao T, et al. Serum antioxidant micronutrients and the risk of oral leukoplakia among Japanese. Oral Oncol. 2000;36(5):466–70.
8. Xu B, Chang SK. Comparative study on antiproliferation properties and cellular antioxidant activities of commonly consumed food legumes against nine human cancer cell lines. Food Chem. 2012;134(3):1287–96.
9. Garavello W, et al. Diet diversity and the risk of oral and pharyngeal cancer. Eur J Nutr. 2008;47(5):280–4.
10. Joury E, et al. Dietary patterns and the risk of oral, pharyngeal and laryngeal cancer in Syria: a case control study. BMC Nutr. 2016;2(1):1.
11. Bosetti C, et al. Influence of the Mediterranean diet on the risk of cancers of the upper aerodigestive tract. Cancer Epidemiol Biomark Prev. 2003;12(10):1091–4.
12. Filomeno M, et al. The role of a Mediterranean diet on the risk of oral and pharyngeal cancer. Br J Cancer. 2014;111(5):981–6.
13. Giacosa A, et al. Cancer prevention in Europe: the Mediterranean diet as a protective choice. Eur J Cancer Prev. 2013;22(1):90–5.
14. Giraldi L, et al. Association between Mediterranean diet and head and neck cancer: results of a large case-control study in Italy. Eur J Cancer Prev. 2016;
15. Taghavi N, Yazdi I. Type of food and risk of oral cancer. Arch Iran Med. 2007;10(2):227–32.
16. Bravi F, et al. Foods, nutrients and the risk of oral and pharyngeal cancer. Br J Cancer. 2013;109(11):2904–10.
17. Jessri M, et al. Macronutrients, vitamins and minerals intake and risk of esophageal squamous cell carcinoma: a case-control study in Iran. Nutr J. 2011;10(1):1.
18. Pavia M, et al. Association between fruit and vegetable consumption and oral cancer: a meta-analysis of observational studies. Am J Clin Nutr. 2006;83(5):1126–34.
19. Marmot M, et al. World Cancer Research Fund/American Institute for Cancer Research Food, Nutrition, Physical Activity, and the Prevention of Cancer: A Global Perspective. Washington DC: AICR, 2007.
20. Parkin D. 5. Cancers attributable to dietary factors in the UK in 2010. Br J Cancer. 2011;105:S24–6.
21. Wilson EA, Demmig-Adams B. Antioxidant, anti-inflammatory, and antimicrobial properties of garlic and onions. Nutr Food Sci. 2007;37(3):178–83.
22. Galeone C, et al. Onion and garlic use and human cancer. Am J Clin Nutr. 2006;84(5):1027–32.
23. Keck A-S, Finley JW. Cruciferous vegetables: cancer protective mechanisms of glucosinolate hydrolysis products and selenium. Integr Cancer Ther. 2004;3(1):5–12.
24. Bosetti C, et al. Cruciferous vegetables and cancer risk in a network of case–control studies. Ann Oncol. 2012;23(8):2198–203. p. mdr604
25. Powolny AA, Singh SV. Multitargeted prevention and therapy of cancer by diallyl trisulfide and related Allium vegetable-derived organosulfur compounds. Cancer Lett. 2008;269(2):305–14.
26. Herr I, Büchler MW. Dietary constituents of broccoli and other cruciferous vegetables: implications for prevention and therapy of cancer. Cancer Treat Rev. 2010;36(5):377–83.
27. Faris MeA, IE, Takruri HR, Issa AY. Role of lentils (*Lens culinaris* L.) in human health and nutrition: a review. Mediterr J Nutr Metab. 2013, 6(1):3–16.
28. Key TJ, et al. Cancer incidence in British vegetarians. Br J Cancer. 2009;101(1):192–7.
29. Mishra A. Head and neck cancer in India–review of practices for prevention policy. Oral Dis. 2009;15(7):454–65.

30. Faris Mo'ez Al-Islam E, et al. Chemopreventive effect of raw and cooked lentils (*Lens culinaris* L) and soybeans (*Glycine max*) against azoxymethane-induced aberrant crypt foci. Nutr Res. 2009;29(5):355–62.
31. Tayyem RF, et al. Consumption of whole grains, refined cereals, and legumes and its association with colorectal cancer among Jordanians. Integr Cancer Ther. 2015;15(3):318–25. doi:10.1177/1534735415620010.
32. Kingsley K, et al. Soy protein extract (SPE) exhibits differential in vitro cell proliferation effects in oral cancer and normal cell lines. J Diet Suppl. 2011;8(2):169–88.
33. Secchi DG, et al. Red meat, micronutrients and oral squamous cell carcinoma of Argentine adult patients. Nutr Hosp. 2015;32(3):1214–21.
34. Xu J, et al. Meat consumption and risk of oral cavity and oropharynx cancer: a meta-analysis of observational studies. PLoS Onc. 2014;9(4):e95048.
35. Samraj AN, et al. A red meat-derived glycan promotes inflammation and cancer progression. Proc Natl Acad Sci. 2015;112(2):542–7.
36. Han Y, et al. Fish consumption and risk of esophageal cancer and its subtypes: a systematic review and meta-analysis of observational studies. Eur J Clin Nutr. 2013;67(2):147–54.
37. Alaarg A, et al. Docosahexaenoic acid liposomes for targeting chronic inflammatory diseases and cancer: an in vitro assessment. Int J Nanomedicine. 2016;11:5027.
38. Sharma G, et al. Apoptosis-mediated chemoprevention by different ratios of fish oil in experimental colon carcinogenesis. Cancer Investig. 2016;34(5):1–11.
39. Algamas-Dimantov A, et al. Prevention of diabetes-promoted colorectal cancer by (n-3) polyunsaturated fatty acids and (n-3) PUFA mimetic. Oncotarget. 2014;5(20):9851.
40. Toporcov TN, Antunes JLF, Tavares MR. Fat food habitual intake and risk of oral cancer. Oral Oncol. 2004;40(9):925–31.
41. Franceschi S, et al. Food groups, oils and butter, and cancer of the oral cavity and pharynx. Br J Cancer. 1999;80(3–4):614.
42. Stark AH, Madar Z. Olive oil as a functional food: epidemiology and nutritional approaches. Nutr Rev. 2002;60(6):170–6.
43. Psaltopoulou T, et al. Olive oil intake is inversely related to cancer prevalence: a systematic review and a meta-analysis of 13,800 patients and 23,340 controls in 19 observational studies. Lipids Health Dis. 2011;10(1):1.
44. Owen R, et al. The antioxidant/anticancer potential of phenolic compounds isolated from olive oil. Eur J Cancer. 2000;36(10):1235–47.
45. Tanaka T, et al. A xanthine oxidase inhibitor 1′-acetoxychavicol acetate inhibits azoxymethane-induced colonic aberrant crypt foci in rats. Carcinogenesis. 1997;18(5):1113–8.
46. Omar SH. Oleuropein in olive and its pharmacological effects. Sci Pharm. 2010;78(2):133–54.
47. Fresco P, et al. New insights on the anticancer properties of dietary polyphenols. Med Res Rev. 2006;26(6):747–66.
48. Arisi MF, et al. All trans-retinoic acid (ATRA) induces re-differentiation of early transformed breast epithelial cells. Int J Oncol. 2014;44(6):1831–42.
49. Chainani-Wu N. Diet and oral, pharyngeal, and esophageal cancer. Nutr Cancer. 2002;44(2):104–26.
50. Soprano DR, Qin P, Soprano KJ. Retinoic acid receptors and cancers. Annu Rev Nutr. 2004;24:201–21.
51. Edefonti V, et al. Vitamin E intake from natural sources and head and neck cancer risk: a pooled analysis in the International head and neck cancer epidemiology consortium. Br J Cancer. 2015;113(1):182–92.
52. Hu J, Qi Q, Zhang Y. Comparative research for the dietary pattern of patients with esophageal cancer at different developing stages and the daily intake of vitamin A, E and β-carotene. Pak J Pharm Sci. 2014;27(4):1093–8.
53. Li Q, et al. Vitamin or mineral supplement intake and the risk of head and neck cancer: pooled analysis in the INHANCE consortium. Int J Cancer. 2012;131(7):1686–99.

54. Edefonti V, et al. Natural vitamin C intake and the risk of head and neck cancer: a pooled analysis in the International head and neck cancer epidemiology consortium. Int J Cancer. 2015;137(2):448–62.
55. Maasland DH, et al. Toenail selenium status and risk of subtypes of head-neck cancer: the Netherlands cohort study. Eur J Cancer. 2016;60:83–92.
56. Hassan CE, Webster TJ. The effect of red-allotrope selenium nanoparticles on head and neck squamous cell viability and growth. Int J Nanomedicine. 2016;11:3641.
57. Chen F, et al. Selenium-binding protein 1 in head and neck cancer is low-expression and associates with the prognosis of nasopharyngeal carcinoma. Medicine. 2016;95(35):e4592.
58. Cai X, et al. Selenium exposure and cancer risk: an updated meta-analysis and meta-regression. Sci Rep. 2016;6:19213.
59. Mainous AG, Gill JM, Everett CJ. Transferrin saturation, dietary iron intake, and risk of cancer. Ann Fam Med. 2005;3(2):131–7.
60. Richie JP, et al. Blood iron, glutathione, and micronutrient levels and the risk of oral cancer. Nutr Cancer. 2008;60(4):474–82.
61. Baharvand M, et al. Serum levels of ferritin, copper, and zinc in patients with oral cancer. Biom J. 2014;37(5):331.
62. O'Doherty MG, et al. Iron intake and markers of iron status and risk of Barrett's esophagus and esophageal adenocarcinoma. Cancer Causes Control. 2010;21(12):2269–79.
63. Fonseca-Nunes A, Jakszyn P, Agudo A. Iron and cancer risk—a systematic review and meta-analysis of the epidemiological evidence. Cancer Epidemiol Biomark Prev. 2013;23(1):12–31.
64. Galeone C, et al. Folate intake and the risk of oral cavity and pharyngeal cancer: a pooled analysis within the International head and neck cancer epidemiology consortium. Int J Cancer. 2015;136(4):904–14.
65. Matsuo K, et al. Folate, alcohol, and aldehyde dehydrogenase 2 polymorphism and the risk of oral and pharyngeal cancer in Japanese. Eur J Cancer Prev. 2012;21(2):193–8.
66. Ibiebele TI, et al. High intake of folate from food sources is associated with reduced risk of esophageal cancer in an Australian population. J Nutr. 2010;141(2):274–83. doi:10.3945/jn.110.131235.
67. Sharp L, et al. Intakes of dietary folate and other B vitamins are associated with risks of esophageal adenocarcinoma, Barrett's esophagus, and reflux esophagitis. J Nutr. 2013;143(12):1966–73. doi:10.3945/jn.113.174664.
68. Xiao Q, et al. Intakes of folate, methionine, vitamin B6, and vitamin B12 with risk of esophageal and gastric cancer in a large cohort study. Br J Cancer. 2014;110(5):1328–33.
69. Tanaka T, Shnimizu M, Moriwaki H. Cancer chemoprevention by carotenoids. Molecules. 2012;17(3):3202–42.
70. Livny O, et al. Lycopene inhibits proliferation and enhances gap-junction communication of KB-1 human oral tumor cells. J Nutr. 2002;132(12):3754–9.
71. Leoncini E, et al. Carotenoid intake from natural sources and head and neck cancer: a systematic review and meta-analysis of epidemiological studies. Cancer Epidemiol Biomark Prev. 2015;24(7):1003–11.
72. de Munter L, et al. Vitamin and carotenoid intake and risk of head-neck cancer subtypes in the Netherlands cohort study. Am J Clin Nutr. 2015;102(2):420–32. doi:10.3945/ajcn.114.106096.
73. Romagnolo DF, Selmin OI. Flavonoids and cancer prevention: a review of the evidence. J Nutr Gerontol Geriatr. 2012;31(3):206–38.
74. Rossi M, et al. Flavonoids, proanthocyanidins, and cancer risk: a network of case-control studies from Italy. Nutr Cancer. 2010;62(7):871–7.
75. Ide R, et al. A prospective study of green tea consumption and oral cancer incidence in Japan. Ann Epidemiol. 2007;17(10):821–6.
76. Maggioni D, et al. Flavonoids in oral cancer prevention and therapy. Eur J Cancer Prev. 2015;24(6):517–28.
77. Chen S-F, et al. Quercetin suppresses drug-resistant spheres via the p38 MAPK–Hsp27 apoptotic pathway in oral cancer cells. PLoS One. 2012;7(11):e49275.

Prevention of Oral Cancer

12

Ahmed Mohamed Malki, Samira Bou Raad, and Rasha Abu-El-Ruz

12.1 Introduction

During the fifteenth century, Desiderius Erasmus, a Dutch scholar and humanist, wisely stated "Prevention is better than cure." On an intuitive and logical level, it does seem more preferable to avoid rather than repair. If we translate this to the health field, we bring forth the implication that maintaining healthy habits and following basic rules of health can prevent certain diseases from occurring. One such disease which has received a tremendous amount of attention in terms of prevention is cancer and in particular oral cancer.

Cancer has been declared as one of the most common causes of mortality and morbidity with more than 10 million new cases and more than 6 million deaths each year worldwide. Oral cancer ranks 12th among all cancers [1]. Data from the Oral Cancer Foundation shows that there are more than 350,000–400,000 new cases of oral cancer each year [1]. In 2004, the World Health Organization (WHO) estimated that 43% of all cancers are a consequence of tobacco use, alcohol consumption, unhealthy diets, unhealthy lifestyles, and infection [2]. Of these, tobacco is the world's most avoidable cause of cancer. Oral cancer is considered a major constituent in the world's burden of cancer. Tobacco and alcohol have been proven to be major risk factors for oral cancer [3]. Other risk factors include chewing betel quid (areca nut mixed with *Piper betle* quid) or gutka, prolonged UV sunlight exposure, long-term irritation of the oral mucous membranes by poor-maintained dentures, immunosuppressive drugs, human papillomavirus 16 (HPV 16) or Epstein-Barr virus (EBV) infection [3], radiation exposure, and untreated lichen planus. Other

A.M. Malki (✉) • R. Abu-El-Ruz
Biomedical Science Department, College of Health Sciences, Qatar University, Doha, Qatar
e-mail: ahmed.malki@qu.edu.qa

S.B. Raad
Human Nutrition Department, College of Health Sciences, Qatar University, Doha, Qatar

A.-E. Al Moustafa (ed.), *Development of Oral Cancer*,
DOI 10.1007/978-3-319-48054-1_12

uncontrollable risk factors include gender, race, age, genetic syndromes such as Fanconi anemia and dyskeratosis congenita, family history, previous cancer disease, and graft-versus-host disease (GVHD) due to stem cell transplant.

Oral cancer, a part of head and neck cancer, is a term used to address the combination of two separate types of cancer: oral cavity cancer and oropharyngeal cancer. The former is comprised of the lips, the inside lining of the lips and cheeks (buccal mucosa), the teeth, the gums, the front two-thirds of the tongue, the floor of the mouth below the tongue, and the bony roof of the mouth (hard palate) [4]. The latter includes the part of the throat just behind the mouth. It begins where the oral cavity stops. It includes the base of the tongue (the back third of the tongue), the soft palate (the back part of the roof of the mouth), the tonsils, and the side and back wall of the throat [3]. The most common type of oral cancer is the squamous cell carcinoma which represents more than 90% of oral cancer cases [3, 5]. Other types include the slow-growing verrucous carcinoma (VC) at 5%, salivary gland carcinoma which takes the benign and malignant forms with several subtypes, and lymphomas and melanomas of the mouth and lips. Leukoplakia and erythroplakia are considered benign or precancerous forms of the oropharyngeal tumors but can lead to harmful cancer if left untreated.

The increased death rate associated with oral cancer is especially high not because oral cancer is complicated when it comes to detection and diagnosis but rather because it is discovered late in its development [3]. Most times oral cancer is detected at the advanced stage at which point prognosis becomes very poor. Additionally, the 5-year survival rate for oral cancer is low, with only 48–55% surviving 5 years compared with 71% survival following prostate cancer, 62% following cervical cancer, 80% following breast cancer, and 78–91% following malignant melanoma [6]. In light of the above facts, prevention becomes a crucial and central weapon in the challenge of oral cancer. Cancer prevention is defined as action taken to lower the chance of getting cancer, consequently lowering the number of new cases of cancer in a population and hopefully decreasing the number of deaths caused by cancer [6]. However, prevention is not a solid concept but rather a state of priorities and stages, the major of which is primary prevention.

Primary prevention aims to decrease the incidence of oral cancer through changing behaviors that may directly contribute to the development of oral cancer. Primary prevention includes but is not limited to cessation of smoking, reduced alcohol consumption, and improved nutrition.

While primary prevention is the gold standard to battling oral cancer, behavioral change takes time and is not always easy to achieve, and hence secondary prevention such as detection of malignant or potentially malignant lesions becomes a key player. Secondary prevention also encompasses HPV vaccination, diagnosis, and treatment of erythroplakia and leukoplakia as well as chemoprevention.

Tertiary prevention is indicated when the patient has previously had cancer which was treated in its acute clinical phase. Tertiary prevention seeks to soften the impact caused by the disease on the patient's function, life expectancy, and quality of life.

12.2 Primary Prevention

12.2.1 Relevant Exposures

As mentioned earlier, primary prevention aims to decrease the incidence of oral cancer by limiting and lowering exposure to certain risk factors through behavior change. The first step in primary prevention is to obtain an in-depth understanding of the relevant exposures and to assess their impact on the risk of the disease within the population [7].

A plethora of research has been conducted on whether behaviors such as tobacco smoking, alcohol consumption, and betel quid and gutka chewing have a causal effect in developing oral cancer. Tsai et al. studied the effect of the abovementioned three factors in a group of males and found that betel quid chewing, tobacco smoking, and alcohol consumption have a noteworthy effect on the age at diagnosis of oral cancer, especially the first two factors [8]. In fact, the International Agency of Research Against Cancer (IARC), in 2003, classified betel quid without tobacco as a group one human carcinogen [8, 9]. Moreover, high usage of tobacco in combination with high consumption of alcohol poses a much greater risk for oral cancer than using either substance alone.

Nutrition and physical activity are also quite high up on the list of determinants for risk of cancer [10]. Unhealthy diets and lack of physical activity are linked to higher risk of cancer in general, which prompted organizations such as the World Cancer Research Fund International and the American Cancer Society to publish guidelines on nutrition and physical activity for cancer prevention [11, 12].

However, if one is to zone in on one specific aspect of a healthy diet that may decrease the risk of developing oral cancer in particular, then the front-runner would be adequate consumption of fruits and vegetables. Many studies have reported on the fact that fruit and vegetable intake is associated with decreased risk of head and neck squamous cell carcinoma (HNSCC) inclusive of oral cancer, with decreasing risk being noted across increasing levels of intake [13–15]. Fruits and vegetables contain a substantial amount of antioxidants, mainly β-Carotene which is a potent antioxidant [1]. Lycopene, a carotenoid and an isomer of β-Carotene, has been highlighted in many epidemiological studies to have potent effect in preventing oral and other cancers [1]. Two theories have been discussed as to the biological effect of lycopene in oral cancer prevention: antioxidative effects and non-antioxidative effects [1]. In its capacity as an antioxidant, lycopene may inactivate free radicals and weaken reactions initiated by free radicals, such as lipid peroxidation and DNA oxidative damage. Consequently, tissue damage and potential cancerization will be prevented. The second theory brought forth adopts the idea that lycopene exerts its bioavailabilities via other non-oxidative effects, such as regulation of gap junction communication (GJC), gene function regulation, hormone and immune modulation, and antiproliferation and prodifferentiation activities [1]. These mechanisms may be interrelated or operate simultaneously to reduce risk for oral precancerous lesions and cancer, thus to provide health benefits [1].

Chronic and prolonged exposure to sun is another behavioral aspect that may raise the risk of oral cancer [16]. Maruccia et al. found a significant association between chronic sun exposure and lip carcinoma in an Italian population [17]. Extended UVB radiation in combination with UVA produces mutations in DNA. Failure to repair these mutations results in tumor formation [17].

The potential association between HPV and oral and oropharyngeal cancer first originated back in 1983. Prior to that, between 1974 and 1977, it was suggested that the HPV viruses could be responsible for cervical cancer [18]. HPV's are "epitheliotropic oncogenic DNA viruses with more than 120 identified genotypes," some of which are called high risk such as HPV-16 and HPV-18 due to the fact that they are conclusively recognized as being strongly linked with cervical cancers [18]. These same HPV strains can bring about oral epithelial transformations which may grow into oral cancer [18]. In fact, research suggests that people who are infected with HPV in the oral cavity are at higher risk of developing oral cancer (odds ratio, 3.7) than those exposed to alcohol and tobacco (odds ratio, 2.6). Current literature regularly points that sexual behavior is closely related to increased oral HPV prevalence, supporting the sexual transmission of the virus [18, 19]. In light of this, risk factors for HPV-induced head and neck squamous cell carcinoma are number of sexual partners, age at first encounter of sexual intercourse, practice of oral sex, and history of genital warts. With respect to sexual behavior and oral cancer, it goes without saying that practicing safe sex and evading multiple partners would be the best method in the way of primary prevention. Vaccination against HPV is also an option and will be discussed further down.

Environmental carcinogens are another set of risk factors that may eventually lead to cancer. In most instances, we do not sense these factors although we embrace their presence. Additionally, seldom are any steps taken to evaluate environmental carcinogens and wisely lessen exposure to them. Multiple agents have been listed and recognized as carcinogens. These bear chemical, biological, or physical natures and are potent enough to induce cancer formation and abnormal cell proliferation. The main mechanism of environmentally induced carcinoma is that the cells undergo several metabolic abnormalities on the cellular and molecular levels upon exposure. These anomalous genetic interactions eventually lead to mutations that result with undesirable cellular genotype and phenotype [20]. The genetic mutations mainly affect two classes of genes: the proto-oncogenes and the tumor suppressor gene. The process involves three phases that are considered and reflected in the level of prevention: initiation of the DNA damage (primary prevention), proliferation of premalignant cells (secondary prevention), and then formation or progression of tumor cells that are potentially invasive or metastatic (tertiary prevention) [20]. Moving away from the environmental-related lifestyle exposure, such as secondhand smoking or excessive exposure to sunlight, certain environmental carcinogens are identified as workplace related. Examples of such workplace-related exposures are plentiful; these include, but are not limited to, solvent aromas, automobile emissions, and volatile organic compounds. The direct contact or inhalation of asbestos is also a well-recognized factor that causes oral cancer [21].

Carcinogens are agents or factors that cause DNA damage or trigger faster cell division than the normal rate [22]. The American Cancer Society identified environmental exposure aspects that influence oral cancer formation and play vigorous roles in envisaging the risks of cancer development. Such aspects are exposure dose or intensity, length of exposure, and the individual's genetic readiness and makeup [22]. Identifying and evaluating the workplace risk factors for oral cancer is indispensable. The IARC monograph volume 1–115 identified more than 400 cancer causative agents in GP1 and GP2A and GP2B, a majority of these chemicals, physical and biological agents, bring into being occupational or industrial [22]. Labrèche et al. enhanced the awareness of work-related carcinogens among Quebec stakeholders by means of statistical correlations through focused epidemiological study in Quebec [22]. The 2002–2006 study indicated buccal cavity cancer annual detection rate of 277 new cases, of which approximately 72 deaths are among males and 41 deaths among females.

All the abovementioned risk factors are controllable since they are all of a behavioral nature; however, it is important to mention that non-modifiable risk factors such as age, gender, and ethnicity exist as well. Historically, discovery and diagnosis of oral cancer occurred for people over the age of 40; however, now it is being seen more in people under this age [23, 24]. There is no evident causative reason for this age shift, but the literature suggests that it could be due to young men and women's sexual choices and the consequent contraction of HPV-16. Similarly, oral cancer used to affect more men than women, but recently the ratio has changed from 6 men to 1 woman to 2–3 men to each woman [3]. Again, we cannot fully conclude the reason behind this occurrence; however, it could potentially be due to an increase in the number of women who have taken up smoking in addition to HPV-16 contraction through sexual behavior. In the United States of America, oral cancer is twice as likely to occur in black populations as it is in white populations. Perhaps if one is to factor in socioeconomic status, level of education, income, and availability of health insurance and health care, one would see that these factors probably play a major role in who develops oral cancer. McClure et al. surveyed two groups of smokers, those who called a commercially funded smoking quit line and others who called a state-funded smoking quit line [25, 26]. Their findings showed that commercially funded (funded through dental insurances) quit line callers had better overall oral healthcare habits. These callers were also predominantly white, of higher socioeconomic and education status, had higher income, and had oral health insurance, compared to state-funded quit line callers [25, 26]. Kulak et al. found results similar to McClure whereby in looking at attempts of smoking cessation among different population cohorts, African Americans had the lowest attempts compared to whites [27]. African Americans were less likely to have health insurance, were of lower socioeconomic status, and were of lower income compared to other white cohorts [27].

At this point suffice it to say that non-modifiable risk factors also revolve closely around lifestyle choices and exposure reduction.

12.2.2 HPV Vaccination as Primary Prevention

Epidemiologic research has shown that there is a strong association between HPV-16 exposure and oropharyngeal cancer, prompting the scientific and medical community to contemplate the efficacy of an HPV vaccine in preventing infection and consequently decreasing the chances of developing HPV-related oropharyngeal cancer. This is particularly important considering that HPV-16 and HPV-18 vaccines have been shown to protect against HPV-induced cervical cancer as well. In fact some countries have mandated that girls be vaccinated at an early age, as young as 11 years, prior to the first sexual encounter. Additionally vaccination against the nine valent HPV (6, 11, 16, 18, 31, 33, 45, 52, and 58) is also itemized in vaccination programs and recommended at an early age for both genders [28]. Data from the Costa Rica Vaccine Trial (CVT) on overall protection efficacy of the HPV 16/18 vaccine (protection at cervical, anal, and oral sites) shows that getting vaccinated protects against multisite infection in women who have never contracted HPV before [29]. Additionally this study also showed that even with the existence of a prior infection, getting vaccinated could protect against a future HPV infection at the oral, cervical, or anal sites.

12.2.3 Approaches to Support Exposure Reduction

In light of the behavioral risk factors mentioned under *relevant exposures*, many government and nongovernment bodies have come together and compiled guidelines on behavioral modifications and lifestyle recommendations that may decrease the risk of oral cancer. In a nut shell, the recommendations state to avoid using tobacco in any form (smoked, chewed, or smokeless), avoid using betel nut even without tobacco, cut down on alcohol with the aim of drinking no more than one standard drink a day for women (2–3 units) and two standard drinks a day for men (3–4), eat at least five servings of fruits and vegetables per day, and last but not least to protect the lips with sunscreen with an SPF of 30 and wear a wide brimmed hat [6, 16].

The abovementioned health messages require behavioral change at the individual level. However, this change may not come about without broader preventive measures such as those which can be presented by government organizations and public health authorities. Examples of such preventive measures are health education on an individual or community basis (e.g., media campaigns, promoting use of sunscreen, creating awareness on the harm of tobacco, safe sex education), regulation of carcinogens in occupational settings and in the environment (e.g., improvement of radiation protection for workers as mandated by the government), price regulation (e.g., imposing of taxes on tobacco and alcohol purchases), advertising restrictions (e.g., banning of tobacco advertising or mandating the printing of healthy warnings on cigarette packages), time and place restrictions (e.g., banning smoking in public areas), and setting up tobacco quit lines which provide motivational and cognitive behavioral counseling for tobacco cessation [7, 25].

While the abovementioned preventive measures are all of equal significance, we live in an innovative and industrial century. Consequently health and safety regulations that protect workers from carcinogens exposure are essential and should be addressed accordingly. In cases where exposure is unavoidable, a minimum exposure in terms of "intensity and frequency" is desired. The availability of personal protective equipment (PPE), safety manuals, and sufficient workers' education are considered the fundamental scopes to decrease work-related oral cancer incidence [22].

12.2.4 Barriers to Primary Prevention

Primary prevention undeniably decreases risk for oral cancer, and the preventive measures needed to support individuals in maintaining their primary prevention behavior are readily available. This begs the following question: why then is primary prevention and behavior change hard to bring about in order to curb oral cancer? In order to answer this question, one must first examine the factors that drive primary prevention.

The motivation for primary prevention on an individual level is deeply interlinked with socioeconomic, psychological, and cultural norms. A pilot study examined the sociocultural factors that affect why people on Guam chew betel nut, their chewing behaviors, perceptions of risks, and probability of changing behaviors [9]. The behavior of chewing betel quid is native practice to South and Southeast Asia, East Africa, and the Western Pacific and is an important expression of social and cultural identity [9]. Reasons for starting betel quid chewing were primarily that it was readily available within the household and, secondly, a preparation (chewing) for family members who had lost their teeth. Others cited that they continued with the practice due to their belief that betel quid has medicinal benefits, in addition to the fact that red-stained teeth (from betel quid chewing) is a sign of beauty (especially among women). Peer pressure and social acceptance were also reported as reasons for the practice. Among the participants who reported decreasing chewing betel quid, expense and medical issues were cited as reasons for diminishing the habit. The above results are consistent with the social cognitive theory which states that people learn through observation of others [9]. People also pick up certain behavioral habits when they perceive positive outcomes. In the above study, participants started chewing betel quid due to peer pressure and the desire to be included in the group. Women also modeled the same behavior since having red-stained teeth due to chewing betel quid is not only preferable but actually desirable. Peer pressure and social acceptance is a repetitive manifestation in terms of reasons for picking up and continuing smoking. Dietz et al. examined young adults' attitudes/beliefs toward smoking [30]. Interestingly, negative messages about tobacco disseminated through antitobacco campaigns had no impact on smoking prevention or cessation. Rather, the number of friends who are smokers had a much more significant impact on their starting or cessation of smoking [30].

When a certain behavior is deeply ingrained into the fabric of sociocultural acceptance, intention to discontinue the behavior diminishes. Little et al. compared intention to quit among two groups of adults: betel quid chewers in Guam and tobacco smokers in Hawaii [31]. Both betel quid and tobacco users cited their motivation to quit; however, the degree of intention was different with the smokers indicating significantly stronger intention to quit, compared to the chewers. Moreover, a higher number of smokers endorsed that they wish they had never started smoking compared to the chewers. Such differences may have several explanatory scenarios. First of all, in the United States of America, there is plenty of awareness on the negative health risks associated with tobacco smoking, whereas on Guam the negative health risks associated with chewing are less widely known [31]. Another explanation is that while in the United States of America smoking usually carries social disapproval, it is not the case with chewing betel quid on Guam. In fact betel quid chewers on Guam worry that they may receive negative social repercussions associated with chewing. It is noteworthy to mention that within both groups, participants who identified themselves as having the intention to quit did not have a plan as to how to quit and when to quit.

In shifting from smoking to HPV-induced oral cancer, knowledge or awareness is a key factor in primary prevention of HPV-induced oral cancer related to sexual behavior. A review of teenage sexual behaviors in China confirmed that sexual knowledge of teenagers was poor and that the media was their main source of information, supporting the need for comprehensive sex education sessions [32].

In summary, primary prevention depends on several factors: awareness of the negative consequences of a certain behavior, how deeply intertwined a certain behavior is with cultural norms and practices, and intention (motivation) to end the negative behavior.

12.3 Secondary Prevention

12.3.1 Understanding Screening

Since the fundamental factors of primary prevention can be hard to attain, consequently making behavior modification difficult, the next best alternative within the prevention spectrum is secondary prevention.

Secondary prevention as defined by the Association of the Faculties of Medicine of Canada “includes procedures that detect and treat pre-clinical pathological changes and thereby control disease progression” [33]. Screening would be one example of secondary prevention. Screening encompasses the application of a relatively easy and inexpensive test to people in order to categorize them as potentials for developing cancer or not. Hence, screening for diagnosis and treatment of precancerous lesions such as leukoplakia, erythroplakia, and lichen planus which may turn into oral cancer is the first line of defense against oral cancer when it comes to secondary prevention. These conditions are characterized by discolored patches in the mouth and on the tongue. Leukoplakia manifests itself as white patches whereas erythroplakia is red areas within the oral cavity. Lichen planus is an itchy rash that can affect the oral cavity. While these lesions are mostly benign, they can become cancerous and so it is imperative that they be screened for, diagnosed and treated.

A mouth cancer screening protocol has been developed. This protocol includes an extra-oral examination, an intra-oral examination, and palpitation of the lymph nodes [34]. Such a protocol is also known as a conventional objective examination (COE). Although this protocol sounds simple, comprehensive and adequate as a screening tool, in reality it can be quite tricky, using this protocol, to determine which abnormalities in the mouth warrant further examination. The fact is that at any one point, a person may have one or more of a number of conditions that mimic potentially malignant lesions [34]. Certain conditions such as aphthous ulcers, herpes simplex, herpes labialis, and a cheek-bite wound or sore spots from ill-fitting dentures all share similar characteristics with perilous lesions [5]. Hence the result of such an examination is highly dependent on the subjective evaluation of the examiner, which in turn is a consequence of his/her experience and knowledge on how to differentiate a malignant occurrence from a nonmalignant one [34].

In light of the above information, COE, although having been practiced for a long time and is considered the mainframe of the oral cancer diagnosis pathway, is often called into question [35]. This is due to the fact that its validity as a screening tool is controversial. Validity is a factor of sensitivity and specificity. Sensitivity measures the number of people with the disease who test positive, while specificity measures the number of people without the disease who test negative [35]. Since many abnormal oral manifestations are similar to a potential cancerous malignancy, the margin for error during a COE can be quite high, thus decreasing the sensitivity and specificity of the examination. This is not to say that a COE is useless and should not be conducted as there is some evidence suggestive of a high sensitivity and specificity to the exam [35]. Regardless of the pros and cons of COEs, routine oral exams should be conducted by dentists on a regular basis especially within high-risk populations such as smokers and alcohol consumers. A trial from India studying the impact of visual oral screening on the reduction of mortality from oral cancer found that among users of tobacco, alcohol, or both, there was a notable 33% reduction in oral cancer mortality following three rounds of visual oral screening [36]. It seems that such information should trigger dentists to routinely perform oral cancer screening on all their patients; however, in reality that is not the case. There is data to suggest that dentists do realize the importance of raising awareness about oral cancer; however, there are some barriers [37]. Three barriers to communication about oral cancer were identified: system factors whereby dentists had no time for discussions with the patient, patient factors whereby dentists did not want to invoke unnecessary fear by discussing oral cancer, and dentist factors whereby dentists felt they did not have the expertise and knowledge to talk about oral cancer [37].

This brings us to the next concept: what are the criteria upon which the scientific community (mainly dentists) place their decision to either act or wait and see upon finding any type of abnormal oral occurrence? Once abnormal or discolored tissue has been observed, a biopsy is warranted in order to definitively diagnose oral cancer [5]. In light of all the tissue abnormalities that dentists see on a daily basis and given that a biopsy is an invasive diagnostic tool, it would be impractical that each discoloration be biopsied. The first step is to wait and see whether the condition subsides on its own or with the help of medication within the span of 14 days. This stems from the fact that herpes simplex ulcerations and aphthous ulcerations, which happen to share almost the same features as oral cancer, normally resolve of their own accord in about 14 days. Another oral abnormality that also closely resembles premalignant lesions and can be diagnosed by dentists is dental irritation. Several studies have looked at dental trauma as a potential carcinogen [38]. These studies advocated the fact that broken, loose-fitting, and rough teeth as well as ill-fitting dentures can potentially cause oral cancer. In comparing the site of origin of oral cancer among smokers and nonsmokers, an Australian study found that nonsmokers develop cancer on the edge of the tongue at twice the rate of smokers [38]. The researches postulated that one of the reasons for such a preferential site of oral cancer occurrence within the nonsmoking cohort is rubbing and irritation caused by dental problems [38].

As previously stated, conventional biopsies are the "gold standard" for the diagnosis of oral cancer; however, due to the cost and invasiveness of this procedure, medical specialists have now turned to oral biopsy brushes. This test is quite noninvasive and painless and can be done at a general practitioner's office and does provide definitive answers as to the need for further examination through a punch biopsy [34]. Other diagnostic tools that can be used in conjugation with visual oral examination are autofluorescence, chemiluminescence, toluidine blue, chemiluminescence alongside toluidine blue, rose bengal, laser-induced fluorescence examination, and 5-aminolevulinic acid (ALA)-induced protoporphyrin IX (PPIX) fluorescence [34].

12.3.2 Treating Chronic Infections

Primary diseases caused by infection may progress to secondary illnesses such as cancer, if not properly treated. The American Cancer Society estimated that more than 15–20% of the overall cancer cases are predominantly caused by infection [39]. These percentages vary from one region to another and often hit their upper limits in developing countries where sanitary and hygienic conditions are at the lowermost. Many microorganisms are identified as biological agents that may eventually cause cancer with no single established concept of how the microorganisms directly or indirectly cause cancer. Some models have been proposed in an attempt to explain the pathway of how microorganisms may cause cancer. Some microorganisms produce genetic alteration and DNA mutation which trigger abnormal proliferation of cells, other microorganisms cause chronic and severe inflammation that damage the tissues, some others produce toxins that mediate cell damage and DNA mutations, and some powerful microorganisms destroy the immune system to hinder it unable to fight against cancer cell formation [39].

Viral infections are the commonest among cancer-triggering infections. Greatest attention was given to the human papillomavirus (HPV-16) which causes genital and oral warts and is primarily classified as sexually transmitted. Its DNA has been detected in precancerous lesions of oral and squamous cell carcinoma. The National Institute for Dental and Craniofacial Research identified other viruses that are linked to oropharyngeal cancer, namely, EBV, Rous sarcoma virus (RSV), herpes simplex virus type 1 (HSV-1), and human immunodeficiency virus (HIV) [40, 41]. RSV has a gene called v-Src which converts the infected cells into malignancy. The HSV-1 causes abnormal cellular changes which further develop into dysplasia and pharyngeal carcinoma. Kaposi sarcoma (KS) is a form of neoplasm that results from acquired immunodeficiency caused by HIV or herpes simplex virus type 8. The formation of KS is associated with CD4 + T impairment. In such infections, the oral cavity exhibits a blue-purplish plaque. Moreover, the immunosuppression due to such viral infections triggers further secondary fungal infections such as paracoccidioidomycosis (PCM) which yield oral lesions and ulcerations that can further develop into carcinoma. Pontes et al. case study shows synergic detection of PCM and KS in HIV-positive buccal biopsy [42]. Early detection and treatment with antivirals, radiation therapy, or chemotherapy yield a better prognosis and lessen the chances of oral cancer proliferation. Oral candidiasis (oral infection with *Candida albicans)* occurs as a primary infection due to poor mouth hygiene or secondary infection due to HIV or other immunodeficiency syndromes or chronic diseases [43]. *Candida albicans* produces nitrosamine which in turn deposits itself through the branching mycelium that extends from the oral mucosal surface and deepens in the epithelial layers. This aforesaid mechanical strategy is a major tactic for dysplastic changes or precancerous lesions and is a process called "endogenous nitrosamine production" [43]. Some studies show that leukoplakia lesions may also exist as a result of mouth cavity *Candida albicans* infection. As mentioned earlier, leukoplakia may further transform to oral carcinoma if not treated; hence, special attention and early detection of leukoplakia can counteract oral cancer development [44]. Bacteria also play an important role in oral cancer development. There is very limited research in this area; nevertheless, what little research exists in this area shows that some oral cavity chronic bacterial infections are also correlated with oral cancer onset [45]. A review article identified some strains that are subjective causes for oral cancer: *Exiguobacterium oxidotolerans*, *Prevotella melaninogenica*, *Staphylococcus aureus*, and *Veillonella parvula*. *Streptococcus anginosus*, although associated with esophageal and pharyngeal cancer, is found to be less significant than the abovementioned bacteria. Moreover, bacteria cause infections through nitrosation or chronic infection that alter the cell cycle through genetic mutation or interfere with the signaling pathway [45]. Either way, both mechanisms may eventually lead to oral cancer [45].

Early detection and treatment for oral infections is a key component in preventing malignant cell transformation. Antivirals and postexposure prophylaxes are crucial steps to prevent the metabolic and molecular pathway alterations due to viral infection. As for bacteria and fungus, many bacterial and fungal infections can be effectively treated through selective or broad-spectrum antibiotics. However broad-spectrum antibiotics should be administered with extra care so as to hinder the development of antibiotic-resistant strains and superinfection due to microbial system imbalance. Anti-inflammatories are also a good option to limit the immune-cellular response and cell destruction, both of which are recognized risk factors for oral cancer development.

Since the topic of this section is infections and oral cancer, it is noteworthy to mention that oral hygiene and adequate dental status have been found to reduce the risk of oral cancer. Certain bacterial, viral, and fungal infections are identified to cause chronic inflammation to the buccal cavity which can eventually lead to DNA damage and further cancer development. Treating these infectious diseases in their early stages is delineated as one of the secondary prevention strategies; therefore, preventing oral infections through practicing healthy lifestyles, vaccinations, and maintaining oral hygiene is virtually the mainstay of oral cancer primary prevention [46].

12.3.3 Secondary Chemoprevention

Candidates for secondary chemoprevention are individuals who smoke, patients with premalignant lesions, or those who are at risk of developing second primary tumor (SPT) due to the past history of aerodigestive malignancy [47]. The success of chemoprevention depends on the risk group, exposure factors, family history, genetic makeup, age, toxicity, biomarkers, complicated health issues, and cost versus efficiency [47].

Chemoprevention is the use of synthetic or natural agents in the suppression or prevention of cancer. Chemoprevention can be further subclassified into three categories: micronutrient, molecular targeting, and green chemoprevention [47].

In terms of oral cancer, initially, chemoprevention started off as micronutrient interventions. Different epidemiological studies pointed in the direction of vitamin A and β-carotene as being associated with decreased risk of head and neck squamous cell carcinoma [47]. Upon closer inspection, it was observed that persons with head and neck squamous cell carcinoma had low vitamin A status. In fact, head and neck squamous cell carcinoma patients with a second primary tumor had the lowest vitamin A status. In all, such results prompted researchers to investigate the efficacy of 13-cis-retinoic acid (13-cRa) as a chemopreventive agent against oral lesions as well as oral cancer [48]. Within such studies, the focus was mainly on using pharmacological doses of 13-cRa which rendered toxicity among the test subjects and, at best, inconclusive results on its efficacy as a chemopreventive agent. Studies on β-carotene demonstrated similar outcomes as 13-cisRa, starting out on a positive note when topical β-carotene was shown to inhibit 7,12-Dimethylbenz(a)anthracene (DMBA)-induced squamous cell carcinoma of the hamster buccal pouch [49]. However, human studies demonstrated an array of results ranging from insignificant improvement in oral lesions, to no effect, to actually being associated with increased relative risk of lung cancer and death from cardiovascular disease [50–52].

When micronutrient interventions proved to be disappointing, interest turned toward molecular targets. At this point, the scientific community had gained sufficient knowledge and understanding of the molecular progression of HNSCC and thus redirected focus toward the abnormal signaling pathways that promote malignant transformation of cells [47]. Molecular target chemoprevention is based on three key signaling molecules (chemoprevention targets): cyclooxygenase-2 (COX-2), epidermal growth factor receptor (EGFR), and peroxisome proliferator-activated receptors (PPARs).

Cyclooxygenase (COX) denotes two isoforms: COX-1 and COX-2; the first isoform is involved with the normal physiologic process; however, COX-2 is usually induced in neoplastic and inflammatory states at different patterns according to different stages [47]. The upregulation of COX-2 is seen on both mRNA level and protein levels and observed in normal epithelials adjacent to HNSCC, leukoplakia, and dysplasia. Some studies show upregulation of COX-2 in mucosa of smokers as well [53]. COX-2 inhibitors can block the prostaglandin E production that influence tumorigenesis and delay the growth of HNSCC cell line. Nonselective COX inhibitors such as aspirin and indomethacin show significant delay in buccal cancer [54, 55]. COX-2 inhibitor drug is found to reduce the risk of SCC, although its safety is questionable, but it has been employed as nonsteroidal anti-inflammatory drugs (NSAIDs). Safety concerns are still under study [55]. The EGFR acts as a proliferative, pro-angiogenetic and anti-apoptotic receptor. It is one of the therapeutic targets for oral cancer. The tyrosine kinase domain of EGFR can be inhibited by Erlotinib chemo-agent. Synergic targeting effect of COX-2 and EGFR was indicated as effective strategy for chemoprevention [47]. The peroxisome proliferator-activated receptors are nuclear receptor proteins that activate genes of cell differentiation and metabolism through their role as transcription factors. The PPARϒ isoform is a differentiation factor, metabolism regulator, and tumor suppressor. It binds to retinoid receptors to downregulate proliferation and angiogenesis. Thiazolidinedione is recognized to activate PPARϒ [47].

Green chemoprevention is a term used to coin interventions that utilize derivatives of natural compounds such as curcumins, resveratrol, green tea extract, luteolin, soybeans, and pomegranate. All these aforementioned plant products have antioxidant properties secondary to the inherent polyphenols present in them [54]. Polyphenol is a subgroup of phytochemicals which inhibit cancer development through different strategies, constrain the intracellular oncoprotein signaling along with the PKC/RAS/MPK or p13-kinase/AKT pathways, downregulate the pro-proliferative anti-apoptotic transcription factors NF-Kb and AP-1, and upregulate the carcinogen-detoxifying enzymes and DNA repair proteins [47]. Different studies show that drinking ten "Japanese size cups" of green tea per day delay cancer onset between 4 and 7 years. Green tea is found to have potent antioxidants called catechins. These catechins are four types and recognized to be the active component to prevent carcinogenesis [56]. The four catechins are epicatechin (EC), epicatechin-3-gallate (ECG), epigallocatechin (EGC), and epigallocatechin-3-gallate (EGCG). One of the greatest advantages of green tea is that it is nontoxic and is outlined as one of the primary, secondary, and tertiary oral cancer prevention strategies. Green tea has a synergic effect when combined with synthetic molecular targeting chemoprevention such as COX-2 [56]. For example, the EGCG and sulindac (nonsteroidal anti-inflammatory drug) exhibit synergic anticancer effect that triggers cell apoptosis and upregulates the G1 growth

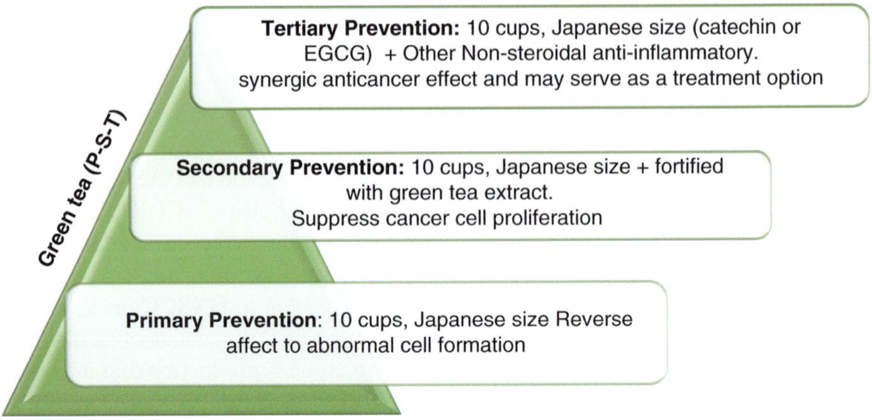

Fig. 12.1 Green tea is a primary, secondary, and tertiary chemoprevention agent

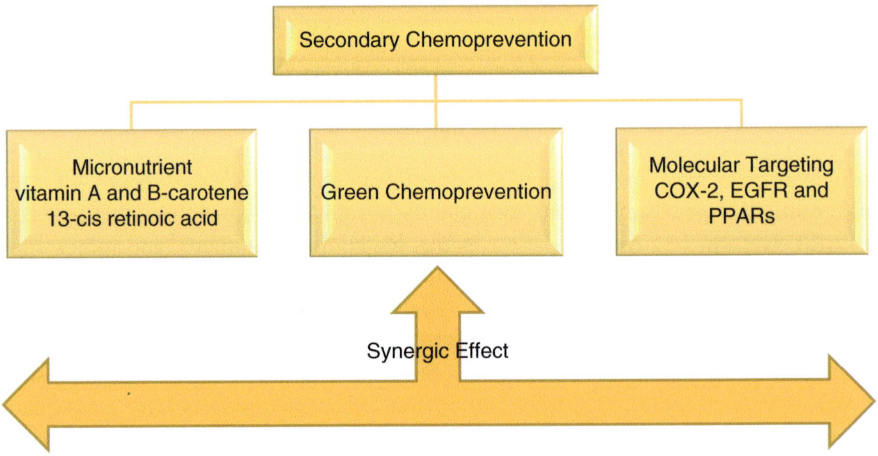

Fig. 12.2 Secondary chemoprevention items and relationship

arrest and DNA damage-inducible gene (GADD 153) [57, 58]. A study revealed a potential of 70.3% reduction in tumor volume after being treated with EGCG green tea catechin with NSAIDs [59] (Figs. 12.1 and 12.2).

12.4 Tertiary Prevention

12.4.1 Genetic Screening and Counseling

Tertiary prevention is the most complicated stage with lesser chances to prevent the disease but rather extends the tactics and methods to pause the disease development, control its progression, reverse its effects, and avoid its reoccurrence [47].

The entire tertiary prevention scheme normally involves the primary and secondary prevention as well; thus, the strategies involved in the aforesaid preventions are complementary to enhancing the overall effectiveness and probabilities of survival [60]. Comprehensive studies concerning the genetic interactions with cancer development have been conducted in the past decades, yet the process is limited in terms of its application and implicit. Many studies show a strong relationship between the cellular functions and genetic makeup in oral cancer development [60]. An oral cancer gene database involved more than 374 cancer-causing genes, of which external hyperlinks and relative information are available for 15 connective genes to oral cancer, yet the specificity of these genes is considered low since the same genes can directly or indirectly lead to other types of cancers [61]. Nonetheless, this database is greatly useful to estimate the risk of oral cancer development especially if other risk factors exist. The database withdrawal information also include useful items such as aliases, description, chromosomal interaction, pathway, interactions, clinical correlations and mutations, single nucleotide polymorphisms (SNPs), messenger ribonucleic acid (mRNA), and proteins [61] (Fig. 12.3).

It was documented that several genetic mutations contribute to oral cancer development. P16 (MTS1, CDKN2, 1N4a) and P53 are tumor suppressor genes that are suspected to be mutated in oropharyngeal cancer. P53 is attributed to major prominence in DNA repair and apoptosis, and mutation in this gene has been linked to smoking or drinking [62]. Likewise, genes encoding glutathione

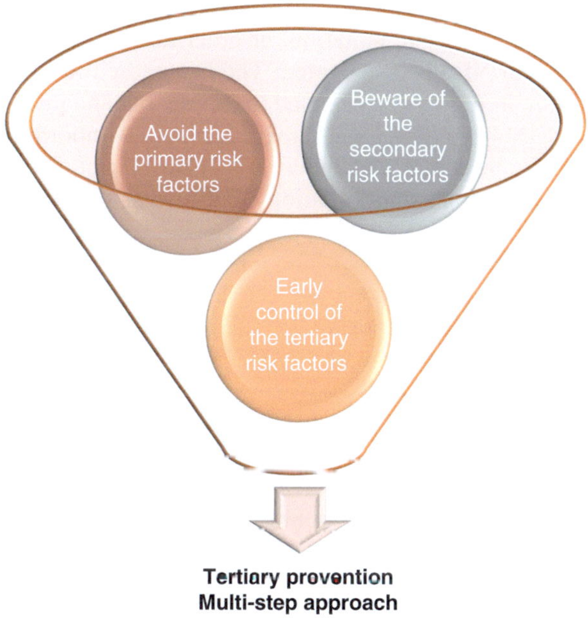

Fig. 12.3 Tertiary prevention, a multistep approach that works in synergy with the primary and secondary prevention

S-transferase enzyme (GST) and its isotypes (GSTM-1 and GSTT) are important for alcohol detoxification and drugs metabolism. GSTM1 polymorphism has been associated with oral cancer risk among smokers [63]. Moreover, a recent meta-analysis study on CYP1A1 gene polymorphism has been associated with oral squamous cell carcinoma (OSCC). This gene has a protective function for the DNA through metabolizing toxic compounds [64]. It is agreed that the overexpression of COX-2 and elevated EGFR gene copies is presumptive for SCC progression. COX-2 play an important role in neoplasm regulation and tumor microenvironment including its formation and metastasis; COX-2 has also been involved in the formation of new blood vessels that support the viability of cancerous cells, malignant progression, and invasion augmentation [47, 65]. Recent studies also suggest that certain genetic variation of PBK/PTEN/AKT/mTOR pathways may identify individuals at higher risk of SPTs. A preclinical study suggests that targeting mTOR pathway may successfully inhibit tumorigenesis. Certain genetic alteration of premalignant tissue, such as loss of heterozygosity (LOH) at either or both loci on chromosome 9p21 and 3p14, can be served as biomarkers for HNSCC cancer risk [54]. Cyclin-dependent kinase inhibitor protein P21, which is encoded by CDKN1A gene on chromosome 6, also called p21WAF1/Cip1, has multiple functions in cell cycle regulation, DNA repair, and apoptosis; thus, individuals with the aforementioned LOH are subject to oral cancer development [66].

Understanding the biochemical interactions and functional pathways of oral cancer provide a solid basis for further analysis; tumor cells become stimulated when the pro-inflammatory cytokines such as TNF-α, IL-1, and IL-6 are induced through infection, aging, gene mutation, or other diseases. As a result, TNF-α gets upregulated and NF-kB is activated. Their increased level alongside with the C-reactive protein (CRP) is correlated to the staging and progression of oral cancer [56, 67]. CD44 is a tumor marker which plays an important role in tumor cell differentiation, invasion, and metastasis. Lifestyle choices are a central aspect of genetic variations and mutations that further trigger oral cancer, for instance, smoking triggers DNA methylations which are associated with oral cancer [68]. The gene-environment interaction between CD44 polymorphism and betel quid chewing or tobacco use increases susceptibility to oral cancer [69]. Similarly, behavioral exposure to environmental carcinogens such as chewing betel quid in the presence of RAGE SNPs gene is associated with the increased risk of oral cancer [70].

In light of the abovementioned examples regarding the genetic interaction with oral cancer development, the National Cancer Institute (NCI) provided factual acquaintances between the individual's genetic alterations and oral cancer risk [71]. It turns out that it is deliberately essential to seek personalized genetic consultation, consider genetic screening and assessment, and seek preventatives and treatment options for individuals who are at a greater risk. Among cancers, hereditary cancer syndrome involves genetic testing to confirm whether a cancer condition is inherited from the family or a mutation has occurred through the same family members. In addition it estimates the personal risk of developing cancer based on the family history and genetic screening. Despite the above, there is no clear indication whether a person who inherited an oral cancer gene is necessarily going to have oral cancer. Many environmental factors play their roles in triggering cancers through gene activation. Cancer-inherited genes can be autosomal dominant, autosomal inherited, or x-linked recessive, and each of the above outlines a different risk rate of cancer development. P53 was found in 40–50% of OSCC cases and is subjective to oral cancer besides other types of cancers [72]. These genetic screenings are done through specialized healthcare providers. The NCI recommends genetic counseling after results are issued to provide structured analysis of the outcomes versus the consequences and provide beneficial recommendations [71, 72]. Genetic cancer screening is an important concept that can be also considered as secondary prevention for high-risk groups. Positive genetic screening indicates an individual's greater risk of developing cancer than the general population, and further steps must be considered such as lifestyle change, planning for younger age screening, bringing other family members for check, reducing the exposure to certain carcinogens, and considering chemoprevention if recommended. Negative results do not necessarily mean that the individual is at no risk of cancer development, since there are other mutagens that may cause DNA damage at any stage of life. Genetic counseling is essential preventative means for, namely, patients with past or current history of any type of cancer, patients who were treated for oral cancer, patients with precancerous lesions, patients with great exposure to oral cancer risk factors, and patients with family history of oral cancer. Genetic testing serves further treatment strategies and broader curative options; it also helps to predict the effectiveness of the treatment strategy and the probable side effects, thus offering advantageous bundle of prevention, detection, treatment, and efficacy.

12.4.2 Chemoprevention, Oncolytic Therapy, and Immunotherapy

As mentioned earlier, chemoprevention using compounds of natural or synthetic origins is given to reduce the risk of developing cancer and halt the transformation of precancerous lesions to cancer. The decision to initiate chemoprevention is based on different molecular biomarker tests such as nuclear organizer region, histo-blood group antigen, and proliferation markers which increased EGFR and decreased the expression of P53 and LOH [73]. Tertiary chemoprevention involves genomic representations and deep understanding for the cell cycle and the process of carcinogenesis. Environmentally induced carcinomas are mainly caused due to DNA damage, followed by unregulated cell proliferation and malignant population formation. Chemoprevention remains to be an option in two different cases. First, the Loss of heterozygosity (LOH) of gp21 due to a mutation in one allele which can lead to malignant transformation from hyperplasia to dysplasia and eventually develop into full carcinoma (studies show that LOH increased the risk of dysplasia transformation to oral cancer within few years) [47]. Second, the occurrence of mutation in one of the cell cycle regulatory genes at P16, 3P14, and 11q13 which includes TP53 [47]. LOH involves a fivefold increase in the chance of cancer development in instances of oral leukoplakia. Erlotinib Prevention of Oral Cancer (EPOC) is indicated upon the validation of LOH as a cancer marker [74]. In addition to the above examples, various chemoprevention agents are being used to inhibit the transcription factors, activate protein 1 pathway AP-1, or inhibit the cell proliferation transcription factor kappa B (NF-kB) [75]. Some of these chemopreventative agents include COX-2 inhibitors, angiogenesis inhibitors, cell cycling inhibitors, and agents that include 6-gingerol and resveratrol beside green tea and curcumin, selenium, and NSAIDS [75].

Oncolytic genetically modified viruses can be used to treat oral cancers; these viruses are specifically directed against the cancer cells and causes lysis to them. Adenoviruses have been considered for this type of therapy and providing hope to prevent oral cancer and further metastatic types of cancer [76]. Clinical trials are still in the process of examining the effectiveness of oncolytic therapy and its relative low toxicity. Adenoviral vectors expressing P53 were used to target HNSCC. Retroviruses, adenoviruses, and herpes viruses are currently under trials to be used as oncolytic agents for cancer cells.

Immunotherapy perceived limited success over the past decades. Some studies used IL-1 to activate T cells and NK cells, which in rerun activate TNF-α to inhibit tumorigenesis. Antisense RNA that inhibits oncogene expression has witnessed low toxicity and high efficacy. Lastly, RNA interference (RNAi)-based gene therapy was used to treat age-related molecular degeneration, but this is still in its preclinical stages [77].

12.4.3 Oral Cancer Prevention and Immunosuppression

The prevention of oral cancer has become an increasing challenge in immunosuppressed patients. Regular oral checkups pre- and post-hematopoietic stem cell transplant (HSCT) and the administration of immunosuppressives are considered an initial step to prevent oral cancer [78].

Some patients develop multi-organ GVHD in the skin, eyes, liver, and oral mucosa after hematopoietic stem cell transplant (HSCT) for chronic myeloid leukemia. This group can later develop oral dysplasia and further squamous cell carcinoma. A case report study revealed that immunosuppressed patients due to hematopoietic stem cell transplant (HSCT) will probably develop multi-organ graft-versus-host disease (GVHD) and are at increasing risk of oral squamous cell carcinoma. GVHD is common in 25–80% of patients who exhibited stem cell transplant. GVHD is an autoimmune syndrome that manifests itself as mouth inflammation, erythema, and ulceration. Autosomal dominant chronic mucocutaneous candidiasis (AD-CMC) is an immunodeficiency disease characterized by mucocutaneous fungal infection which leads to oropharyngeal and esophageal cancer. The disease is characterized by STAT1 mutation and T helper 17 deficiency [79]. Fanconi anemia (FA) is an autosomal recessive DNA repair disorder, whereas dyskeratosis congenita (DC) is a bone marrow failure syndrome; both syndromes are characterized by increasing folds of head and neck squamous cell carcinoma due to immunosuppression [80].

The above mentioned hereditary and immune disorders are normally treated with immunosuppressives following a bone marrow transplant to inhibit the immune response which in return reduces the impact of inflammation and cell destruction. Unfortunately, some of the treatment options for these disorders induce oral cancer development; azathioprine is a mutagenic agent and cyclosporine induces phenotypic changes and promotes tumor growth [81]. Corticosteroids promote solid tumors of epithelial origin (pro-tumorigenic) [82]. These Immunosuppressed patients may be managed by chemotherapy to counteract cancer cell proliferation. Radiation is also considered for patients with GVHD due to stem cell transplant to shrink the tumor and kill cancer cells [78].

12.4.4 Barriers to Secondary and Tertiary Preventions

Secondary and tertiary preventions are challenging in some cases. Patients at these stages are usually at increased risk of oral cancer development and many factors intercalate with each other. This in turn makes for difficult management and limited options. It's quite impossible to point the finger at one single risk factor or reason for cancer development; however, applying the best practices to reduce the effect of the risk factors for cancer development is warranted. Chemoprevention with micronutrients can be characterized with substantial toxicity and poor long-term efficacy [47]. In some studies, β-carotene proved to be associated with increased risk of lung cancer and death from cardiovascular disease, whereas the nonselective COX-2 inhibitors have been associated with hemorrhagic and gastrointestinal complications [47]. Chemoprevention can also correlate with heterogeneous transformation and spontaneous regression on the basis of LOH. Nonetheless, in some cases, the chemoprevention reversal effect for OPL doesn't correlate to complete cancer prevention [47]. Other barriers also include dose toxicity, tolerance, cost-effectiveness, preexistence of other chronic diseases, and availability of treatment. Furthermore, the lack of specific biomarkers for oral cancers and the limited clinical trials in this field are some of the major challenges encountered [47].

Summary table

Headline	Primary prevention	Secondary prevention	Tertiary prevention
Risk factors	*Controllable risk factors*: Tobacco, betel quid, gutka, UV/tanning, poor diet and lack of healthy physical activities, exposure to environmental or occupational carcinogenic agents [8–10, 20] *Uncontrollable*: Age, gender, ethnicity [3, 23, 24, 27]	• Predisposition to infections through lack of oral hygiene, immunosuppression, unsafe sexual behavior, environmental exposure to infectious agents [18, 19, 46] • Presence of primary diseases that possibly cause cancer such as autoimmune syndromes and chronic infections [79] • Family history high incidence of oral cancer [71, 72] • Excessive mouth irritation due to chronic inflammation [38]	• Patient history of oral cancer or any other type of cancer *(even if successfully treated)* [71] • Presence of oncogenes that may cause oral cancer through screening [71] • Existence of problematic chronic diseases that probably cause cancer [71] • Treating existing cancers, inherited immune disorders with immunosuppressives, bone marrow transplant or organ transplant [78]
Prevention strategy	• Controllable risk factors avoidance: smoking cessation, quit drinking alcohol, use sunscreens, avoid chewing betel quid and avoid gutka consumption, practice healthy lifestyle, and eat healthy diet that is rich in antioxidants [1, 8, 11, 17] • Lifestyle choices, early check and dental follow-up [46], consult doctors to assess the uncontrollable risk factors and obtain personalized prevention plan, take decisions regarding lifestyle changes such as accommodation, improve the socioeconomic status and education	• Early dental screening for erythroplakia and leukoplakia [34, 44] • Treat inflammation and mouth ulceration and inhibit mouth irritation [34] • Vaccination [46] • Chemoprevention (micronutrient, molecular targeting, and green chemoprevention) [47]	• Seek professional genetic counseling, obtain personalized prevention plan, and conduct further tests [71, 72] • Regular specific screening and check is required for high-risk group • Treat the precancerous conditions though chemotherapy and radiation [78]
Limitation	• Cultural norms, resistance to change the unhealthy lifestyles, unwillingness to quit joyful habits, limitation of the governmental regulations [7, 9]	• Lack of knowledge or education about the secondary risk factors, poor healthcare support and dental insurance coverage, limited public health support and awareness campaigns about the secondary risks factors [25, 26, 32]	• Toxicity and side effects of the treatment options [47] • Developing channel of complications through treating multiple diseases at the same time • Poor physiological responsiveness to treatment [50, 51]

Conclusion

Oral cancer is a disease that is preventable and controllable but habitually has been given little significance by both healthcare providers and the public. Additionally, although there is a plethora of research on therapeutic modalities for oral cancer, not enough attention has been paid to early detection and prevention. Early detection and prevention can no longer be considered one's own responsibility but rather a matter of public health specialists, nutritionists, dentists, doctors, psychologists, biomedical scientists, and policy makers. Prevention of oral cancer should become a public health topic with manifestations in dental schools, health ministries, and councils as well as awareness campaigns. We firmly believe that healthcare professionals such as doctors, psychologists, nutritionists, and dentists should be trained to assess and converse with high-risk patients in order to create awareness on the impact of negative habits such as smoking, drinking excessive alcohol, and poor nutrition quality in developing oral cancer. These healthcare professionals need to work as a team in changing a person's behavior. Perhaps future directives could include setting up team meetings with high-risk patients. For example, when a high-risk patient sees a dentist for a routine checkup, the dentist should suggest an informative sit in with other professionals who may enable and help the patient in changing his behavior. However, if a person has no insurance to visit a dentist or doctor in the first place, such a team approach may not be feasible. At this point, we need to draw on the ability of policy makers and health ministries to promote and enforce some form of policy on initiation of dental insurance similar to policies that have been enforced in order to decrease exposure to risk factors. On the topic of insurance, another future directive could be to include biomedical scientists into the scope of coverage for people who may benefit from gene mapping and genetic recommendations.

References

1. Lu R, Dan H, Wu R, Meng W, Liu N, Jin X, et al. Lycopene: features and potential significance in the oral cancer and precancerous lesions. J Oral Pathol Med. 2011;40(5):361–8.
2. Petersen PE. Oral cancer prevention and control – the approach of the World Health Organization. Oral Oncol. 2009;45(4–5):454–60.
3. Rivera C. Essentials of oral cancer. Int J Clin Exp Pathol. 2015;8(9):11884–94.
4. Sand L, Jalouli J. Viruses and oral cancer. Is there a link? Microbes Infect. 2014;16(5):371–8.
5. Anderson WD 3rd, Treister NS, Mayeaux EJ Jr, Nalliah RP. Oral lesions you can't afford to miss. J Fam Pract. 2015;64(7):392–9.
6. Speight P, Warnakulasuriya S, Ogden G. Early detection and prevention of oral cancer: a management strategy for dental practice. London: The British Dental Association; 2010.
7. Dos Santos Silva I. Cancer prevention. In: Cancer epidemiology: principles and methods. France: International Agency for Research on Cancer, 1999. p. 355–80.
8. Tsai KY, CC S, Lin YY, Chung JA, Lian Ie B. Quantification of betel quid chewing and cigarette smoking in oral cancer patients. Community Dent Oral Epidemiol. 2009;37(6):555–61.
9. Murphy KL, Herzog TA. Sociocultural factors that affect chewing behaviors among betel nut chewers and ex-chewers on Guam. Hawaii J Med Public Health. 2015;74(12):406–11.

10. Mayne ST, Playdon MC, Rock CL. Diet, nutrition, and cancer: past, present and future. Nat Rev Clin Oncol. 2016;13:504–15.
11. Kushi LH, Doyle C, McCullough M, Rock CL, Demark-Wahnefried W, Bandera EV, et al. American Cancer Society guidelines on nutrition and physical activity for cancer prevention: reducing the risk of cancer with healthy food choices and physical activity. CA Cancer J Clin. 2012;62(1):30–67.
12. WCRF/AICR. Food, nutrition, physical activity and the prevention of cancer: a global perspective. 2nd ed. Washington: WCRF/AICR; 2007.
13. Bradshaw PT, Siega-Riz AM, Campbell M, Weissler MC, Funkhouser WK, Olshan AF. Associations between dietary patterns and head and neck cancer: the Carolina head and neck cancer epidemiology study. Am J Epidemiol. 2012;175(12):1225–33.
14. Sapkota A, Hsu CC, Zaridze D, Shangina O, Szeszenia-Dabrowska N, Mates D, et al. Dietary risk factors for squamous cell carcinoma of the upper aerodigestive tract in central and eastern Europe. Cancer Causes Control. 2008;19(10):1161–70.
15. Bravi F, Bosetti C, Filomeno M, Levi F, Garavello W, Galimberti S, et al. Foods, nutrients and the risk of oral and pharyngeal cancer. Br J Cancer. 2013;109(11):2904–10.
16. Scully C, Kirby J. Statement on mouth cancer diagnosis and prevention. Br Dent J. 2014;216(1):37–8.
17. Maruccia M, Onesti MG, Parisi P, Cigna E, Troccola A, Scuderi N. Lip cancer: a 10-year retrospective epidemiological study. Anticancer Res. 2012;32(4):1543–6.
18. Khot KP, Deshmane S, Choudhari S. Human papilloma virus in oral squamous cell carcinoma – the enigma unravelled. Chin J Dent Res. 2016;19(1):17–23.
19. Dalla Torre D, Burtscher D, Solder E, Widschwendter A, Rasse M, Puelacher W. The impact of sexual behavior on oral HPV infections in young unvaccinated adults. Clin Oral Investig. 2016;20:1551–7.
20. Maru GB, Hudlikar RR, Kumar G, Gandhi K, Mahimkar MB. Understanding the molecular mechanisms of cancer prevention by dietary phytochemicals: from experimental models to clinical trials. World J Biol Chem. 2016;7(1):88–99.
21. Smith AJ, Oertle J, Prato D. Environmental carcinogens and the kinds of cancers they cause. Open J Oncol. 2014;3(1).
22. Labreche F, Duguay P, Boucher A, Arcand R. But other than mesothelioma? An estimate of the proportion of work-related cancers in Quebec. Curr Oncol. 2016;23(2):e144–9.
23. Joseph LJ, Goodman M, Higgins K, Pilai R, Ramalingam SS, Magliocca K, et al. Racial disparities in squamous cell carcinoma of the oral tongue among women: a SEER data analysis. Oral Oncol. 2015;51(6):586–92.
24. Saba NF, Goodman M, Ward K, Flowers C, Ramalingam S, Owonikoko T, et al. Gender and ethnic disparities in incidence and survival of squamous cell carcinoma of the oral tongue, base of tongue, and tonsils: a surveillance, epidemiology and end results program-based analysis. Oncology. 2011;81(1):12–20.
25. McClure JB, Riggs KR, St John J, Cerutti B, Zbikowski S. Understanding oral health promotion needs and opportunities of tobacco quitline callers. Public Health Rep. 2012;127(4):401–6.
26. McClure JB, Riggs K, St John J, Catz SL. [more] evidence to support oral health promotion services targeted to smokers calling tobacco quitlines in the United States. BMC Public Health. 2013;13:336.
27. Kulak JA, Cornelius ME, Fong GT, Giovino GA. Differences in quit attempts and cigarette smoking abstinence between whites and African Americans in the United States: literature review and results from the International tobacco control US survey. Nicotine Tob Res. 2016;18(Suppl 1):S79–87.
28. Campos-Outcalt D. Immunization update: this year's changes. J Fam Pract. 2016;65(3):198–200.
29. Beachler DC, Kreimer AR, Schiffman M, Herrero R, Wacholder S, Rodriguez AC, et al. Multisite HPV16/18 vaccine efficacy against cervical, anal, and oral HPV infection. J Natl Cancer Inst. 2016;108(1).
30. Dietz NA, Sly DF, Lee DJ, Arheart KL, McClure LA. Correlates of smoking among young adults: the role of lifestyle, attitudes/beliefs, demographics, and exposure to anti-tobacco media messaging. Drug Alcohol Depend. 2013;130(1–3):115–21.

31. Little MA, Pokhrel P, Murphy KL, Kawamoto CT, Suguitan GS, Herzog TA. Intention to quit betel quid: a comparison of betel quid chewers and cigarette smokers. Oral Health Dent Manag. 2014;13(2):512–8.
32. Vlantis AC. Human papilloma virus and oropharyngeal carcinoma – lessons from history. Chin J Dent Res. 2016;19(1):9–16.
33. Basic concepts in prevention, surveillance, and health promotion [Internet]. phprimer.afmc.ca. The Association of Faculties of Medicine of Canada; [cited 2017 May 19]. Available from: http://phprimer.afmc.ca/Part1-TheoryThinkingAboutHealth/Chapter4BasicConceptsInPreventionSurveillanceAndHealthPromotion.
34. Giovannacci I, Vescovi P, Manfredi M, Meleti M. Non-invasive visual tools for diagnosis of oral cancer and dysplasia: a systematic review. Med Oral Patol Oral Cir Bucal. 2016;21:e305–15.
35. Lingen MW, Kalmar JR, Karrison T, Speight PM. Critical evaluation of diagnostic aids for the detection of oral cancer. Oral Oncol. 2008;44(1):10–22.
36. Sankaranarayanan R, Ramadas K, Thomas G, Muwonge R, Thara S, Mathew B, et al. Effect of screening on oral cancer mortality in Kerala, India: a cluster-randomised controlled trial. Lancet. 2005;365(9475):1927–33.
37. Awojobi O, Newton JT, Scott SE. Why don't dentists talk to patients about oral cancer? Br Dent J. 2015;218(9):537–41.
38. Perry BJ, Zammit AP, Lewandowski AW, Bashford JJ, Dragovic AS, Perry EJ, et al. Sites of origin of oral cavity cancer in nonsmokers vs smokers: possible evidence of dental trauma carcinogenesis and its importance compared with human papillomavirus. JAMA Otolaryngol Head Neck Surg. 2015;141(1):5–11.
39. Mueller NE. Cancers caused by infections: unequal burdens. Cancer Epidemiol Biomark Prev. 2003;12(3):237s.
40. Xu C, Chen YP, Ma J. Clinical trials in nasopharyngeal carcinoma-past, present and future. Chin Clin Oncol. 2016;5(2):20.
41. Xu W, Liu Z, Bao Q, Qian Z. Viruses, other pathogenic microorganisms and esophageal cancer. Gastrointest Tumors. 2015;2(1):2–13.
42. Pontes HA, Guimaraes DM, Pontes FS, Paiva HB, Pinto LC, de Freitas Silva BS, et al. Kaposi sarcoma and paracoccidioidomycosis in the same fragment of oral mucosa biopsy: a rare association in human immunodeficiency virus-positive patient. A case report. Diagn Microbiol Infect Dis. 2011;69(2):196–9.
43. Krogh P, Hald B, Holmstrup P. Possible mycological etiology of oral mucosal cancer: catalytic potential of infecting Candida albicans and other yeasts in production of N-nitrosobenzylmethylamine. Carcinogenesis. 1987;8(10):1543–8.
44. Sankari SL, Gayathri K, Balachander N, Malathi L. Candida in potentially malignant oral disorders. J Pharm Bioallied Sci. 2015;7(Suppl 1):S162–4.
45. Chocolatewala N, Chaturvedi P, Desale R. The role of bacteria in oral cancer. Indian J Med Paediatr Oncol. 2010;31(4):126–31.
46. Mangalath U, Aslam SA, Abdul Khadar AH, Francis PG, Mikacha MS, Kalathingal JH. Recent trends in prevention of oral cancer. J Int Soc Prev Community Dent. 2014;4(Suppl 3):S131–8.
47. Sheth SH, Johnson DE, Kensler TW, Bauman JE. Chemoprevention targets for tobacco-related head and neck cancer: past lessons and future directions. Oral Oncol. 2015;51(6):557–64.
48. de Vries N, Snow GB. Relationships of vitamins A and E and beta-carotene serum levels to head and neck cancer patients with and without second primary tumors. Eur Arch Otorhinolaryngol. 1990;247(6):368–70.
49. Schwartz J, Shklar G. Regression of experimental hamster cancer by beta carotene and algae extracts. J Oral Maxillofac Surg. 1987;45(6):510–5.
50. Garewal HS, Meyskens FL Jr, Killen D, Reeves D, Kiersch TA, Elletson H, et al. Response of oral leukoplakia to beta-carotene. J Clin Oncol. 1990;8(10):1715–20.
51. Mayne ST, Cartmel B, Baum M, Shor-Posner G, Fallon BG, Briskin K, et al. Randomized trial of supplemental beta-carotene to prevent second head and neck cancer. Cancer Res 2001;61(4):1457–63.

52. Omenn GS. Chemoprevention of lung cancers: lessons from CARET, the beta-carotene and retinol efficacy trial, and prospects for the future. Eur J Cancer Prev. 2007;16(3):184–91.
53. Moraitis D, Du B, De Lorenzo MS, Boyle JO, Weksler BB, Cohen EG, et al. Levels of cyclooxygenase-2 are increased in the oral mucosa of smokers: evidence for the role of epidermal growth factor receptor and its ligands. Cancer Res. 2005;65(2):664–70.
54. Saba NF, Haigentz M Jr, Vermorken JB, Strojan P, Bossi P, Rinaldo A, et al. Prevention of head and neck squamous cell carcinoma: removing the "chemo" from "chemoprevention". Oral Oncol. 2015;51(2):112–8.
55. Trelle S, Reichenbach S, Wandel S, Hildebrand P, Tschannen B, Villiger PM, et al. Cardiovascular safety of non-steroidal anti-inflammatory drugs: network meta-analysis. BMJ. 2011;342:c7086.
56. Fujiki H, Imai K, Nakachi K, Shimizu M, Moriwaki H, Suganuma M. Challenging the effectiveness of green tea in primary and tertiary cancer prevention. J Cancer Res Clin Oncol. 2012;138(8):1259–70.
57. Igase M, Okura T, Nakamura M, Takata Y, Kitami Y, Hiwada K. Role of GADD153 (growth arrest- and DNA damage-inducible gene 153) in vascular smooth muscle cell apoptosis. Clin Sci (Lond). 2001;100(3):275–81.
58. Fujiki H, Sueoka E, Watanabe T, Suganuma M. Primary cancer prevention by green tea, and tertiary cancer prevention by the combination of green tea catechins and anticancer compounds. J Cancer Prev. 2015;20(1):1–4.
59. Fujiki H, Sueoka E, Watanabe T, Suganuma M. Synergistic enhancement of anticancer effects on numerous human cancer cell lines treated with the combination of EGCG, other green tea catechins, and anticancer compounds. J Cancer Res Clin Oncol. 2015;141(9):1511–22.
60. Ashworth A, Lord CJ, Reis-Filho JS. Genetic interactions in cancer progression and treatment. Cell. 2011;145(1):30–8.
61. Gadewal NS, Zingde SM. Database and interaction network of genes involved in oral cancer: version II. Bioinformation. 2011;6(4):169–70.
62. Hsieh L-L. Characteristics of mutations in the p53 gene in oral squamous cell carcinoma associated with betel quid chewing and cigarette smoking in Taiwanese. Carcinogenesis. 2001; 22(9):1497–503.
63. Kruger M, Pabst AM, Mahmoodi B, Becker B, Kammerer PW, Koch FP. The impact of GSTM1/GSTT1 polymorphism for the risk of oral cancer. Clin Oral Investig. 2015;19(8): 1791–7.
64. Xie S, Luo C, Shan X, Zhao S, He J, Cai Z. MspI polymorphism and the risk of oral squamous cell carcinoma: evidence from a meta-analysis. Mol Clin Oncol. 2016;4(4):660–6.
65. Santoro A, Bufo P, Russo G, Cagiano S, Papagerakis S, Bucci P, et al. Expression and clinical implication of cyclooxygenase-2 and e-cadherin in oral squamous cell carcinomas. Cancer Biol Ther. 2015:0.
66. Karimian A, Ahmadi Y, Yousefi B. Multiple functions of p21 in cell cycle, apoptosis and transcriptional regulation after DNA damage. DNA Repair (Amst). 2016;42:63–71.
67. Jablonska E, Piotrowski L, Grabowska Z. Serum levels of IL-1b, IL-6, TNF-a, sTNF-RI and CRP in patients with oral cavity cancer. Pathol Oncol Res. 1997;3(2):126–9.
68. Guerrero-Preston R, Baez A, Blanco A, Berdasco M, Fraga M, Esteller M. Global DNA methylation: a common early event in oral cancer cases with exposure to environmental carcinogens or viral agents. P R Health Sci J. 2009;28(1):24–9.
69. Chou YE, Hsieh MJ, Hsin CH, Chiang WL, Lai YC, Lee YH, et al. CD44 gene polymorphisms and environmental factors on oral cancer susceptibility in Taiwan. PLoS One. 2014;9(4):e93692.
70. Su S, Chien M, Lin C, Chen M, Yang S. RAGE gene polymorphism and environmental factor in the risk of oral cancer. J Dent Res. 2015;94(3):403–11.
71. Singh RD, Patel KR, Patel PS. p53 mutation spectrum and its role in prognosis of oral cancer patients: a study from Gujarat, West India. Mutat Res. 2016;783:15–26.
72. Chandra A, Singh A, Sebastian BT, Agnihotri A, Bali R, Verma PK. Oral squamous cell carcinomas in age distinct population: a comparison of p53 immunoexpression. J Cancer Res Ther. 2013;9(4):587–91.

73. Tanaka T, Tanaka M. Oral carcinogenesis and oral cancer chemoprevention: a review. Patholog Res Int. 2011;2011:431246.
74. William WN Jr, El-Naggar AK. A novel target for oral cancer chemoprevention? Notch quite, yet. Cancer Prev Res (Phila). 2015;8(4):262–5.
75. Baliga KA, Kini R, Naik V, Kini S. Chemopreventive agents; its role in oral cancer prevention. Int J Adv Health Sci. 2015;2(1):22–7.
76. Shilpa P, Kaul R, Bhat S, Sultana N, Pandeshwar P. Oncolytic viruses in head and neck cancer: a new ray of hope in the management protocol. Ann Med Health Sci Res. 2014;4(Suppl 3):S178–84.
77. Bali A, Bali D, Sharma A. An overview of gene therapy in head and neck cancer. Indian J Hum Genet. 2013;19(3):282–90.
78. Naidu MU, Ramana GV, Rani PU, Mohan IK, Suman A, Roy P. Chemotherapy-induced and/or radiation therapy-induced oral mucositis – complicating the treatment of cancer. Neoplasia. 2004;6(5):423–31.
79. van de Veerdonk FL, Netea MG. Treatment options for chronic mucocutaneous candidiasis. J Infect. 2016.
80. Alter BP, Giri N, Savage SA, Quint WG, de Koning MN, Schiffman M. Squamous cell carcinomas in patients with Fanconi anemia and dyskeratosis congenita: a search for human papillomavirus. Int J Cancer. 2013;133(6):1513–5.
81. de Araujo RL, Lyko Kde F, Funke VA, Torres-Pereira CC. Oral cancer after prolonged immunosuppression for multiorgan chronic graft-versus-host disease. Rev Bras Hematol Hemoter. 2014;36(1):65–8.
82. Azher S, Azami O, Amato C, McCullough M, Celentano A, Cirillo N. The non-conventional effects of glucocorticoids in cancer. J Cell Physiol. 2016;231:2368–73.

MIX
Papier aus verantwortungsvollen Quellen
Paper from responsible sources
FSC® C105338

If you have any concerns about our products, you can contact us on
ProductSafety@springernature.com

In case Publisher is established outside the EU, the EU authorized representative is:
Springer Nature Customer Service Center GmbH
Europaplatz 3, 69115 Heidelberg, Germany

Printed by Libri Plureos GmbH
in Hamburg, Germany